RURAL NURSING

Charlene A. Winters, PhD, APRN, ACNS-BC, is a professor in the College of Nursing at Montana State University-Bozeman, Missoula Campus. Dr. Winters teaches in the graduate program and has played an active role in curriculum development. She has served as a project director for the Clinical Nurse Leader and Clinical Nurse Specialist graduate options. Her research interests focus on the health of rural populations—rural nursing practice, rural nursing theory development, and adaptation to and self-management of chronic illness(es) by rural dwellers. She is an active member of the Rural Nurse Organization, the Western Institute of Nursing, the Montana and National Associations of Clinical Nurse Specialists, Sigma Theta Tau International, the Council for the Advancement of Nursing Science, the American Association of Critical Care Nurses, and is a charter member of the International Council of Nursing—Rural and Remote Nurses Network. Dr. Winters is the coeditor of two previous editions of *Rural Nursing: Concepts, Theory, and Practice*. She holds a doctorate degree in nursing from Rush University, College of Nursing, Chicago, Illinois, and bachelor and master of Science degrees in nursing from California State University, Long Beach.

RURAL NURSING
Concepts, Theory, and Practice

Fourth Edition

Charlene A. Winters, PhD, APRN, ACNS-BC

Editor

SPRINGER PUBLISHING COMPANY
NEW YORK

Copyright © 2013 Springer Publishing Company, LLC

All rights reserved.

No part of this publication may be reproduced, stored in a retrieval system, or transmitted in any form or by any means, electronic, mechanical, photocopying, recording, or otherwise, without the prior permission of Springer Publishing Company, LLC, or authorization through payment of the appropriate fees to the Copyright Clearance Center, Inc., 222 Rosewood Drive, Danvers, MA 01923, 978-750-8400, fax 978-646-8600, info@copyright.com or on the Web at www.copyright.com.

Springer Publishing Company, LLC
11 West 42nd Street
New York, NY 10036
www.springerpub.com

Acquisitions Editor: Allan Graubard
Production Editor: Michael O'Connor
Composition: Techset

ISBN: 978-0-8261-7085-9
e-book ISBN: 978-0-8261-7086-6

13 14 15 16 / 5 4 3 2 1

The author and the publisher of this Work have made every effort to use sources believed to be reliable to provide information that is accurate and compatible with the standards generally accepted at the time of publication. The author and publisher shall not be liable for any special, consequential, or exemplary damages resulting, in whole or in part, from the readers' use of, or reliance on, the information contained in this book. The publisher has no responsibility for the persistence or accuracy of URLs for external or third-party Internet websites referred to in this publication and does not guarantee that any content on such websites is, or will remain, accurate or appropriate.

Library of Congress Cataloging-in-Publication Data

Rural nursing : concepts, theory, and practice / Charlene A. Winters, editor. — 4th ed.
  p. ; cm.
  Includes bibliographical references and index.
  ISBN 978-0-8261-7085-9 (alk. paper) — ISBN 978-0-8261-7086-6 (alk. paper)
  I. Winters, Charlene A.
  [DNLM: 1. Community Health Nursing. 2. Rural Health Services. 3. Rural Health. 4. Rural Population. WY 106]
  610.73'43—dc23

2012046369

Special discounts on bulk quantities of our books are available to corporations, professional associations, pharmaceutical companies, health care organizations, and other qualifying groups. If you are interested in a custom book, including chapters from more than one of our titles, we can provide that service as well.

For details, please contact:

Special Sales Department, Springer Publishing Company, LLC

11 West 42nd Street, 15th Floor, New York, NY 10036-8002

Phone: 877-687-7476 or 212-431-4370; Fax: 212-941-7842

E-mail: sales@springerpub.com

Printed in the United States of America by Bang Printing.

To my mentor, Dr. Helen J. Lee, whose dedication to the health of rural persons, rural nursing practice and education, and rural nursing theory development is unwavering. I am proud to call Helen my friend and colleague.

CONTENTS

Contributors **xi**
Foreword Pamela Stewart Fahs, RN, DSN **xv**
Preface **xvii**

Part I The Rural Nursing Theory Base

1. Rural Nursing: Developing the Theory Base   1
   Kathleen Ann Long and Clarann Weinert

2. Updating the Rural Nursing Theory Base   15
   Helen J. Lee and Meg K. McDonagh

3. Exploring Rural Nursing Theory Across Borders   35
   Charlene A. Winters, Elizabeth H. Thomlinson,
   Chad O'Lynn, Helen J. Lee, Meg K. McDonagh,
   Dana S. Edge, and Marlene A. Reimer

4. The Rural Nursing Theory: A Literature Review   49
   Deana L. Molinari and Ruiling Guo

Part II Perspectives of Rural Persons

5. Health Needs and Perceptions of Rural Persons   65
   Ronda L. Bales, Charlene A. Winters, and Helen J. Lee

6. Assessing Resilience in Older Frontier Women   79
   Gail M. Wagnild and Linda M. Torma

7. Rural and Remote Women and Resilience: Grounded
   Theory and Photovoice Variations on a Theme: An Update   95
   Beverly D. Leipert

8. Palliative Care at the End of Life: A Rural Family Perspective   119
   Dorothy M. "Dale" Mayer and Rebecca Murphy

Part III The Rural Dweller and Response to Illness

9. Patterns of Responses to Symptoms in Rural Residents: The Symptom–Action–Timeline Process *131*
   Janice A. Buehler, Maureen Malone, and Janis M. Majerus-Wegerhoff

10. Beyond the Symptom–Action–Timeline Process: Explicating the Health-Needs–Action Process *141*
    Andrea D. Rasmussen, Chad O'Lynn, and Charlene A. Winters

11. Chronic Illness Experience of Isolated Rural Women: Use of an Online Support Group Intervention *159*
    Charlene A. Winters and Therese Sullivan

12. Negotiation of Constructed Gender Among Rural Male Caregivers *173*
    Chad O'Lynn

13. Complementary Therapy and Health Literacy in Rural Dwellers *205*
    Jean M. Shreffler-Grant, Elizabeth Nichols, Clarann Weinert, and Bette Ide

14. Acceptability: One Component in Choice of Health Care Provider *215*
    Jean M. Shreffler-Grant

15. Health Disparities in Rural Populations Across the Life Span *225*
    Angeline Bushy

Part IV Rural Nursing Practice and Education

16. The Distinctive Nature and Scope of Rural Nursing Practice: Philosophical Bases *241*
    Jane Ellis Scharff

17. Men Working as Rural Nurses: Land of Opportunity *259*
    Chad O'Lynn

18. Rural Nurses' Attitudes and Beliefs Toward Evidence-Based Practice *275*
    Brenda D. Koessl, Charlene A. Winters, Helen J. Lee, and Lori Hendrickx

19. The Use of Rural Hospitals for Clinical Placements in Nursing Education *293*
    Lori Hendrickx, Heidi Mennenga, and Laurie Johansen

20. U.S.–Mexico Border: Challenges and Opportunities in Rural and Border Health   303
    Eva M. Moya, Guillermina Solis, Rebeca L. Ramos, Mark W. Lusk, and Carliene S. Quist

21. Reestablishing Nursing Education in Haiti: Nurses Helping Nurses After Complex Humanitarian Emergencies   335
    Michele V. Sare

Part V Rural Public Health

22. Environmental Risk Reduction for Rural Children   357
    Wade G. Hill and Patricia Butterfield

23. The Culture of Rural Communities: An Examination of Rural Nursing Concepts at the Community Level   367
    Nancy E. Findholt

24. Community Resiliency and Rural Nursing: Canadian and Australian Perspectives   377
    Judith C. Kulig, Desley Hegney, and Dana S. Edge

25. Influence of the Rural Environment on Children's Physical Activity and Eating Behaviors   393
    Nancy E. Findholt, Linda J. Jerofke, Yvonne L. Michael, and Victoria W. Brogoitti

26. Public Health Accreditation in Rural and Frontier Counties: A Montana Perspective   401
    Michele V. Sare

27. Nurses in Occupational Practice in Agricultural and Rural Communities in New York State: Providing Occupational Health and Safety Education and Prevention Services   421
    Bernadette D. Hodge, Diana E. Gaetano, Susan B. Ackerman, Connie A. Jastremski, and Terry Fulmer

Part VI Looking Ahead

28. Implications for Education, Practice, and Policy   439
    Jean M. Shreffler-Grant and Marlene A. Reimer

29. Nursing Workforce Development, Clinical Practice, Research, and Nursing Theory: Connecting the Dots   449
    Angeline Bushy and Charlene A. Winters

30. An Analysis of Key Concepts for Rural Nursing   469
    Helen J. Lee, Charlene A. Winters, Robin L. Boland, Susan J. Raph, and Janice A. Buehler

Index   481

CONTRIBUTORS

Susan B. Ackerman, RN, BS, Bassett Healthcare Network, New York Center for Agricultural Medicine and Health (NYCAMH), Cooperstown, New York

Ronda L. Bales, MN, APRN, FNP-BC, Adjunct Assistant Professor, College of Nursing, Montana State University-Bozeman, Billings, Montana

Robin L. Boland, MN, RN, FNP-C, Nurse Practitioner, Primary Care Associates, Great Falls, Montana

Victoria W. Brogoitti, BS, Director, Union County Commission on Children and Families, La Grande, Oregon

Janice A. Buehler, PhD, RN, Associate Professor (retired), College of Nursing, Montana State University-Bozeman, Billings, Montana

Angeline Bushy, PhD, RN, FAAN PHCNS-BC, Professor and Bert Fish Chair, College of Nursing, University of Central Florida, Daytona Beach, Florida

Patricia Butterfield, PhD, RN, FAAN, Professor and Dean, College of Nursing, Washington State University, Washington

Dana S. Edge, PhD, RN, Associate Professor, School of Nursing, Queen's University, Kingston, Ontario, Canada

Nancy E. Findholt, PhD, RN, Associate Professor, School of Nursing, Oregon Health and Science University, La Grande, Oregon

Terry Fulmer, PhD, RN, FAAN, Dean, Bouve College of Health Sciences, Northeastern University, Boston, Massachusetts

Diana E. Gaetano, RN, BS, COHN-S, Bassett Healthcare Network, New York Center for Agricultural Medicine and Health (NYCAMH), Cooperstown, New York

Ruiling Guo, MLIS, AHIP, Associate Professor and Health Sciences Librarian, Health Sciences Library, Idaho State University, Pocatello, Idaho

Desley Hegney, PhD, RN, Professor, School of Nursing and Midwifery, Curtin Health Innovation Research Institute, Curtin University, Perth, Western Australia, Australia

Lori Hendrickx, EdD, RN, CCRN, Professor, College of Nursing, South Dakota State University, Brookings, South Dakota

Wade G. Hill, PhD, RN, Associate Professor, College of Nursing, Montana State University-Bozeman, Bozeman, Montana

Bernadette D. Hodge, MS, RN, MLS, Bassett Healthcare Network, New York Center for Agricultural Medicine and Health (NYCAMH), Cooperstown, New York

Bette Ide, PhD, RN, Professor (retired), College of Nursing, University of North Dakota, Great Forks, North Dakota

Connie A. Jastremski, MS, MBA, RN, ANP-CS, FCCM, Chief Nursing Officer, Bassett Healthcare Network, Cooperstown, New York

Linda J. Jerofke, PhD, Assistant Professor, Department of Anthropology and Sociology, Eastern Oregon University, La Grande, Oregon

Laurie Johansen, MS, RN, PHN, Instructor, College of Nursing, South Dakota State University, Brookings, South Dakota

Brenda D. Koessl, MN, APRN, FNP-BC, Director of Nursing, Frances Mahon Deaconess Hospital, Glasgow, Montana

Judith C. Kulig, Phd, RN, Professor, School of Health Sciences, University of Lethbridge, Monarch, Canada

Helen J. Lee, PhD, RN, Professor Emeritus, College of Nursing, Montana State University-Bozeman, Missoula, Montana

Beverly D. Leipert, PhD, RN, Associate Professor, Arthur Labatt Family School of Nursing, University of Western Ontario, London, Ontario, Canada

Kathleen Ann Long, PhD, APRN, FAAN, Associate Provost, Dean and Professor, College of Nursing, University of Florida, Gainesville, Florida

Mark W. Lusk, EdD, LMSW, Professor and Chair, Department of Social Work, University of Texas, El Paso, Texas

Janis M. Majerus-Wegerhoff, MN, RN, Calgary, Alberta, Canada

Maureen Malone, MN, RN, Public Health Nurse (retired), Indian Health Service, Hardin, Montana

Dorothy M. "Dale" Mayer, PhD, APRN, ACNS-BC, Assistant Professor, College of Nursing, Montana State University-Bozeman, Missoula, Montana

Meg K. McDonagh, MN, FNP, Senior Instructor, Faculty of Nursing, University of Calgary, Calgary, Alberta, Canada

Heidi Mennenga, PhD, RN, Assistant Professor, College of Nursing, South Dakota State University, Brookings, South Dakota

Yvonne L. Michael, ScD, Associate Professor, School of Public Health, Department of Epidemiology and Biostatistics, Drexel University, Philadelphia, Pennsylvania

Deana L. Molinari, PhD, RN, CNE, Professor (retired), School of Nursing, Idaho State University, Blackfoot, Idaho

Eva M. Moya, PhD, LMSW, Assistant Professor, Department of Social Work, College of Health Sciences, University of Texas, El Paso, Texas

Rebecca Murphy, BSN, MN, APRN, FNP-BC, Family Nurse Practitioner, Bozeman Deaconess Palliative Care Consultants, Bozeman, Montana

Elizabeth Nichols, DNS, RN, FAAN, Professor Emeritus, College of Nursing, Montana State University-Bozeman, Bozeman, Montana

Chad O'Lynn, PhD, RN, RA, Assistant Professor, University of Portland, Portland, Oregon

Carliene S. Quist, Graduate Student, Department of Social Work, University of Texas at El Paso, El Paso, Texas

Rebeca L. Ramos, MPH, MPA, Executive Director, The Alliance of Border Collaboratives, El Paso, Texas

Susan J. Raph, MN, RN, CNAA-BC, Campus Director and Associate Clinical Professor, College of Nursing, Montana State University-Bozeman, Great Falls, Montana

Andrea D. Rasmussen, BSN, RN, Graduate Student, College of Nursing, Montana State University-Bozeman, Missoula, Montana

Marlene A. Reimer, RN, PhD, CNN(C) (deceased), Professor, Faculty of Nursing, University of Calgary, Calgary, Alberta, Canada

Michele V. Sare, MSN, RN, Adjunct Assistant Professor, College of Nursing, Montana State University-Bozeman and CEO, Nurses for Nurses International, Hall, Montana

Jane Ellis Scharff, MN, RN, Campus Director and Associate Clinical Professor, College of Nursing, Montana State University-Bozeman, Billings, Montana

Jean M. Shreffler-Grant, PhD, RN, Professor, College of Nursing, Montana State University-Bozeman, Missoula, Montana

Guillermina Solis, PhD, RN, F/GNP-C, Postdoctoral Fellow, College of Nursing, University of Texas at El Paso, El Paso, Texas

Therese Sullivan, PhD, RN, Associate Professor (retired), College of Nursing, Montana State University-Bozeman, Helena, Montana

Elizabeth H. Thomlinson, PhD, RN (deceased), Associate Dean and Associate Professor, Undergraduate Programs, Faculty of Nursing, University of Calgary, Calgary, Alberta, Canada

Linda M. Torma, PhD, APRN, GCNS-BC, Assistant Professor, College of Nursing, Montana State University-Bozeman, Missoula, Montana

Gail M. Wagnild, PhD, RN, Principal, The Resilience Center, Worden, Montana

Clarann Weinert, SC, PhD, RN, FAAN, Sister of Charity (Cincinnati, Ohio) and Professor Emeritus, College of Nursing, Montana State University-Bozeman, Bozeman, Montana

Charlene A. Winters, PhD, APRN, ACNS-BC, Professor, College of Nursing, Montana State University-Bozeman, Missoula, Montana

FOREWORD

It is indeed an honor to be asked to write the Foreword for the fourth edition of *Rural Nursing: Concepts, Theory, and Practice*. This book has been a staple on my own bookshelf from its inception in 1998. I have introduced the book to many nurses over the past decade and a half and plan to continue this tradition with the latest edition. I have the pleasure of teaching in a PhD program in rural nursing here at Binghamton University and I find that this book meets the needs of students, practitioners, and scholars in rural nursing. I believe this rural nursing book is valuable for many reasons, but in particular I value both its depth and breadth of topics.

As rural nursing has grown as a specialty, so has this book, which encapsulates the major concepts, beginning theory, and enriching practice of rural nursing. Early in the history of this critical text, the majority of chapters focused on a concept analysis of the major concepts in rural nursing. Today's text goes far beyond concept analysis, as areas pertinent to practice in the many realms of rural and frontier nursing are developed, tested, and revised.

The editor, Charlene A. Winters, PhD, APRN, ACNS-BC, has done an excellent job of including the seminal work in rural nursing and adding new material, both chapters updated from previous editions and new works in areas that need expansion. *Rural Nursing* has always republished the classic article by Long and Weinert (1989) on the development of the rural nursing theory base (Chapter 1), which in my opinion is timeless and an excellent introduction to the classic concepts of interest in rural nursing. The section on rural nursing practice and education begins with a seminal chapter on the distinctive nature and scope of rural nursing (Chapter 16) and also expands the rural geographical regions represented in this book, moving from a North American focus to include new chapters on work in Haiti and along the U.S.–Mexico border. The last section, "Looking Ahead," includes one of my favorite chapters, "An Analysis of Key Concepts for Rural Nursing" (Chapter 30) by Lee, Winters, Boland, Raph, and Buehler. This final chapter in the book is a wonderful synopsis of critical rural theory concepts and the relational statements that tie them together. Whether you are a doctoral student or seasoned scholar, this chapter can give you both a quick overview as well as an idea of where work needs to be done in developing rural nursing theory.

The Contents of *Rural Nursing: Concepts, Theory, and Practice* (4th ed.) reads like a Who's Who of rural nursing. I have had the pleasure of hearing many of these authors speak about their work at national and international conferences, have read many of their previous works, and value their expertise in rural nursing. Dr. Winters has done an excellent job of pulling together the work of those who gave rural nursing its start as well as authors who will move us forward in the care of rural populations in the future. Whether you are a nurse working in acute care, community health, nursing education, or research, there is something in this book for you.

—Pamela Stewart Fahs, RN, DSN
Professor and Endowed Decker Chair in Rural Nursing
Binghamton University
Decker School of Nursing
Binghamton, New York

PREFACE

This book, *Rural Nursing: Concepts, Theory, and Practice*, is the fourth edition of a text focusing on the health of rural dwellers, the provision of health care in rural settings, and what is required for effective nursing practice, education, and research in this context. The first edition, titled *Conceptual Basis for Rural Nursing*, was edited by Dr. Helen J. Lee. I joined Helen as a coeditor for the second and third editions, retitled *Rural Nursing: Concepts, Theory, and Practice*, but now find myself as the sole editor for this latest edition. Helen has chosen to relinquish her role as the coeditor to focus on her roles of contributor and mentor. As I began to write the Preface, I knew immediately that I wanted to capture Helen's reflections of the genesis of the rural text. Luckily, Helen agreed and, as she reminisced about the book's development, some experiences along the journey emerged that I will share with you here.

A native Montanan, Helen graduated from what was then Montana State College School of Nursing (now Montana State University College of Nursing), and proceeded to seek employment in a variety of places, both rural (Ridgecrest, CA; Aberdeen, SD) and urban (Tacoma, WA; Dallas, TX, Copenhagen, Denmark). After these multiple travel experiences in both practice and educational positions, she recalls being interested in returning to education and to a rural environment, and so she scheduled interviews in Montana, Washington, and Oregon.

Helen vividly remembered coming to the Bozeman and Great Falls campuses of Montana State University (MSU) for a faculty interview. She stated,

> I recall talking with Dean Anna Shannon on the Bozeman campus. She had arrived the previous year and voiced exciting plans for the future of the school. Educated at the University of California at San Francisco, Dean Shannon had a vision for the school's direction. She was well aware of the early work on nursing theories and noted that little emphasis was put on environment. Also, in examining the literature, she found an absence of rural nursing articles; any articles found were a few research studies from sociology that explored the characteristics of young women entering nursing.

Accepting a position in Montana, I became part of the faculty participating in the development of a master's degree program in rural nursing. The program evolved through the teachings of Dr. Jacqueline Taylor (ethnography) and Dr. Ruth Ludeman (sociology). The theory development process grew through the efforts of graduate students, faculty, administration, and help from consultants. Interviews of rural persons throughout the state of Montana were examined for concepts that frequently emerged from the data. This qualitative material, linked with quantitative studies, led to the theory article published in 1989 by Drs. Kathleen Long and Clarann Weinert (see Chapter 1).

The first edition consisted of chapters written by faculty and students of Montana State University (MSU) College of Nursing. The second edition included material written by authors across the United States and Canada. The Canadian alliance was initiated by Meg McDonagh, a master's student at the University of Calgary nursing program who visited MSU because of her interest in the rural theory development. Included in the content in the third edition was a new chapter written by authors from Canada and Australia. The fourth edition expands with 13 new chapters; among them is one on U.S.–Mexico border issues and one focused on Haiti.

More than four decades have passed since the College of Nursing developed a master's program that focused on the care of individuals living in a rural/remote environment. The published editions have recorded the progress of our work and the expansion of content beyond Montana to the United States and beyond our borders. The extension of the content areas and the countries represented demonstrate the book's importance to nurse educators, researchers, clinicians, and policy makers (Helen J. Lee, July 1, 2012, personal communication).

As Dr. Lee recounted, the fourth edition of *Rural Nursing: Concepts, Theory, and Practice* continues to expand our understanding of the rural health care environment. As with the first three editions, the quest continues to provide an evidence base and theory structure to help nurses and other providers address the health needs of persons living in rural communities. New chapters have been added on topics important to rural providers, educators, and researchers including: a review of literature on rural nursing theory; promoting healthy aging and resilience; palliative care; individual responses to health needs; vulnerability and health disparities across the life span; the use of rural hospitals in nursing education; health issues at the U.S.–Mexico border; nurses helping nurses in Haiti after a humanitarian emergency; accreditation of rural and frontier public health agencies; environmental risks for rural children; occupational health and safety in agricultural communities; and rural nursing workforce development. The fourth edition continues the tradition of including seminal chapters from previous editions; several chapters retained from the third edition were updated with references to the latest literature or newly collected data.

Part I contains the seminal article on the rural nursing theory base, followed by three chapters in which the authors examine the rural theory base and related literature. Part II includes chapters about the perspectives of rural persons, and Part III focuses on rural dwellers and their response to illness. Part IV begins with the seminal article about rural nursing practice and follows with reports of studies conducted with nurses in differing rural nurse practice and educational settings. Part V has greatly expanded and contains chapters devoted to rural public health. Part VI, the final section, contains three chapters: In the first, the authors outline implications for rural nursing education, practice, and policy; in the second, the authors address workforce issues critical to rural practice, research, and theory development; and in the last one, the authors provide an analysis of the key concepts introduced in the first edition.

I wish to acknowledge the work of my colleagues, students, and study participants whose contributions made this text possible. Hopefully, readers will find the latest edition thought-provoking and useful in their clinical practice, teaching efforts, and research activities. I look forward to the comments and critiques of my rural colleagues.

Charlene A. Winters

RURAL NURSING

Chapter 1

RURAL NURSING: DEVELOPING THE THEORY BASE
Kathleen Ann Long and Clarann Weinert

A LOGGER SUFFERING FROM "HEART LOCK" does not have a cardiovascular abnormality. He is suffering from a work-related anxiety disorder and can be assisted by an emergency room nurse who accurately assesses his needs and responds with effective communication and a supportive interpersonal relationship. A farmer who has lost his finger in a grain thresher several hours earlier does not have time during the harvesting season for a discussion of occupational safety. He will cope with his injury assisted by a clinic nurse who can adjust the timing of his antibiotic doses to fit with his work schedule in the fields.

Many health care needs of rural dwellers cannot be adequately addressed by the application of nursing models developed in urban or suburban areas, but require unique approaches emphasizing the special needs of this population. Although nurses are significant, and frequently the sole health care providers for people living in rural areas, little has been written to guide the practice of rural nursing. The literature provides vignettes and individual descriptions, but there is a need for an integrated, theoretical approach to rural nursing.

Rural nursing is defined as the provision of health care by professional nurses to persons living in sparsely populated areas. Over the last 8 years, graduate students and faculty members at the Montana State University College of Nursing have worked toward developing a theory base for rural nursing. Theory development has used primarily a retroductive approach, and data have been collected and refined using a combination

---

K. A. Long and C. Weinert (1989). From Rural nursing: Developing the theory base. *Scholarly Inquiry for Nursing Practice: An International Journal*, 3, 113–127. Copyright 1989 by Springer Publishing Company. Reprinted with permission.

of qualitative and quantitative methods. The experiences of rural residents and rural nurses have guided the identification of key concepts relevant to rural nursing. The goal of the theory-building process has been to identify commonalities and differences in nursing practice across all rural areas and the common and unique elements of rural nursing in relation to nursing overall. The implications of developing a theory of rural nursing for practice have been examined as a part of the ongoing process.

The theory-building process was initiated in the late 1970s. At that time, literature and research related to rural health care were limited and focused primarily on the problem of retaining physicians in rural areas and providing assessments of rural health care needs and prescriptions for rural health care services based on models and experiences from urban and suburban areas (Coward, 1977; Flax, Wagenfeld, Ivens, & Weiss, 1979). The unique health problems and health care needs of extremely sparsely populated states, such as Montana, had not been addressed from the perspective of the rural consumer. No organized theoretical base for guiding rural health care practice in general, or rural nursing in particular, existed.

QUALITATIVE DATA

The target population for qualitative data collection was the people of Montana. Montana, the fourth largest state in the United States, is an extremely sparsely populated state, with nearly 800,000 people and an average population density of approximately five persons per square mile. One-half of the counties in Montana have three or fewer persons per square mile, with six of those counties having less than one person per square mile. There is only one metropolitan center in the state; it is a city of nearly 70,000 people, with a surrounding area that constitutes a center of approximately 100,000 (Population Profiles, 1985).

Qualitative data were collected through ethnographic study by Montana State University College of Nursing graduate students. These data provided the initial ideas about health and health care in Montana. Since general propositions about rural health and rural health care did not exist, gathering of concrete data was the first step toward subsequent development of more general theoretical propositions.

Graduate students used ethnographic techniques as described by Spradley (1979) to gather information from individuals, families, and health care providers. Interview sites were selected by students on the basis of specific interest and convenience. During a 6-year period, data were gathered from approximately 25 locations. In general, each student worked in depth in one community, collecting data from 10 to 20 informants over a period of at least 1 year. Data were gathered primarily from persons in ranching and farming areas and from towns of less than

2,500 persons. In some instances, student interest led to extensive interviews with specific rural subgroups, such as men in the logging industry or older residents in a rural town (Weinert & Long, 1987). Open-ended interview questions were developed using Spradley's guidelines. The questions emphasized seeking the informants' views without superimposing the cultural biases of the interviewer. The opening question in the interview was, "What is health to you . . . from your viewpoint? . . . your definition?" Interviewers used standard probes and a standard format of questions regarding health beliefs and health care preferences.

Spradley (1979) indicated that the goal of ethnographic study is to "build a systematic understanding of all human cultures from the perspective of those who have learned them" (p. 10). The goal of data collection in Montana was to learn about the culture of rural Montanans from rural Montanans. Emphasis in the cultural learning process was on understanding health beliefs, values, and practices. Rigdon, Clayton, and Diamond (1987) have noted that understanding the meaning that persons attach to subjective experiences is an important aspect of nursing knowledge. The ethnographic approach captured the meanings that rural dwellers ascribe to the subjective states of health and illness and facilitated the development of a rich database.

As the database developed, the following definitions and assumptions were accepted as a foundation for theory development. *Rural* was defined as meaning sparsely populated. Within this context, states such as Montana, which are sparsely populated overall, are viewed as rural throughout, despite the existence of some population centers within them. Further, based on this definition, rural regions or areas can be identified within otherwise heavily populated states. An assumption is made that, to some degree, health care needs are different in rural areas from those of urban areas. Also, all rural areas are viewed as having some common health care needs. Finally, another assumption is made that urban models are not appropriate to, or adequate for, meeting health care needs in rural areas.

Retroductive Theory Generation

Faculty work groups were developed to examine and organize the qualitative data. The work groups involved three to five nursing faculty members, each with rural nursing experience, but with varied backgrounds and expertise. Thus, a work group included experts from various clinical areas, as well as persons with direct experience either in small rural hospitals or in larger metropolitan centers within rural states. Standard ethnographic content analysis (Spradley, 1979) was used to sort and categorize the ethnographic data. Groups worked toward consensus about the meaning and organization of specific data. Recurring themes were identified and viewed as having relevance and importance for the rural informants in relation to their views of health.

A retroductive approach, as originally described by Hanson (1958), was used for examining the initial ethnographic data and to build the theory base. Specific concepts and relational statements were derived from the data, and more general propositions were induced from these statements. The new propositions were then used for developing additional specific statements which could be supported by existing data or which were categorized for later testing. The retroductive approach was literally a "back and forth" process that permitted persons familiar with the data to move between the data and beginning-level theoretical propositions. The process was orderly and consistent, and required group consensus about data interpretation and the relevance of derived propositions. The retroductive process continued in work groups over several years as additional ethnographic data were gathered. Consultants participated at key points in the process, to raise questions, add insights, and critically evaluate the group's theory-building approach. Walker and Avant (1983) have noted that the retroductive process "adds considerably to the body of theoretical knowledge. It is, in fact, the way theory develops in the 'real world'" (p. 176).

QUANTITATIVE DATA

Following several years of ethnographic study, the faculty members involved in theory development wished to enrich the qualitative database by collecting relevant quantitative data. Kleinman (1983) stated, "Qualitative description, taken together with various quantitative measures, can be a standardized research method for assessing validity. It is especially valuable in studying social and cultural significance, e.g., illness beliefs interaction norms, social gain, ethnic help seeking, and treatment responses" (p. 543). Hinds and Young (1987) noted, "The combination of different methodologies within a single study promotes the likelihood of uncovering multiple dimensions of a phenomenon's empirical reality" (p. 195).

A survey developed by Weinert in 1983 attempted to validate some of the rural health concepts that had emerged from the ethnographic data. These concepts were health status and health beliefs, isolation and distance, self-reliance, and informal health care systems. Survey instruments with established psychometric properties were selected to measure the specific concepts of interest. A mail questionnaire completed by the respondents included the Beck Depression Inventory (Beck, 1967) and the Trait Anxiety Scale (Spielberger, Gorsuch, & Lushene, 1970) to tap mental health status, and the General Health Perception Scale (Davies & Ware, 1981) to measure physical health status and health beliefs. A background information form assessed demographic variables, including the period of residence and geographic locale. The Personal Resource Questionnaire

(Brandt & Weinert, 1981) assessed the use of informal systems for support and health care.

The convenience sample of survey participants was located through the Agricultural Extension Service, social groups, and informal networks. All the participants lived in Montana, completed the questionnaires in their homes, and returned them by mail to the researcher. The 62 survey participants were middle-class Whites, with an average of 13.5 years of education and a mean age of 61.3 years, who had lived in Montana for an average period of 45.6 years. The survey sample consisted of 40 women and 22 men residing in one of 13 sparsely populated Montana counties. The most populated county has a population density of 5.9 persons per square mile, and one town of nearly 6,000 people. In the most sparsely populated county, there is one town with 600 people and an average population density of 0.5 persons per square mile.

Findings from the quantitative study were used throughout the theory development process to support or refute concept descriptions and relational statements derived from the ethnographic data. Survey findings are discussed in the following section as they relate to key concepts and relational statements.

REFINING THE BUILDING BLOCKS OF THEORY

To order the data and foster the formation of relational statements, an organizational scheme for theory development was adopted. Using the paradigm first described by Yura and Torres (1975) and later by Fawcett (1984), ethnographic data were categorized under the four major dimensions of nursing theory: person, health, environment, and nursing. The data were then ordered from the more general to the more specific. This process led to the identification of constructs, concepts, variables, and indicators.

An example helps in illustrating this process. Ethnographic data had been gathered from "gypo" loggers. These men are independent logging contractors from northwestern Montana who work in rugged isolated areas, usually living in trailers or tents while working. Examples of quotes from these loggers and their associates as found in the data are: A logger states, "We worry about the here and now"; a local physician says, "Loggers enter the health care system during times of crisis only"; the public health nurse in the area says, "Loggers don't want to hear about health care problems; they don't return until the next accident." Table 1.1 shows the scheme used for organizing these data. The concepts "present time" orientation and crisis orientation to health are identified. These are placed under the person dimension. In this example, the constructs are not fully developed, but are viewed as either psychological or sociocultural, or both. The important variables identified thus far are definitions of time

TABLE 1.1 Data Ordering Scheme

Dimension	Psychological/sociocultural
Concept	"Present time" orientation Crisis orientation to health
Variable	Definitions of time Definitions of crisis
Indicators	Hours, minutes, days Seasons, work seasons Number of injuries Number of illnesses

and of crisis. Possible indicators are measures of time, such as hours or seasons, and measures of crisis, such as numbers of illnesses or injuries.

Key Concepts

In the process of data organization it was noted that some concepts appeared repeatedly in ethnographic data collected in several different areas of the state. In addition, aspects of several of these concepts were supported by the quantitative survey data (Weinert, 1983). Using Walker and Avant's (1983) model of concept synthesis, these concepts were identified as key concepts in relation to understanding rural health needs and rural nursing practice. These key concepts are as follows: work beliefs and health beliefs, isolation and distance, self-reliance, lack of anonymity, outsider/insider, and old-timer/newcomer.

As key concepts in this theory, work beliefs and health beliefs are viewed differently in rural dwellers as contrasted with urban or suburban residents. These two sets of beliefs appear to be closely interrelated among rural persons. Work or fulfilling one's usual functions is of primary importance. Health is assessed by rural people in relation to work role and work activities, and health needs are usually secondary to work needs.

The related concepts of isolation and distance are identified as important in understanding rural health and nursing. Specifically, they help in understanding health-care-seeking behavior. Quantitative survey data indicated that rural informants who lived outside towns traveled a distance of almost 23 miles, on an average, for emergency health care and over 50 miles for routine health care. Despite these distances, ethnographic data indicated that rural dwellers tended to see health services as accessible and did not view themselves as isolated.

Self-reliance and independence of rural persons are also seen as key concepts. The desire to do for oneself and care for oneself was strong among the rural persons interviewed; this has important ramifications in relation to the provision of health care.

Two key concept areas, lack of anonymity and outsider/insider, have particular relevance to the practice of rural nursing. Lack of anonymity, a hallmark of small towns and surrounding sparsely populated areas, implies a limited ability for rural persons to have private areas of their lives. Rural nurses almost always reported being known to their patients as neighbors, as part of a given family, as members of a certain church, and so on. Similarly, these nurses usually know their patients in several different social and personal relationships beyond the nurse–patient relationship. The old-timer/newcomer concept, or the related concept of outsider/insider, is relevant in terms of the acceptance of nurses and of all health care providers in rural communities. The ethnographic data indicated that these concepts were used by rural dwellers in organizing their view of the social environment and in guiding their interactions and relationships. Survey data revealed that those who had lived in Montana for over 10 years, but less than 20, still considered themselves to be "newcomers" and expected to be viewed as such by those in their community (Weinert & Long, 1987).

Relational Statements

In an effort to move from a purely descriptive theory to a beginning level explanatory one, some initial relational statements were generated from the qualitative data and were supported by the quantitative data that had been collected thus far. The statements are in the early stages of testing.

The first statement is that rural dwellers define health primarily as the ability to work, to be productive, and to do usual tasks. The ethnographic data indicate that rural persons place little emphasis on the comfort, cosmetic, and life-prolonging aspects of health. One is viewed as healthy when he or she is able to function and is productive in one's work role. Specifically, rural residents indicated that pain was tolerated, often for extended periods, so long as it did not interfere with the ability to function. The General Health Perception Scale indicated that rural survey participants reported experiencing less pain than an age-comparable urban sample (Weinert & Long, 1987). Further, scores on the Beck Depression Inventory and the Trait Anxiety Scale (Weinert, 1983) revealed that they experienced less anxiety and less depression.

The second statement is that rural dwellers are self-reliant and resist accepting help or services from those seen as "outsiders" or from agencies seen as national or regional "welfare" programs. A corollary to this statement is that help, including needed health care, is usually sought through an informal rather than a formal system. Ethnographic data supported both the second statement and its corollary. Numerous references were found to show, for example, a preference for "the 'old doc' who knows us" over the new specialist who was unfamiliar. Data from the Personal Resource Questionnaire (Weinert, 1983) indicated that rural dwellers relied primarily on family, relatives, and close friends for help and support. Further, the rural survey respondents reported using health care professionals and formal human service agencies much less frequently than did comparable urban respondents in previous studies.

A third statement is that health care providers in rural areas must deal with a lack of anonymity and a much greater role diffusion than providers in urban or suburban settings. This statement has a marked significance for rural nursing practice. Although limited ethnographic and survey data have been collected from rural nurses thus far, some emerging themes have been identified. In addition to identifying a sense of isolation from professional peers, rural nurses emphasize their lack of anonymity and a sense of role diffusion. There is an inability to keep separate the activities and the behaviors of the individual nurse's various roles. In a small town, for example, the nurse's behavior as a wife, a mother, and a church attendee are all significantly related to her effectiveness as a health care professional in that community. Further, in their professional role, nurses reported experiencing role diffusion. Nurses are expected to perform a variety of diverse and unrelated tasks. During a single shift, a nurse may work in obstetrics delivering a baby, care for a dying patient on the medical–surgical unit, and initiate care of a trauma patient in the emergency room. Likewise, during an evening shift or on weekends, a nurse may be required to carry out tasks reserved for the pharmacist or dietitian on the day shift.

RELATIONSHIP OF CONCEPTS AND STATEMENTS TO THE LARGER BODY OF NURSING KNOWLEDGE

How people define health and illness has a direct impact on how they seek and use health care services and is a key concept in understanding client behavior and in planning intervention.

Definition of Health

The rural Montana dwellers primarily defined health as the ability to work and to be productive. The work of other researchers supports the finding that residents of sparsely populated areas view health in terms of ability to work and to remain productive. Ross (1982), a nurse anthropologist, studied the health perceptions of women living in the Lake District along the coast of Nova Scotia. She conducted in-depth interviews with 60 women of both British and French backgrounds in small coastal fishing communities. Similar to the rural dwellers in Montana, these women described good health as being "able to do what you want to do" and to be "able to work." Lee's (1991) recent work in Montana supports earlier findings, on which the rural nursing theory was built. She found that work and health practices were closely related among farmers and ranchers; health is viewed as a functional state in relation to work. Scharff's (1987) interviews with nurses practicing in small rural hospitals in eastern Washington, northern Idaho, and western Montana indicated that they viewed the health needs of rural people as overlapping those of people living in urban situations in many instances. The nurse informants, however, noted that rural people equate health with the ability to work or function in their daily activities. Rural people were viewed as delaying health care until they were very ill, thus often needing hospitalization at the point of seeking care.

Self-Reliance

The statement derived from the Montana data that "rural dwellers resist accepting help from outsiders or strangers" has been supported by data from research in rural Maryland (Salisbury State College, 1986). People living in the rural eastern shore area were described as highly resistant to care from persons viewed as outsiders, and rural shore residents often refused to go "across the bridge" to Baltimore to seek health care, even though this was a trip of less than 100 miles and would allow access to sophisticated, specialized treatment. Like the rural people in Montana, these Maryland residents sought health care information and assistance from local, and often informal, sources. The self-reliance of rural persons and their resistance to outside help were also reported by Counts and Boyle (1987) in relation to the residents of the Appalachian area. Self-reliance was noted as a major feature that must be considered in planning nursing care services for this population.

The rural Nova Scotia women studied by Ross (1982) indicated informal personal networks of family, friends, and neighbors as important sources of health information who also provided the physical, financial, emotional, and social support that contributes to well-being. When these women were asked what connection there was between health and the availability of hospitals, doctors, and other medical care, 42% indicated that it was the individual's responsibility for health knowledge and care; 25% thought professionals were useful to a certain point in providing advice and services such as routine physical exams; 19% indicated that these services were for sick persons, not healthy persons; and 9% felt the formal health care system had no relationship to health (Ross, 1982, p. 311). One woman commented, "Health is not a topic to discuss with doctors and nurses" (Ross, 1982, p. 309).

Rural Nursing

The Montana data and the theory derived from it indicate that nurses and other health care providers in rural areas must deal with a lack of anonymity. Nurses are known in a variety of roles to their patients, and in turn, know their patients in a variety of roles. Most of the nurses interviewed by Scharff (1987) felt that by knowing their patients personally they could give better care. Other nurses, however, noted that providing professional care for family or friends can be a frightening experience. Nurses indicated that there was no anonymity for them in the rural community, which at times was reassuring and at other times, constricting (Scharff, 1987).

The concept of role diffusion in the rural hospital setting was very apparent in Scharff's (1987) work. She reported that a rural hospital nurse must be a jack-of-all-trades who often practices within the realm of numerous other health care disciplines, including respiratory therapy, laboratory technology, dietetics, pharmacy, social work, psychology, and medicine. Examples of the intersections between rural nursing and other disciplines include doing EKGs (electrocardiography or elektrokardiogramm), performing arterial punctures, running blood gas machines, drawing blood, setting up cultures, going to the pharmacy to pour drugs, going to the local drugstore to get medications for patients, ordering x-rays and medications, delivering babies, directing the actions of physicians, and cooking meals when the cook gets snowed in. As Scharff noted, some of these functions are carried out by urban nurses practicing in particular settings such as a trauma center or an intensive care unit. Rural nurses, however, are usually not circumscribed by assignment to a particular unit or department and are expected to function in multiple roles, even during one work shift.

This generalist work role and the lack of anonymity of rural nurses are substantiated by findings and descriptions from several other rural areas of the United States (Biegel, 1983; St. Clair, Pickard, & Harlow, 1986). A study of nurses in rural Texas noted, "Nurses play roles as nurse, friend, neighbor, citizen, and family member" within a community; further, rural nurses in their work roles were described as needing to be "all things to all people" (St. Clair et al., 1986, p. 28).

Generalizability

The issue of a situation or locale-specific theory and its relationship to the larger body of nursing knowledge needs serious consideration. The work of Scharff (1987) indicated that the core of rural nursing is not different from that of urban nursing. The intersections, however, those "meeting points at which nursing extends its practice into the domains of other professions"; the dimensions, that is, the "philosophy, responsibilities, functions, roles, and skills"; and the boundaries, which "respond to new and growing needs and demands from society" (American Nurses Association, 1980), appear to be very distinct for rural nursing practice.

Questions still remain as to how generalizable findings from Montana residents are to other rural populations. Clearly, there is a need for more organized and rigorous data collection in relation to rural nursing before these questions can be answered. A sound theory base for rural practice requires a continued research, conducted across diverse rural settings.

IMPLICATIONS FOR NURSING PRACTICE

The findings from the Montana research about people living in sparsely populated areas have implications for nursing practice in rural areas. Since work is of major importance to rural people, health care must fit within work schedules. Health care programs or clinics that conflict with the rural economic cycle such as haying or calving will not be used. Since health is defined as the ability to work, health promotion must address the work issue. For example, health education related to cardiovascular disease should highlight strategies for preventing conditions that involve long-term disability such as stroke. These aspects will be more meaningful to rural dwellers than preventive aspects that emphasize a longer, more comfortable life.

The self-reliance of rural dwellers has specific nursing implications. Rural people often delay seeking health care until they are gravely ill or incapacitated. Nursing approaches need to address two distinct aspects: nonjudgmental intervention for those who undergo a delayed treatment and a strong emphasis on imparting knowledge of preventive health. If the nurse can provide adequate information regarding health, the rural dwellers' desire for self-reliance may lead to health-promotion behaviors. With a good information base, rural people can make appropriate decisions regarding self-care versus the need for professional intervention.

Health care services must be tailored to suit the preferences of rural persons for family and community help during periods of illness. Nurses can provide instruction, support, and relief to family members and neighbors, who are often the primary care providers for sick and disabled persons.

The formal health care system needs to fit into the informal helping system in rural areas. A long-term community resident, such as the drugstore proprietor, can be assisted in providing accurate advice to residents through the provision of reference materials and a telephone backup system. One can anticipate greater acceptance and use by rural residents of an updated but old and trusted health care resource, rather than a new professional but "outsider" service (Weinert & Long, 1987).

Nurses who enter rural communities must allow for extended periods prior to acceptance. Involvement in diverse community activities, such as civic organizations and recreational clubs, may assist the nurse in being known and accepted as a person. In rural communities, acceptance as a health care professional is often tied to personal acceptance. Thus, it appears that rural communities are not appropriate practice settings for nurses who prefer to maintain entirely separate professional and personal lives.

The stresses that appear to affect nurses in rural practice settings have particular importance. Rural nurses see themselves as cut off from the professional mainstream. They are often in situations where there is no collegial support to assist in defining an appropriate practice role and its boundaries. The educational preparation of those who wish to practice in rural settings needs to emphasize not only generalist skills, but also a strong base in change theory and leadership techniques. Nurses in rural practice need a sound orientation to techniques for accessing diverse sources of current information. If the closest library is several hundred miles away, for example, can all arrangements for interlibrary loan and access to material via telephone, bus, or mail be arranged? Networks that link together nurses practicing in distant rural sites are particularly useful, both for information exchange and for mutual support.

SUMMARY

It is becoming increasingly clear that rural dwellers have distinct definitions of health. Their health care needs require approaches that differ significantly from urban and suburban populations. Subcultural values, norms, and beliefs play key roles in how rural people define health and from whom they seek advice and care. These values and beliefs, combined with the realities of rural living—such as weather, distance, and isolation—markedly affect the practice of nursing in rural settings. Additional ethnographic and quantitative data are needed to further define both the common and the locale-specific conditions and characteristics of rural populations. Continued research can provide a more solid base for the nursing theory that is required to guide the practice and the delivery of health care to rural populations.

ACKNOWLEDGMENTS

Qualitative data collected and analyzed by the Montana State University College of Nursing graduate students and faculty form the basis for a substantial portion of this chapter. Ethnographic data collection and analysis was supported, in part, by a U.S. Department of Health and Human Services, Division of Nursing, and Advanced Training Grant to the Montana State University College of Nursing (#1816001649AI). The project that provided the survey data was funded by a Montana State University Faculty Research/Creativity Grant. This chapter is based partially on a paper presented at the Western Society for Research in Nursing Conference, Tempe, AZ Arizona, May 1987.

REFERENCES

American Nurses Association. (1980). *Nursing. A social policy statement (No. NP-6320M 9/82R)*. Kansas City, MO: Author.

Beck, A. (1967). *Depression: Causes and treatment*. Philadelphia: University of Pennsylvania Press.

Biegel, A. (1983). Toward a definition of rural nursing. *Home Health Care Nursing, 1*, 45–46.

Brandt, P., & Weinert, C. (1981). The PRQ: A social support measure. *Nursing Research, 30*, 277–280.

Counts, M., & Boyle, J. (1987). Nursing, health and policy within a community context. *Advances in Nursing Science, 9*, 12–23.

Coward, R. (1977). Delivering social services in small towns and rural communities. In R. Coward (Ed.), *Rural families across the life span: Implications for community programming* (pp. 1–17). West Lafayette: Indiana Cooperative Extension Services.

Davies, A., & Ware, J. (1981). *Measuring health perceptions in the health insurance experiment*. Santa Monica, CA: Rand.

Fawcett, J. (1984). *Analysis and evaluation of conceptual models of nursing*. Philadelphia, PA: F. A. Davis.

Flax, J., Wagenfeld, M., Ivens, R., & Weiss, R. (1979). *Mental health and rural America: An overview, and annotated bibliography*. Rockville, MD: U.S. Government Printing Office.

Hanson, N. (1958). *Patterns of discovery*. Cambridge: Cambridge University Press.

Hinds, P., & Young, K. (1987). A triangulation of methods and paradigms to study nurse-given wellness care. *Nursing Research, 36*, 195–198.

Kleinman, A. (1983). The cultural meanings and social uses of illness: A role for medical anthropology and clinically oriented social science in the development of primary care theory and research. *Journal of Family Practice, 16*, 539–545.

Lee, H. J. (1991). Relationship of hardiness and current life events to perceived health and rural adults. *Research in Nursing and Health, 14*(5), 351–359.

Montana State University Center for Data Systems and Analysis (1985). *Population profiles of Montana counties: 1980*. Bozeman, MT: Author.

Rigdon, I., Clayton, B., & Diamond, M. (1987). Toward a theory of helpfulness for the elderly bereaved: An invitation to a new life. *Advances in Nursing Science, 9*, 32–43.

Ross, H. (1982). *Women and wellness: Defining, attaining, and maintaining health in Eastern Canada*. Dissertation Abstracts International, 42, DEO 82–12624.

Salisbury State College. (1986, June). Discussion of Salisbury State College rural health findings. Presented at the Contemporary Issues in Rural Health Conference, Salisbury, MD.

Scharff, J. (1987). *The nature and scope of rural nursing: Distinctive characteristics.* Unpublished master's thesis, Montana State University–Bozeman.

Spielberger, C., Gorsuch, R., & Lushene, R. (1970). *STAI manual for the State-Trait Anxiety Questionnaire.* Palo Alto, CA: Consulting Psychologist.

Spradley, J. (1979). *The ethnographic interview.* New York: Holt, Rinehart, & Winston.

St. Clair, C., Pickard, M., & Harlow, K. (1986). Continuing education for self-actualization: Building a plan for rural nurses. *Journal of Continuing Education in Nursing, 17,* 27–31.

Walker, L., & Avant, K. (1983). *Strategies for theory construction in nursing.* Norwalk, CT: Appleton-Century-Crofts.

Weinert, C. (1983). *[Social support: Rural people in their new middle years].* Unpublished raw data.

Weinert, C., & Long, K. (1987). Understanding the health care needs of rural families. *Journal of Family Relations, 36,* 450–455.

Yura, H., & Torres, G. (1975). *Today's conceptual frameworks with the baccalaureate nursing programs* (NLN Pub. No. 15–1558, pp. 17–75). New York, NY: NLN.

Chapter 2

UPDATING THE RURAL NURSING THEORY BASE

Helen J. Lee and Meg K. McDonagh

HISTORICAL PERSPECTIVES

"Sparsely populated areas: Toward nursing theory" was the title of a 1982 symposium at the Western Council on Higher Education for Nursing (now Western Institute of Nursing). In her introductory remarks, Montana State University-Bozeman (MSU-B) College of Nursing Dean Anna Shannon stated that the presentation would demonstrate how a school could "maximize its resources, provide opportunities for faculty and student research and contribute . . . to the development of an empirically based theory of rural nursing" (pp. 70–71). She noted a lack of literature and research about rural nursing and the infrequent inclusion of environment within nursing theories.

Faculty and graduate students' studies about (a) the role of distance in home dialysis, (b) sodium in drinking water and adolescent blood pressure, and (c) beliefs and practices of Crow Indian women, Hmong refugees, and Hutterite colony members were presented within the symposium. Concluding remarks included a plan for theory construction and testing using retroduction, a process involving both inductive and deductive reasoning. Theory development activity continued at MSU-B College of Nursing, resulting in this text's seminal article (see Chapter 1, "Rural Nursing: Developing the Theory Base").

Our present chapter includes a summary of the rural nursing theory structure explicated by Long and Weinert in 1989 and a review of the literature supporting or refuting the viability of the theoretical statements and concepts. Based on the review, we propose changes in the rural nursing theory structure and make suggestions for future work.

THE RURAL NURSING THEORY STRUCTURE

Many disciplines exist to generate, test, and apply theories that will improve the quality of people's lives. (Fawcett, 1999, p. 1)

The quality of the lives of rural persons and the lack of empirical studies about their health care was of concern to MSU-B nursing researchers. A middle-range theory emerged from a recognized need for a practice framework that acknowledges the unique perceptions of rural persons and the generalist experience of nurses who practice in rural settings. Prior to the development of the theory, it was assumed that nursing care of rural persons was similar to the care of persons living in urban environments.

The resulting descriptive theory is the "most basic type of middle range theory" (Fawcett, 1999, p. 15). Middle range theory focuses "on a limited dimension of the reality of nursing" and grows at the "intersection of practice and research to provide guidance for everyday practice and scholarly research rooted in the discipline of nursing" (Smith & Liehr, 2003, p. xi). It emerged from observations gathered through qualitative and quantitative descriptive studies conducted in the sparsely populated rural setting of Montana. It describes specific characteristics and observations made of rural persons seeking health care and their health care providers. The published theory contains several key concepts and three theoretical statements (Long & Weinert, 1989).

The first statement is descriptive and states that *"rural dwellers define health primarily as the ability to work, to be productive, to do usual tasks"* (Long & Weinert, 1989, p. 120). Key concepts associated with this statement are work beliefs and health beliefs. The second statement is relational and proposes that *"rural dwellers are self-reliant and resist accepting help or services from those seen as 'outsiders' or from agencies seen as national or regional 'welfare' programs"* (Long & Weinert, 1989, p. 120). Rural persons preferred to seek health care from insiders, persons with whom they were familiar. Additional key concepts pertaining to this statement are old-timer and newcomer. A corollary to the second statement is that "help, including needed medical care, is usually sought through an informal rather than a formal system" (p. 120). The third statement is relational and focuses on health care providers; it indicates that *lack of anonymity and role diffusion are experienced more acutely among rural providers than among providers in urban or suburban settings.* Lack of anonymity also applies to the recipients of health care in rural areas, as all persons in that environment have a "limited ability . . . to have private areas of their lives" (Long & Weinert, 1989, p. 119).

In addition to the above three statements, an understanding of the concepts "isolation" and "distance" is important in the health care-seeking behavior of rural residents. Isolation refers to separation from or being placed alone (Lee, Hollis, & McClain, 1998). Distance is measurable time, physical space between places, and personal perception of that space (Henson, Sadler, & Walton, 1998). Qualitative data upon which the theoretical work was based indicated that rural residents did not feel isolated, despite the fact that they averaged 23 miles of travel to their nearest emergency room and over 50 miles to their primary health care source (Long & Weinert, 1989, p. 119).

RELATED NURSING LITERATURE

The content of Long and Weinert's (1989) rural nursing theory article was and is widely quoted in nursing literature, including community health and rural nursing texts, and in presentations given about rural nursing. However, periodic rural nursing literature reviews contain few citations specifically focusing on health perceptions and needs of rural persons. We located three qualitative studies through conference proceedings, the contents of which were subsequently published (Bales, Winters, & Lee, 2006 [see Chapter 5]; Lee & Winters, 2004; Thomlinson, McDonagh, Reimer, Crooks, & Lees, 2004). Other sources included two nursing master's theses (Bales, 2006; Moran, 2005), a study that focused on the health care meanings, values, and practices of Anglo-American male population in the rural American Midwest (Sellers, Poduska, Propp, & White, 1999), a study exploring rurality and health in mid-life women (Thurston & Meadows, 2003), and a study examining the health-information-seeking experiences of rural women in Ontario, Canada (Wathen & Harris, 2006, 2007). We also located several journal articles, mostly qualitative rural research, that included rural concepts found in Long and Weinert's article. In the following sections, each theoretical statement is followed by findings from the literature supporting or refuting the statement.

Theoretical Statement #1 (Descriptive)

> ...[R]ural dwellers define health primarily as the ability to work, to be productive, to do usual tasks. (Long & Weinert, 1989, p. 120)

Four qualitative studies conducted in the United States examined health perceptions; one with rural men aged 25 to 49 years, one with rural men and women aged 28 to 63 years, and two with older rural persons aged 60 to 85. Three provided support for the above descriptive statement that defines health as the ability to carry out important functions (Niemoller, Ide, & Nichols, 2000; Pierce, 2001; Sellers et al., 1999). In the fourth study, Averill (2002) found that definitions of health varied across her southwest U.S. sample that included older retirees, more recent retirees, and Hispanic elders. The older retirees from mining and ranching communities viewed health in a similar manner to the original qualitative theory development samples, while more recent retirees focused on strategies to remain healthy—proper diet, regular exercise, and regular health exams. The Hispanic elders in Averill's sample frequently mentioned incorporating home remedies and herbal preparations into their health maintenance practices.

Participants in the six health perceptions and needs studies (Bales, 2006; Bales et al., 2006; Lee & Winters, 2004; Moran, 2005; Thomlinson et al., 2004; Winters et al., 2006b) conducted in the United States and Canada were more likely to define health holistically. Lee and Winters (2004) found that for rural persons working in service occupations, being able to function included being physically, mentally, and emotionally fit. Participants in a study conducted by Bales et al. (2006) thought that being healthy meant being mentally and physically active, eating well, and having an overall sense of well-being. Thomlinson and her colleagues (2004) interpreted their participants' responses by saying that health was a "holistic relationship between the physical, mental, social and spiritual aspects of their lives" (p. 261). This same view of health was echoed by Canadian middle-aged women in Thurston and Meadows' (2003) study and by the older adults residing in Appalachia who completed surveys and participated in focus groups (Goins, Spencer, & Williams, 2010).

Australian women in de la Rue and Coulson's (2003) study, aged 73 to 87, equated health with not being ill. They knew maintenance of their health was influenced by their geographical location and their desire to remain living on the land.

Summary

The literature both supports and refutes the first theoretical statement. Support appears in studies of rural male adults and of older persons and retirees from the extractive industries (mining, farming). Lack of support for the functional definition of health emerges from a variety of settings and from differing rural samples. It may be that age, the rural environmental setting, the influence of the work ethic, and culture are factors in defining health (de la Rue & Coulson, 2003). Potentially, younger rural participants may be influenced by increased media exposure and its emphasis on health promotion and the use of preventive health practices. In addition, health care providers may be expanding their view of health beyond the illness care model and may be sharing this with their clients.

Theoretical Statement #2 (Relational)

> ...[R]ural dwellers are self-reliant and resist accepting help or services from those seen as "outsiders" or from agencies seen as national or regional welfare programs. (Long & Weinert, 1989, p. 120)

The attribute of self-reliance dominates the literature about rural persons and their health-seeking behaviors (Davis & Magilvy, 2000; Jirojwong & MacLennan, 2002; Lee & Winters, 2004; Niemoller et al., 2000; Sellers et al., 1999; Thomlinson et al., 2004; Wathen & Harris, 2006, 2007; Winters et al., 2006b). Care was sought by rural residents after first "consulting books" (Jirojwong & MacLennan, 2002, p. 251) and trying "to deal with an illness themselves" (Thomlinson et al., 2004, p. 10). Because of the presence of chronic illnesses, older adults were knowledgeable about nearby medical care resources, including physicians, physician's assistants, and nurse practitioners (Niemoller et al., 2000; Pierce, 2001; Roberto & Reynolds, 2001), and if available, would use them "to achieve their desired level of independence" (Niemoller et al., p. 39). However, if the desired resources were not available, these same older adults stated they would "manage" (Niemoller et al., p. 39).

Canadian women (aged 20–82) in the study conducted by Wathen and Harris (2006) shared differing strategies when faced with an urgent health situation. Some would visit a hospital emergency room while others would self-medicate and wait until the next morning to contact their family doctor. Decision making was influenced by perception of the knowledge and skills of available professional practitioners and, in some situations, by the results of previous interactions with regard to managing their chronic illnesses. In addition, decisions were affected by the distances they needed to travel, especially during the winter.

Corollary to Relational Statement #2

> ...[H]elp, including needed health care, is usually sought through an informal rather than a formal system. (Long & Weinert, 1989, p. 120)

The literature revealed a variety of findings related to the relational statement corollary. Bales (2006) found that mothers living in U.S. frontier settings would seek advice from family, friends, and neighbors and would initiate self-care activities if health care situations were not considered serious. However, if the illness or injury was gauged as serious, professional health care was immediately accessed no matter the distance involved. Bypassing the informal for the formal system because of the seriousness of the illness or injury also was found in studies conducted by Buehler, Malone, and Majerus (1998) and Thomlinson and colleagues (2004).

Participants in two Canadian studies (Thomlinson et al., 2004; Wathen & Harris, 2006, 2007) indicated that family, friends, and neighbors were cited as a major source of support, particularly during the information-gathering phase (Wathen & Harris, 2006). Those particularly valued were persons who held a health care professional role or had experienced a disease or illness first hand (Wathen & Harris, 2006). Although older rural women in the U.S. study conducted by Pierce (2001) stated they were eager to help neighbors and the less fortunate, they also shared their reluctance to tell family and neighbors about their own needs unless really necessary.

Help gained through accessing informal knowledge via the media, popular magazines, books, libraries, and the Internet was cited in three studies (Roberto & Reynolds, 2001; Thomlinson et al., 2004; Wathen & Harris, 2007). A sample of older women living in the United States actively sought information about living with their osteoporosis (Roberto & Reynolds, 2001): Members of a Canadian sample stated that they frequently made use of formal information sources through libraries, books, and computers (Thomlinson et al., 2004; Wathen & Harris, 2007).

Summary

The second theoretical statement and its corollary are both sustained and refuted by the findings in the literature. Self-reliance remains a characteristic attribute of rural persons and influences the way they respond to illness or injury and their subsequent care-seeking behaviors. The informal system (family, friends, and neighbors) is still frequently used as a resource. However, the rural cultural barrier to accessing care through formal resources appears to be changing. The increased knowledge and the need to have information about health and the chronic illnesses they are experiencing may be removing the cultural barrier of approaching "outsiders" for health and medical care. In part, this may be occurring because desired health information can now be obtained through use of computers while maintaining anonymity. Prior to the current age of information technology, maintaining anonymity while seeking health information was not an option.

Theoretical Statement #3 (Relational)

> ...[H]ealth care providers in rural areas must deal with a lack of anonymity and much greater role diffusion than providers in urban or suburban settings. (Long & Weinert, 1989, p. 120)

The findings for the two concepts forming this relational statement—lack of anonymity and role diffusion—are sustained in the literature about health care providers from Australia, New Zealand, and the United States. In relation to the lack of anonymity, authors stated that "in close knit communities ... news travels fast" (Lau, Kumar, & Thomas, 2002, Results and Discussion, paragraph 7) and that "social life realities in small communities frequently blur professional boundaries" (Blue & Fitzgerald, 2002, pp. 319–320). Social factors pertaining to practice in rural communities include privacy issues for both the professional and the clients for whom they give care (Lau et al., 2002). Health care practitioners in rural environments who are known by their clients may find that older women prefer receiving professional care from a familiar person (Courtney, Tong, & Walsh, 2000; Pierce, 2001), whereas middle-aged women prefer to go elsewhere for care because of that familiarity (Brown, Young, & Byles, 1999; Lee & Winters, 2004). Lee and Winters found this particularly true for women's health care and mental health.

Role diffusion was found in studies conducted with psychiatrists and nurses in Australia (Lau et al., 2002) and by Rosenthal (1996) in her study of rural nursing in America. Hegney (1997) described role diffusion in both generalist and extended roles in her study of Australian rural nursing practice. Role diffusion was evident in the practice of hospice nurses in New Zealand (McConigley, Kristjanson, & Morgan, 2000). The reality in sparsely populated areas is that with fewer persons available to perform multiple tasks, more tasks must be undertaken by the individuals who practice in these areas.

Summary

The third theoretical statement about lack of anonymity and role diffusion is well supported in the literature. Familiarity, the opposite of anonymity, can be a facilitator or a barrier to seeking health and illness care from local health care practitioners. Familiarity is a distinguishing feature of rural nursing that allows rural nurses a special knowledge of those for whom they provide care within their communities (Hegney, 1997).

The lack of anonymity that health care providers experience in rural communities is in itself a paradox. On the one hand, it is often the familiarity and knowing of community members and the lack of anonymity that draws health care professionals to rural areas. Yet, it is often these same attributes that can later drive them away.

Conclusion

The review of the literature pertaining to the descriptive middle range rural nursing theory base revealed a variety of findings. The rural residents' definition of health in the first descriptive statement is changing from that of a functional nature to a more holistic view that includes physical, mental, social, and spiritual aspects. The self-reliance of rural residents in the second relational statement is broadly supported; however, the resistance to seeking help from those seen as "outsiders" is changing. The third relational statement pertaining to health care providers and their lack of anonymity and role diffusion is supported. The findings for the concept of distance in the original rural theory development work are not supported. This literature appraisal of the rural nursing theory base structure supports a need for change.

THE REVISED RURAL NURSING THEORY STRUCTURE

Based on the review of the literature, we recommended the following revisions to the first two theoretical statements originally proposed by Long and Weinert in 1989.

Theoretical Statement #1 (Descriptive)

> Rural residents define health as being able to do what they want to do; it is a way of life and a state of mind; there is a goal of maintaining balance in all aspects of their lives. (Lee & McDonagh, 2006, p. 314)

> Older rural residents and those with ties to extractive industries are more likely to define health in a functional manner—to work, to be productive, and to do usual tasks. (Lee & McDonagh, 2006, p. 314)

Essential to understanding rural persons' motivation for illness treatment, health maintenance, and health promotion is knowledge of their health perceptions (Long, 1983). The above replacement statements provide a broader view of the health perceptions that have been found with more recent research among rural individuals, families, and communities. They reflect both the earlier emphasis on role performance that is evident among older residents and among those employed in extractive industries and the expanded view of health perception definitions elicited from other individuals living in rural communities.

Theoretical Statement #2 (Relational)

> Rural residents are self-reliant and make decisions to seek care for illness, sickness, or injury depending on their self-assessment of the severity of their present health condition and of the resources needed and available. (Lee & McDonagh, 2006, p. 315)

> Rural residents with infants and children who experience illness, sickness, or injury will seek care more quickly than for themselves. (Lee & McDonagh, 2006, p. 315)

These theoretical statements refer to the health-seeking behaviors of rural residents. Key concepts from the 1989 model included self-reliance, seeking care from insiders, and the use of the informal system. Research findings continue to assert that self-reliance is a key characteristic identified in the management of health care situations by rural persons. However, changes were seen in the health-seeking behaviors of these residents as they seek advice and care from insiders and outsiders and also make use of both informal and formal systems of care.

Additional concepts emerged from the comparative research about rural persons' health behaviors: *health-seeking behaviors* and *choice* (Winters et al., 2006b). *Health-seeking behaviors*, defined as "conscious behaviors designed to promote healthy relationships among physical, mental, social and spiritual aspects of one's life so that life balance is maintained" (Winters et al., 2006b, Chapter 3, p. 34), include three subthemes: symptom–action–timeline process (SATL; Buehler et al., 1998), resources, and self-reliance.

Conscious *choice* is made in at least two domains of rural persons' lives. The first is the choice to live in a rural environment; the second is in accessing health care resources. Choosing to live in a rural environment is closely associated with the concept of place (see discussion later in this chapter).

Theoretical Statement #3 (Relational)

Health care providers continue to experience lack of anonymity and role diffusion. Because the original statement was well supported in the literature review, no changes are recommended.

FUTURE DIRECTIONS

Exploration of the literature regarding rural health perceptions and needs revealed many new avenues for future exploration. Themes of *distance* and *resources* were identified repeatedly in the literature reviewed. Newly proposed concepts emerging from the literature review included *health-seeking behaviors, choice, environmental context,* and *social capital.* Each of these concepts is addressed in the following sections.

Distance

Although *distance* was not part of any of the three theoretical statements making up the rural nursing theory base, the content of the rural literature we accessed for this review frequently touched on the concept. In the seminal article by Long and Weinert (1989), the participants included in the multiple studies tended to see health services as accessible and did not view themselves as isolated. Canadian authors MacLeod, Browne, and Leipert (1998) stated that distance may not be a problem but said the concept exerts a strong influence in providing health care in rural areas. This view affirms Johnson, Ratner, and Bottorff's (1995) assertion that one's geographic location may influence or even determine the form of health-seeking behaviors rural residents demonstrate. In an article cited earlier, the older women described distance and geographical barriers with concern; yet, they seemed to take problems with accessibility "in stride" (Pierce, 2001, p. 52). However, the study participants did express concern about the quality of nearby health services.

The remainder of the research all refuted the initial findings about distance and access to health care in Long and Weinert's (1989) theory-based article. Fitzgerald, Pearson, and McCutcheon (2001), Moran (2005), and Racher and Vollman (2002) stated that access to health care services is a major concern for residents across North America's rural and remote areas and for the health professionals serving them. Access to care is particularly a concern for rural individuals with chronic illness; an expressed problem was finding the "best" doctor (Fitzgerald et al., 2001). Buehler and Lee (1992) found the more rural the caregivers of persons with cancer, the more limited were formal health care resources available to assist them and their families. Distance to emergency care was an expressed concern of service providers in rural areas (Lee & Winters, 2004) and of mothers of children living in frontier areas (Bales, 2006). In a survey of middle-aged women, Brown and colleagues (1999) concluded that experiencing difficulties with accessing health care results in greater reliance on self-treatment and self-care, thereby leading to development of "attitudes of independence and self-reliance [sic]" (p. 151).

Resources

In addition to distance, *resources* is a concept that directly impacts access to health care services. Gulzar (1999) and Racher and Vollman (2002) discuss the complexity of accessing health services. The rurality or remoteness of a given place affects access to health services. Within the rural environment, such factors as geography, politics, and economics, as well as the acceptability and the education of health care providers, all influence the residents' access to and choice of health resources. Studying patterns of health care use and feedback loops among residents may add to the understanding of the complexity of accessing health care services in rural and remote areas (Racher & Vollman, 2002). Delivery of health services across sparsely populated areas presents unique challenges because of the vast distances involved and the scarcity of health professionals. For example, the greater the nurse-to-patient or physician-to-patient ratio and the more rural or remote the community, the more limited the health resources are for rural and remote community members.

Health-Seeking Behaviors

Health-seeking behaviors were defined as "conscious behaviors designed to promote healthy relationships among physical, mental, social and spiritual aspects of one's life so that life balance in maintained" (Winters et al., 2006b, Chapter 3, p. 34). The authors included three subthemes, SATL process, resources, and self-reliance, as part of health-seeking behaviors. The SATL process (Buehler et al., 1998) is used to describe the social process and to identify symptoms of sickness, illness, or injury and then seek the appropriate level of requisite care. The level of care sought may be self, lay, or professional, depending upon the perceived seriousness and type of symptom. Accessing resources is a part of the SATL process. Self-reliance, defined as behaviors to promote or maintain health without seeking assistance from others, was prevalent in the data from Montana and the Canadian provinces of Alberta and Manitoba. Winters et al. (2006b, p. 35) considered self-reliance a subtheme of health-seeking behavior because of its paramount influence on a person's seeking health care in sparsely populated rural areas.

Choice

Choice, the making of conscious decisions to live in a rural environment and access health care resources, was a new theme that emerged from the comparison study (Winters et al., 2006b). Explicitly evident in the Montana data and implicitly identified in the Canadian study through the participants' expressions of the benefits of living in rural environments, the theme of choice is associated with the concept of "place." Although we think of place in a geographical context, it is a broader entity that shapes one's political, economic, spatial, geographic, and cultural views of the world (Kelly, 2003). De la Rue and Colson (2003) found that rural participants' well-being and health were influenced by the "geographical location of living on the land" (p. 5). "Place" provided these rural residents with a kind of emotional or spiritual connectedness that affected the outcomes of their health experiences.

Wathen and Harris (2007) thought that rural living affected the choice of resources that members of their Canadian study would consult about a chronic health concern or an acute medical problem. If the available rural doctor "might not be the best or too up to date" (p. 643), they preferred their informal system (colleagues, friends, family), medical books, pharmacists, and/or the veterinarian.

Choice in making decisions related to accessing health care can be affected by several factors. Questions often asked to aid in determining a course of action are: Where is the closest facility that will provide the health care needed? What are the qualifications of the persons who staff that facility? What level of confidence is there in the local health care providers? Does familiarity with the professionals who staff the facility make a difference in making the choice of where to go? Is anonymity an important factor in this situation? Does the health care facility accept the insurance [true in the U.S. health care system] carried by the individual or family seeking care (Moran, 2005)? What hours does the facility stay open? What are the weather conditions? During stormy conditions, what roads are better maintained (freezing rain, snow, and ice; summer rain, wind, and flooding). In an acute emergency, can a fixed-wing aircraft or helicopter land nearby? These represent only a fraction of the factors and questions that may play a role in the decision making for accessing health care.

Environmental Context

Appearing repeatedly throughout the literature reviewed were terms like "*place*," "*geographical location*," "*context*," or "*environmental context*." According to Jones and Ross (2003, p. 16), nursing practice is "shaped by its situatedness" (p. 16). Authors speak of the context of a place and the resources needed that are particular to a context or place (Andrews, 2002, 2003; Andrews & Moon, 2005; MacLeod et al., 2008; Poland, Leboux, Holmes, & Andrews, 2005; Thurston & Meadows, 2004; Winters et al., 2006a). According to Lauder, Reel, Farmer, and Griggs (2008), "'Context' is an important unit of analysis.... A rural heath context is both physical and relational and aspects of rural environments ... may enhance or impede health" (p. 75).

Health perceptions, needs, and actions of rural persons are also influenced by the environmental context. This was particularly evident in the research reported by de la Rue and Coulson (2003), Thomlinson and colleagues (2004), and Winters et al. (2006a). In their intervention study of rural women with chronic illnesses, Winters and her colleagues found that four themes emerged through the "overarching theme of distance: (a) physical setting, (b) social/cultural/economic environment, (c) nature of women's work, and (d) accessibility/quality of health care" (pp. 284–285).

Social Capital

Social capital is a concept that comes from sociology and has come into increasing importance over the last 20 years (Shookner, Scott, & Vollman, 2008). Rooker (2002, as cited in Lauder et al., 2006) defines the term as "forms of association that express trust and norms of reciprocity" (p. 75). The Policy Research Initiative for the government of Canada (PRI; 2005 as cited in Shookner et al., 2008) further clarifies social capital as the "networks of social relations that may provide individuals and groups with access to resources and supports" (p. 87). "Creating supportive environments is about building social capital" (p. 87) and is similar to the notion of building "rural health services research capacity" (Hartley, 2005 p. 12).

Nurses practicing in rural settings tend to be more actively engaged professionally and personally in the rural communities in which they live and work (Bushy, 2000; Scharff, 1998). However, the present role of nurses in creating supportive health care environments is not well understood; recognition, conceptualization, and measurement are needed "to more fully appreciate the impact nurses have on rural health access and services" (Lauder et al., 2008, p. 74).

Three qualitative studies about nurses spoke to the necessity of developing social capital within rural communities (Conger & Plager, 2008; Gibb, Livesey, & Zyle, 2003; MacKinnon, 2008). Advanced Practice Registered Nurse (APRN) graduates realized the importance of "rural connectedness" through development of support networks with other health care providers, relationships with urban health care centers, connections with local communities, and support through electronic means (Conger & Plager, 2008). Nurses providing maternity care realized that they needed to know "their community—who lives in their community, what their skills are, and whether they are available to address local health needs or respond to emergency situations" (MacKinnon, 2008, p. 6). Nurses in solo mental health practice recognized the necessity of assisting rural and remote clients "to achieve a level of social functioning to integrate the person back into their community network" (Gibb, 2003, p. 248). To do this they found that they needed to work more closely with the potential support structures identified within the clients' community. This was best achieved by fostering a caring home environment, trying to keep people with their families and in their place of employment (Gibb et al., 2003). By having such a support structure, rural mental practitioners can avoid sending the mental health client to a psychiatric institution when a crisis occurs.

SUMMARY

Theories are developed for the purposes of describing, explaining, and predicting phenomena (Fawcett, 2000). The intent of the early theory development work at the College of Nursing at MSU-B was to use the descriptive research data collected in sparsely populated rural areas to develop a middle range theory, one that would provide a framework for nurses providing care to rural dwellers (Shannon, 1982). What evolved was a descriptive theory, the most basic type of middle range theory (Fawcett, 1999).

Although controversy exists about the placement and abstraction level of middle range theories within the hierarchical structure of nursing theories (Peterson & Bredow, 2004), the basic theory structure, regardless of level, is similar—theoretical statements that describe or link key concepts (Fawcett, 1999). The interweaving of those concepts and statements provides a pattern of ideas, which provide a new perspective on phenomena (Smith & Liehr, 2003). The pattern, once published and subjected to testing, should remain open to scrutiny, debate, and if necessary, to change and the incorporation of new ideas.

By subjecting the middle range rural nursing theory to testing in several studies (Bales, 2006; Bales et al., 2006; Lee & Winters, 2004;

Moran, 2005; Thomlinson et al., 2004; Winters et al., 2006b) and in the findings from several related studies, it has become evident that change has occurred over the past 30 years that has altered the applicability of the original published rural nursing theory base by Weinert and Long (1989). This change is demonstrated by the revisions to theoretical statements and the new emerging concepts.

Vision for the Future

Because of the descriptive nature of the middle range rural nursing theory, additional descriptive research is needed (Fawcett, 1999). Analysis methods can take several approaches, including the Wilson method (Walker & Avant, 1995), the evolutionary method (Rogers, 1993), the empirical or inductive approach (Morse, 1995), or a combination thereof. Testing of the proposed changes to the rural nursing theory relational statements through qualitative studies (ethnography, grounded theory, phenomenology, narrative inquiry, historical inquiry, and photovoice) and participatory action research needs to take place in other sparsely populated areas. Development and testing of instruments to measure the concepts are also needed. Conducting surveys to measure attributes, attitudes, knowledge, and opinions using open-ended and semi-structured interviews and questionnaires is required (Fawcett, 1999). With a compilation of these focused research efforts can emerge a model, a schema, or a list of logically ordered statements that, when present, will provide guidance for the care of rural dwellers (Smith & Liehr, 2003).

Moving the Work Forward

A core group of nurse researchers from Montana and Alberta periodically met to review and critique theoretical material and models. Members of this North American Study (NAS) group discussed and planned projects to further rural nursing theory development while offering research and educational opportunities to graduate students within their courses or independent studies. A rural nursing and theory listserv group, initiated several years ago, provided a mechanism for online discussion for furthering rural nursing research and theory development. While this listserv is now dormant, two resources are potentially available for reestablishment of communication: (a) Nursing Theory Link Page, www.nrsing.clayton.edu/eichelberger/nursing.htm, (b) The International Council of Nurses (ICN) Rural and Remote Nursing Network, www.icn.ch/rrn_network.htm, and Improving Health Among Rural and Vulnerable Populations www.facebook.com/#!/groups/395662340465359/.

The NAS and listserv members did identify the following questions for continued exploration of rural health care behaviors: (a) Are these health-seeking behaviors unique to rural residents? (b) Will health-seeking behavior activities of the SATL process fit under the same middle range theory framework as those for health promotion? (c) How do illness variables affect rural persons' health-seeking behaviors? (d) How to illness variables affect rural people's choices of health care providers? (e) Are rural dwellers more accepting of "outsiders" if they are health care professionals working in partnerships with the rural community and local health professionals?

CONCLUSION

Revised statements for the middle range rural nursing theory as published by Long and Weinert (1989) are ready for testing. The emerging concepts identified in the review of the rural nursing literature are also ready for exploration, testing, and tool development. Continued research and theoretical development efforts will increase the potential for a middle range theory that can provide a structure for acceptable, adaptable, and appropriate nursing care for rural persons.

REFERENCES

Andrews, G. J. (2002). Towards a more place-sensitive nursing: An invitation to medical and health sensitive health geography. *Nursing Inquiry, 9*(4), 221–238.

Andrews, G. J. (2003). Locating a geography of nursing: Space, place, and the progress of geographical thought. *Nursing Philosophy, 4*, 231–248.

Andrews, G. J., & Moon, G. (2005). Space, place, and the evidence base: Part I – An introduction to health geography. *Worldviews on Evidence Based Nursing, 2*, 55–62.

Averill, J. B. (2002). Voices from the Gila: Health care issues for rural elders in south-western New Mexico. *Journal of Advanced Nursing, 40*, 654–662.

Bales, R. L. (2006). Health perceptions, needs, and behaviors of remote rural women of childbearing and childrearing age. In H. J. Lee, & C. A. Winters (Eds). *Rural nursing: Concepts, theory and practice* (2nd ed., pp. 66–78). New York, NY: Springer Publishing.

Bales, R. L., Winters, C. A., & Lee, H. J. (2006). Health needs and perceptions of rural persons. In H. J. Lee, & C. A. Winters (Eds). *Rural nursing: Concepts, theory and practice* (2nd ed., pp. 53–65). New York, NY: Springer Publishing.

Blue, I., & Fitzgerald, M. (2002). Interprofessional relations: Care studies of working relationships between registered nurses and general practitioners in rural Australia. *Journal of Clinical Nursing, 11*, 314–321.

Brown, W. J., Young, A. F., & Byles, J. E. (1999). Tyranny of distance? The health of mid-age women living in five geographical areas of Australia. *Australian Journal of Rural Health, 7,* 148–154.

Buehler, J. A., & Lee, H. J. (1992). Exploration of home care resources for rural families with cancer. *Cancer Nursing, 15,* 299–308.

Buehler, J. A., Malone, M., & Majerus, J. M. (1998). Patterns of responses to symptoms in rural residents: The symptom-action-time-line process. In H. J. Lee (Ed.), *Conceptual basis for rural nursing* (pp. 318–328). New York, NY: Springer Publishing.

Bushy, A. (2000). *Orientation to nursing in the rural community.* Thousand Oaks, CA: Sage.

Conger, M. M., & Plager, K. A. (2008). Advanced practice nursing practice in rural areas: Connectedness versus disconnectedness. *Online Journal of Rural Nursing and Health Care, 8*(1), 24–38. Retrieved January 24, 2009 from http://rno.org

Courtney, M., Tong, S., & Walsh, A. (2000). Older patients in the acute care setting: Rural and metropolitan nurses' knowledge, attitudes and practices. *Australian Journal of Rural Health, 8,* 94–102.

Davis, R., & Magilvy, J. K. (2000). Quiet pride: The experience of chronic illness by rural older adults. *Journal of Nursing Scholarship, 32,* 385–390.

de la Rue, M., & Coulson, I . (2003). The meaning of health and well-being: Voices from older rural women. *The International Electronic Journal of Rural and Remote Health Research, Education, Practice, and Policy, 3*(192), 1–10. Retrieved October 4, 2003 from http://rrh.deakin.edu.au

Fawcett, J. (1999). *The relationship of theory and research* (3rd ed.). Philadelphia, PA: Davis.

Fawcett, J. (2000). *Analysis and evaluation of contemporary nursing knowledge: Nursing models and theories.* Philadelphia, PA: Davis.

Fitzgerald, M., Pearson, A., & McCutcheon, H. (2001). Impact of rural living on the experience of chronic illness. *Australian Journal of Rural Health, 9,* 235–240.

Gibb, H. (2003). Rural community mental health nursing: A grounded theory account of sole practice. *International Journal of Mental Health Nursing, 12,* 243–250.

Gibb, H., Livesey, L., & Zyla, W. (2003). At 3 am who the hell do you call? Case management issues in sole practice as a rural community mental health nurse. *Australasian Psychiatry, 11*(Suppl.), S127–S130.

Goins, R. T., Spencer, S. M., & Williams, K. (2010). Lay meanings of health among rural older adults in Appalachia. *The Journal of Rural Health, 27,* 13–20.

Gulzar, L. (1999). Access to health care. *Journal of Nursing Scholarship, 31,* 13–19.

Hartley, D. (2005). Rural health research: Building capacity and influencing policy in the United States and Canada. *Canadian Journal of Nursing Research, 37*(1), 7–13.

Hegney, D. (1997). Rural nursing practice. In L. Siegloff (Ed.), *Rural nursing in the Australian context* (pp. 25–43). Deacon Act, Australia: Royal College of Nursing.

Henson, D., Sadler, T., & Walton, S. (1998). Distance. In H. J. Lee (Ed.), *Conceptual basis for rural nursing* (pp. 51–60). New York, NY: Springer Publishing.

Jirojwong, S., & MacLennan, R. (2002). Management of episodes of incapacity by families in rural and remote Queensland. *Australian Journal of Rural Health, 10,* 249–255.

Johnson, J. L., Ratner, P. A., & Bottorff, J. L. (1995). Urban–rural differences in the health-promoting behaviors of Albertans. *Canadian Journal of Public Health, 86,* 103–108.

Jones, S., & Ross, J. (2003). *Describing your scope of practice: A resource for rural nurses.* Christchurch, NZ: Centre for Rural Health. Retrieved February 6, 2008 from http:/www.moh.govt.nz

Kelly, S. E. (2003). Bioethics and rural health: Theorizing place, space, and subjects. *Social Science & Medicine, 56,* 2277–2288.

Lau, T., Kumar, S., & Thomas, D. (2002). Practicing psychiatry in New Zealand's rural areas: Incentives, problems and solutions. *Australasian Psychiatry, 10*(1), 33–38.

Lauder, W., Reel, S., Farmer, J., & Griggs, H. (2006). Social capital, rural nursing and rural nursing theory. *Nursing Inquiry, 13*(1), 73–79.

Lee, H. J., Hollis, B. R., & McClain, K. A. (1998). Isolation. In H. J. Lee (Ed.), *Conceptual basis for rural nursing* (pp. 61–75). New York, NY: Springer Publishing.

Lee, H. J., & McDonagh, M. K. (2010). Updating the rural nursing theory base. In C. A. Winters, & H. J. Lee (Eds), *Rural nursing: Concepts, theory, and practice* (3rd edition, pp. 19–39). New York, NY: Springer Publishing.

Lee, H. J., & Winters, C. A. (2004). Testing rural nursing theory: Perceptions and needs of service providers. *Online Journal of Rural Nursing and Health Care, 4*(1). Retrieved September 16, 2004, from http://www.rno.org/journal/issues/vol-4/issue.1/Lee_article.htm

Long, K. A. (1983). The concept of health: Rural perspectives. *Nursing Clinics of North America, 28,* 123–130.

Long, K. A., & Weinert, C. (1989). Rural nursing: Developing the theory base. *Scholarly Inquiry for Nursing Practice: An International Journal, 3,* 113–127.

MacKinnon, K. A. (2008). Labouring to nurse: The work of rural nurses who provide maternity care. *Rural and Remove Health Care, 8,* 1–15. Retrieved January 20, 2008, from http://www.rrh.org.au

MacLeod, M., Browne, A. J., & Leipert, B. (1998). International perspective: Issues for nurses in rural and remote Canada. *Australian Journal of Rural Health, 6,* 72–78.

MacLeod, M. L. P., Misener, R. M., Banks, K., Morton, A. M., Vogt, C., & Bentham, D. (2008). "I'm a different kind of nurse": Advice from nurses in rural and remote Canada. *Canadian Journal of Nursing Leadership, 21*(3), 40–53.

McConigley, R., Kristjanson, L., & Morgan, A. (2000). Palliative care nursing in rural Western Australia. *International Journal of Palliative Nursing, 6*(2), 80–90.

Moran, C. A. (2005). *Replication study of rural nursing theory: A Missouri perspective.* Unpublished thesis, Central Missouri State University.

Morse, M. J. (1995). Exploring the theoretical basis of nursing using advanced techniques of concept analysis. *Advances in Nursing Science, 17*(3), 31–46.

Niemoller, J. K., Ide, B. A., & Nichols, E. G. (2000). Issues in studying health-related hardiness and use of services among older rural adults. *Texas Journal of Rural Health, 18,* 35–43.

Peterson, S. J., & Bredow, T. S. (2004). *Middle range theories: Application to nursing research.* Philadelphia, PA: Lippincott Williams & Wilkins.

Pierce, C. (2001). The impact of culture of rural women's descriptions of health. *The Journal of Multicultural Nursing and Health, 7,* 50–53, 56.

Poland, B., Lehoux, P., Holmes, D., & Andrews, G. J. (2005). How place matters: Unpacking technology and power in health and social care. *Health & Social Care in the Community, 13,* 170–180.

Racher, F. E., & Vollman, A. R. (2002). Exploring the dimensions of access to health services: Implications for nursing research and practice. *Research and Theory for Nursing Practice: An International Journal, 16,* 77–90.

Roberto, K. A., & Reynolds, S. G. (2001). The meaning of osteoporosis in the lives of rural women. *Health Care for Women International, 22,* 599–611.

Rogers, B. L. (1993). Concept analysis: An evolutionary view. In B. L. Rogers, & K. A. Kraft (Eds), *Concept development in nursing: Foundations, techniques and application* (pp. 73–92). Philadelphia, PA: Saunders.

Rosenthal, K. A. (1996). *Rural nursing: An exploratory narrative description.* Unpublished dissertation, University of Colorado, Denver.

Scharff, J. (1998). The distinctive nature and scope of rural nursing practice: Philosophical bases. In H. Lee (Ed.), *Conceptual basis for rural nursing* (pp. 19–38). New York, NY: Springer Publishing.

Sellers, S. C., Poduska, M. D., Propp, L. H., & White, S. E. (1999). The health care meanings, values, and practices of Anglo-American males in the rural midwest. *Journal of Transcultural Nursing, 10,* 320–330.

Shannon, A. (1982). Introduction: Nursing in sparsely populated areas. In J. Taylor (Ed.), *Sparsely populated areas: Toward nursing theory. Western Journal of Nursing Research,* 4(3, Suppl.), 70–71.

Shookner, M., Scott, C. M., & Vollman, A. R. (2008). Creating supportive environments for health: Social network analysis. In A. R. Vollman, E. T. Anderson, & J. McFarlane (Eds), *Canadian community as partner: Theory & multidisciplinary practice* (2nd ed.). Philadelphia, PA: Lippincott Williams & Wilkins.

Smith, M. J., & Liehr, P. R. (Eds.). *Middle range theory of nursing.* New York, NY: Springer Publishing.

Thomlinson, E., McDonagh, M. K., Reimer, M., Crooks, K., & Lees, M. (2004). Health beliefs of rural Canadians: Implications for practice. *Australian Journal of Rural Health, 12,* 258–263.

Thurston, W. E., & Meadows, L. M. (2003). Rurality and health: Perspectives of mid-life women. *The International Electronic Journal of Rural and Remote Health Research, Education, Practice, and Policy,* 3(219), 1–12. Retrieved November 6, 2003, from http://rrh.deakin.edu.au

Walker, L., & Avant, K. (1995). *Strategies for theory construction in nursing* (3rd ed.). Norwalk, CT: Appleton-Century-Crofts.

Wathen, C. N., & Harris, R. M. (2006). An examination of the health information seeking experiences of women in rural Ontario, Canada. *Information Research,* 11(4). Retrieved October 26, 2008 from http: information.net/ir/11-4/paper267.html

Wathen, C. N., & Harris, R. M. (2007). "I try to take care of it myself." How rural women search for health information. *Qualitative Health Research,* 17(5), 639–6651.

Winters, C. A., Cudney, S. A., Sullivan, T., & Thuesen, A. (2006a). The rural context and women's self-management of chronic health conditions. *Chronic Illness, 2,* 273–289.

Winters, C. A., Thomlinson, E. H., O'Lynn, C., Lee, H. J., McDonagh, M. K., Edge, D. S. et al. (2006b). Exploring rural nursing theory across borders. In H. J. Lee, & C. A. Winters (Eds), *Rural nursing: Concepts, theory, and practice* (2nd ed., pp. 27–39). New York, NY: Springer Publishing.

Chapter 3

EXPLORING RURAL NURSING THEORY ACROSS BORDERS

Charlene A. Winters,
Elizabeth H. Thomlinson, Chad O'Lynn,
Helen J. Lee, Meg K. McDonagh,
Dana S. Edge, and Marlene A. Reimer

THE DESCRIPTIVE RURAL NURSING THEORY first published by Long and Weinert in 1989, and republished in 1999, is widely accepted and frequently quoted in presentations and articles. However, the theory hardly has been tested. Recently, the authors, nurse scientists from the United States and Canada, joined forces to validate the rural theory concepts. Lee and Winters (2004) conducted a qualitative study to explore rural people's health perceptions and needs in the state of Montana, and Thomlinson, McDonagh, Reimer, Crooks, and Lees (2002) did the same in the Canadian provinces of Alberta and Manitoba. Then we compared the findings from these two studies. Our specific aims in the comparison were to (a) validate existing rural nursing theory concepts, (b) identify new emerging concepts, and (c) determine areas for further theoretical development and research.

BACKGROUND AND SIGNIFICANCE

Rural nursing is the provision of health care by professional nurses to people living in sparsely populated areas (Long & Weinert, 1989, 1999). Rural nursing theory evolved because of a recognized need for a framework for practice that considers the special needs of this population. The theory-building process began in the late 1970s with the collection of qualitative and quantitative data by the Montana State University-Bozeman College of Nursing graduate students and faculty. A rich database resulted in the identification of several key concepts and the development of three theoretical statements related to understanding rural health needs and rural nursing practice. The first statement was that "rural dwellers define health primarily as the ability to work, to be productive, to do usual tasks" (Long & Weinert, 1989, p. 120). Two closely interrelated concepts associated with this statement pertain to work beliefs and health beliefs. Health is defined in relation to work, and health needs are secondary to work needs.

The second theoretical statement was that "rural dwellers are self-reliant and resist accepting help or services from those seen as 'outsiders' or from agencies seen as national or regional 'welfare' programs" (Long & Weinert, 1989, p. 120). Closely associated to this statement is the tendency of rural dwellers to rely on informal social networks for health care. Key concepts pertaining to this statement are self-reliance, outsider, insider, old-timer, and newcomer. Rural dwellers tend to engage in self-care and prefer the familiarity of the people and professionals who know them in contrast to the newcomer, or specialist, who is unfamiliar. Other concepts identified as important in understanding the health care-seeking behavior of rural residents are distance, isolation, and lack of anonymity, which are descriptive of the rural context in which these people live and work. The qualitative data from Montana, upon which the theoretical work was based, indicated that rural residents accepted distance as a normal part of living in a rural area. The degree of distance involved, whether actual or perceived, led some rural dwellers to experience a sense of isolation. Lastly, a lack of anonymity implies a limited ability for rural people to have private areas in their lives, a phenomenon common to small towns and sparsely populated areas.

The third theoretical statement was that health care providers in rural areas "must deal with a lack of anonymity and much greater role diffusion than providers in urban or suburban settings" deal with (Long & Weinert, 1989, p. 120). In a small community, everyone knows who the nurse is and this knowledge affects the nurse's effectiveness as a health care professional in that community. Furthermore, nurses are expected to function as expert generalists. For example, on a given day, a nurse working during the day shift in a rural hospital may care for a laboring woman, recover an older man following surgery, triage in the emergency room, and/or prepare a pediatric trauma patient for transport to a regional medical center.

When the theory-building process began, literature and research related to rural health care were limited and focused primarily on rural health care delivery and access to service issues (Long & Weinert, 1989). A theoretical base for guiding rural health care did not exist. This prompted the faculty and students of the Montana State University-Bozeman College of Nursing to begin the development of a theory base for rural nursing practice. Although rural nursing theory concepts are now widely accepted, a limited number of researchers have reported their efforts to test these initial findings. Our recent research of the literature resulted in only two citations for work that specifically focused on rural nursing theory

(Nichols, 1989, 1999). Both were response articles to Long and Weinert's theory-based article. Much of the published rural literature and research continues to focus on issues related to health care delivery and access. Given the paucity of research, we designed a study to test the rural nursing concepts described nearly 30 years ago.

METHODS AND PROCEDURES

The Montanan study and the Canadian study were similar in design and purpose (Lee & Winters, 2004; Thomlinson et al., 2002), but were planned and carried out separately. In both studies, we used an ethnographic approach (Miles & Huberman, 1994; Morse & Field, 1995; Rossman & Rallis, 2003). In an ethnographic study, researchers describe and interpret phenomena of interest in a cultural or social group or system (Creswell, 1998). Consistent with this approach, we collected data through open-ended interviews of rural people and observational field notes (Rossman & Rallis, 2003) that documented our insights, interactions with participants, and the physical and cultural context of the communities in which the participants lived. Through these activities, Lee and Winters and Thomlinson and her colleagues were able to identify the perceptions of the rural people and learn what they understood about their health and how they managed their day-to-day health care situations. Using this open-ended approach, we found that themes emerged from the interview narratives (Miles & Huberman, 1994), allowing us to make comparisons with the concepts and statements contained in the rural nursing theory proposed by Long and Weinert (1989).

The Montana Study

Montana is the fourth largest state in the United States, covering 147,042 square miles of area and stretching across 641 miles from the east to west. The state is sparsely populated, with a density of 6.2 persons per square mile (Census 2000 Data for the State of Montana, n.d.). According to the 2000 Census, 90.6% of the state's residents are Caucasian; the principal minority population of 6.2% is Native American. Farming, fishing, and forestry occupations occupy 2.2% of the population, whereas 42.4% of the population is employed in service, sales, and office occupations (Census 2000 Data for the State of Montana). The Rocky Mountains run north and south through the western part of the state, whereas eastern Montana is characterized by its rolling plains.

Lee and Winters (2004) conducted the Montanan study according to the guidelines set forth by the Montana State University-Bozeman Human Subject Committee. They recruited participants through word of mouth (snowball sampling). Each participant signed a consent form that emphasized that only aggregate data would be reported. Lee and Winters maintained confidentiality of participants by removing names and identifiers. All the participants were older than 18 years of age, employed in service occupations, and had lived in their respective communities for at least 5 years (see Table 3.1).

Graduate nursing students enrolled in a rural nursing course conducted 38 interviews in the fall semesters of 2000 and 2001 with individuals living in rural towns with populations of 1500 individuals or less. Using open-ended questions, they asked participants about their perceptions of health and how they responded to illness and injury. Interviews lasted from 30 to 60 minutes and were audio taped. Once interviews were transcribed, the students analyzed the narratives for themes. The students recorded observational field notes to document their activities, interactions, and insights. They wrote individual papers addressing the themes emerging from their interviews and field observations. Working separately, Lee and Winters (2004) coded the transcripts and field notes, identifying common themes. They then met to compare their findings with those identified by the students. They continually compared data supporting the emerging themes until they arrived at a consensus on the findings. Four major themes emerged from the analysis of the Montana data: (a) Definitions of health, (b) health-seeking behaviors, (c) choices, and (d) distances and access to resources.

The Canadian Study

The provinces of Alberta and Manitoba are approximately equal in size, with each province covering 250,000 square miles of area or roughly one and three-quarters of the size of the state of Montana. The geography of Alberta closely parallels that of Montana, with rolling prairie and the Rocky Mountains bordering the western edge of the province. The terrain in Manitoba varies from flat farmlands in the south to the Cambrian Shield, an area of granite rock with thin soil, in the north. In the north are large tracts of land covered with muskeg and forest. A major geographic difference between the two provinces is that 17% of Manitoba is covered with water compared with 3% of Alberta (Statistics Canada, 2004). The geographic diversity was a major reason for selecting these two distinct sites for the study.

In Alberta, the industries of farming, logging, ranching, and oil production employ 7% of the population, with sales, service, business, and finance employing 41% of Albertans. Similarly, in Manitoba, farming, logging, mining, and fishing employ 7% of the population, whereas sales, service, business, and finance employ 41.6% of Manitobans (Statistics Canada, 2004).

Following ethical approval by the Conjoint Health Research Ethics Board at the University of Calgary, Thomlinson et al. (2002) sought

TABLE 3.1 Demographics

	Montana Sample	Canadian Sample
Men	14	13
Women	24	42
Ethnicity		
Caucasian	35	52
Native American	3	
Aboriginal		3
Age range, years	22–85 ($m = 49$)	18–84*
Education	7–18 ($m = 13$)	8–16*
Marital status		
Married	26	37
Divorced	5	5
Single	7	9 (5 widow/widower)
Unknown		4
Occupation		
Grocery store clerks	4	
Secretaries	3	
Hospital workers	3	
Restaurant workers	3	
Beauty shop workers	2	
Animal care workers	2	
Museum operators	2	
County employees	2	
Window treatment	2	
Post office workers	2	
Retirees		9
Ranchers		7
Education		19
Health care		3
Accountant		1
Bookkeeper		1
Other	13	15

(continued)

TABLE 3.1 Demographics (*Continued*)

	Montana Sample	Canadian Sample
Time in rural community (years)	5–84 (*m* = 34)	3+*
Size of community (persons)	70–1728	50–5000
County density (persons per square mile)	0.8–29.8	Not calculated
Distance to the nearest large town (miles)	12–250 (*m* = 60)	Not asked
Distance to the nearest emergency care (miles)	0.1–110 (*m* = 30)	3–90*
Self-reported health status		
Excellent	5	Not asked
Very good	3	
Good	17	
Fair	8	
Poor	1	
Did not respond	4	
Health insurance		
Yes	29	All have health care insurance
No	8	
No response	1	

*Means not available.
m = mean.

participants through newspaper advertisements and through word of mouth from other participants. In the first stage of the study, they selected 29 participants from municipal districts and small towns within 300 km of Calgary. In the second stage, they sought 26 participants living in central and northern Manitoba for interviews (see Table 3.1). As with the Montana study, all participants were over 18 years of age and signed consent forms that emphasized that only aggregate data be reported. The confidentiality of participants was maintained through the removal of names and identifiers. Thomlinson and colleagues and nursing student research assistants conducted face-to-face, semi-structured interviews lasting 45 to 60 minutes. Participants selected the locations for interviews, which were usually held in their homes.

Initially, four researchers (E. Thomlinson, M. McDonagh, K. Crooks, and M. Lees) coded five interview transcripts separately, and then compared their findings. Two of the researchers (E. Thomlinson and

M. McDonagh) completed the analysis of the remainder of the transcripts. The major themes that emerged from the transcripts included definitions of health, health-seeking behaviors, resources that were accessed, and definitions of rural and northern.

DATA ANALYSIS

In June 2003, the authors of the Montana and Canadian studies met at the University of Calgary, Alberta. We developed agreements regarding steps in the process of data comparison, responsibilities of team membership, dissemination of findings, and authorship. Subsequent meetings were conducted via teleconference.

We began the process by viewing and comparing the demographic characteristics of the two samples. We compared the concepts, themes, salient characteristics, and relevant qualitative data excerpts from both studies and then displayed them using a concept-ordered matrix (Miles & Huberman, 1994). Concepts and themes having the same or very similar defining attributes were collapsed into a common theme. We further evaluated concepts and themes for differences in sample and methods and then added them to the matrix, resulting in a combined dataset. We then compared findings with rural nursing theory concepts and theoretical statements. In this manner, we maintained methodological rigor of consistency, neutrality, truth-value, and applicability (Morse & Field, 1995).

FINDINGS

After much analysis and discussion, we identified by consensus four common themes and nine subthemes (see Table 3.2) and summarized them below.

TABLE 3.2 Common Themes and Sub-themes

Theme	Sub-theme
Definitions of Health	a. Sickness b. Illness
Health-Seeking Behaviors	a. SATL b. Resources c. Self-reliance
Choices	a. Residence b. Health care provider
Distance	a. Rural b. Northern

Common Themes

Definition of Health

We identified the theme *definition of health* in both studies. In the Montana study, health was described primarily as the absence of conditions that would interrupt work or play and included physical, mental, and emotional fitness. In the Canadian study, the definition of health was similar but included the importance of spiritual and environmental considerations.

Participants from both studies spoke of health as a concept that was to some degree related to age and the absence of chronic illness, with comments such as, "I'm healthy for my age." Following further examination of the transcripts and discussion, we agreed upon the common theme *definition of health* as a holistic perspective in which optimal ability to function at work or play and to pursue desired activities is maintained. Optimal ability is obtained through health-seeking and health-promoting behaviors to achieve holistic balance, resolution of short-term disruptions, and adaptation to long-term health challenges.

In addition, Canadian participants differentiated between sickness and illness, noting that sickness is short in duration and is curable; whereas illness is either chronic in nature or serious and life threatening. We then determined that sickness and illness were subthemes of definition of health.

Health-Seeking Behaviors

The theme symptom–action–timeline (SATL) emerged from the Montana data and was used to describe the social process of identifying symptoms and seeking self-care, lay care, or professional health care for illness and injuries (Buehler, Malone, & Majerus, 1998). SATL was similar to the theme health-seeking behaviors, which emerged from the Canadian data. We discussed the similarities and differences between these two themes, noting that SATL focused on obtaining health resources once a health disruption is noted. Furthermore, the theme health-seeking behaviors incorporated SATL as well as behaviors designed to promote health and prevent health disruptions. We determined that health-seeking behavior was a common theme and SATL was a subtheme of health-seeking behavior. Health-seeking behavior is defined as conscious behavior designed to promote healthy relationships among physical, mental, social, and spiritual aspects of one's life so that life balance is maintained.

A theme identified in the Canadian data and defined as people and other sources of information and assistance one uses in health-seeking behaviors was named *resources*. Examples of resources that were provided by Canadian participants included community elders, trusted traditional healers, libraries, the Internet, and health care professionals who really listen. The Montana researchers also noted resources as a component of

SATL. As a result, we determined resources to be an additional sub-theme of health-seeking behaviors.

In reviewing the data, we noted a number of excerpts that described the self-reliance of rural dwellers. Participants engaged in self-care when managing illness and injury and, when needed, chose to seek care first from friends and family members prior to seeing a health care professional. Participants commented that they kept their "medicine cabinets stocked," and when injured they would pull the edges of the wound together if only a "couple of inches long." They would see a health care provider for injuries they did not think they "could put a Band-Aid on" or handle themselves. Because of its prevalence in the data and the context in which the term appeared, we determined that self-reliance was a subtheme under health-seeking behaviors.

Choices

The conscious life choices one makes in terms of residence and accessing health services was a theme we identified as choices. The theme emerged from the Montana data, based on participants' comments regarding their choice to live in rural areas and their decision-making processes regarding when and which health resources they access when ill or injured. Generally, participants expressed satisfaction with living in rural areas and commented on the benefits of rural living. The Canadian researchers did not initially identify choices as a theme. However, they did find that the participants exhibited a "taking charge" attitude, which we believed to be equated with making choices. And because the Canadian participants made comments similar to Montana participants regarding the benefits of rural living and how living in sparsely populated areas shaped their health care decision making, we reached a consensus in identifying choices as a theme.

Distance

Thomlinson et al. (2002) classified participants in their study as either rural or northern, and asked the participants to describe what these terms meant to them. They noted that the Canadian government has six definitions of rural and defines northern as the region north of a north-and-south line determined by 16 combined social, biotic, economic, and climatic aspects of geography (McNiven, 1999). Distance was the factor that differentiated rural from northern for Canadian participants, in that northern residents are more isolated and distances to all services, not just health services, are much farther than those for rural residents. Distance was also described by the Montana participants, with comments focusing on distance to services, lack of service availability, and travel times to services. Thus, we determined that distance was a theme and rural and northern were sub-themes of distance. Distance was defined as separation (space, time, and behavior) between the rural population and health care resources.

DISCUSSION

The definition of health we identified in this study, although more holistic than the original definition, continues to support the interrelatedness of work and health and provides partial support for the first theoretical statement identified by Long and Weinert (1989). Furthermore, the new definition of health adds to the original definition by including "ability to play," identifying the importance of mental and emotional fitness, and including the notion that health is qualified by age and the presence of illness. In addition, we determined health-seeking and health-promoting behaviors to be foundational to the maintenance of health.

Although variations existed within groups, health-seeking behaviors were demonstrated by participants from both countries. Therefore, we identified *health-seeking behaviors* as a common theme and described the processes participants used to promote healthy relationships among physical, mental, social, and spiritual aspects of their lives. Underlying the overall theme of health-seeking behavior were three subthemes: (a) SATL, (b) resources, and (c) self-reliance.

The acronym SATL, described previously by Buehler et al. (1998), is the social process of identifying symptoms and seeking self-care, lay care, or professional health care for illness and injuries. With this process, participants choose the resources that they believe will be effective in promoting their health status or managing their health concern. We defined *resources* as people, other sources of information, and assistance one uses in health-seeking behaviors.

Self-reliance is described by Chafey, Sullivan, and Shannon (1998) as behaviors of accomplishing tasks without the help of others, stemming from values (such as autonomy) or contextual variables (such as barriers to resource access). Accordingly, we identified *self-reliance* in this collaborative study. Findings indicate that participants preferred to engage in self-care for illness and injuries and sought assistance from informal resources prior to seeking the services of health care professionals. The findings support the second theoretical statement of Long & Weinert (1989), and the addition of three subthemes to health-seeking behaviors contributes to the expansion of the rural nursing theory base.

The theme *choices* refers to the participants' conscious decision-making processes regarding their places of residence and patterns of accessing health services. During data analysis, we realized that participants were constantly making choices, and these decisions affected their lifestyle, their personal health and health practices and that of their families, and their livelihood. Examples of such choices include decisions regarding when, where, and from whom to seek care for an injury, where they should reside (stay on the farm or move into town), and what kind of foods they should be eating to maintain health and yet stay within their allotted budget. Long and Weinert (1989) did not previously identify *choices* as part of rural nursing theory.

Distance was an important concept that Long and Weinert (1989) identified in their original descriptive theory, and we also found it important in the comparison study. We defined it as separation (space, time, and behavior) between the rural population and health care resources, and then further broke it down on the basis of the degree of remoteness, recognizing that distances to all services, not just health services, are much greater for isolated rural residents. Expanding the concept of distance to include definitions of rural and northern is one way that degrees of remoteness can be used to extend rural nursing theory. The identification and explication of the themes *definition of health, health-seeking behaviors, choices,* and *distance* have implications for furthering health care providers' understanding of the health care-seeking behaviors, practices, and preferred resources of rural dwellers.

Implications for Rural Nursing Theory and Practice

The findings of this comparison study validate and expand upon existing rural nursing theory concepts and provide partial support for the first and second theoretical statements identified by Long and Weinert (1989). As the focus of this study was on the health perceptions and needs of rural people, it is beyond the scope of this project to address the rural nursing theory concepts germane to the third theoretical statement that rural health care providers must deal with a lack of anonymity and much greater role diffusion than providers in urban or suburban settings.

Through the expansion of the previous understanding of health, educators and practitioners are provided the opportunity to view their specific rural population's health needs in a broader context. The data also reveal that a variety of health-seeking and health-promoting behaviors is important to rural dwellers. The information gained from this study about SATL, choices, and distance has significant implications for further rural nursing theory development and practice. By increasing the amount of information gathered and the breadth of the rural population sampled, the theory base solidifies its applicability to rural nurses and thus has the potential to positively affect the health care delivery to rural dwellers in North America. Understanding the health care decision-making processes used by rural dwellers will assist nurses to provide care appropriate to their clients' needs and rural lifestyle.

Although distance is not a new concept in the rural nursing theory base, our understanding of distance and what it means to specific rural groups has been expanded in this study. The data support the notion that distance is not constant; it is variable among specific populations and their contexts. This has implications for how the context of rural dwellers is understood by rural nurses and has the potential to affect future programs for health education and health-program delivery.

While each of the four themes and nine subthemes requires further examination, the aforementioned findings suggest that major tenets of rural nursing theory can be applied across the western United States–Canadian border. This finding provides contextual information important to the further development of rural nursing theory. Additional research that compares and contrasts the health perceptions and needs of people living in differing rural environments is necessary to further build upon the theory base. In addition, replication of this study is needed internationally as well as in other North American rural and remote areas to provide the necessary rigor and applicability of rural nursing theory. Finally, studies are needed that address the third theoretical statement, which focuses on the issues facing nurses practicing in rural and remote areas. A more solid base for rural nursing theory is required to guide the delivery of nursing care to rural and remote populations.

ACKNOWLEDGMENTS

This research was funded by the Montana State University—Bozeman College of Nursing Block Grant; Sigma Theta Tau International, Zeta Upsilon Chapter; and Visiting Scholar, University of Calgary, Alberta, Canada.

REFERENCES

Buehler, J., Malone, M., & Majerus, J. (1998). Patterns of response to symptoms in rural residents: The symptom–action–time-line process. In H. J. Lee (Ed.), *Conceptual basis for rural nursing* (pp. 318–328). New York, NY: Springer Publishing.

Census 2000 data for the state of Montana. (n.d.). Retrieved December 15, 2002, from http://www.census.gov/census2000/states/mt.html

Chafey, K., Sullivan, T., & Shannon, A. (1998). Self-reliance: Characterization of their own autonomy by elderly rural women. In H. J. Lee (Ed.), *Conceptual basis for rural nursing* (pp. 156–177). New York, NY: Springer Publishing.

Creswell, J. (1998). *Qualitative inquiry and research design: Choosing among five traditions*. Thousand Oaks, CA: Sage.

Lee, H. J., & Winters, C. A. (2004). Testing rural nursing theory: Perceptions and needs of service providers. *Online Journal of Rural Nursing and Health Care,*

4. Retrieved July 5, 2004 from http://www.rno.org/journal/issues/Vol-4/issue-1/Lee_article.htm

Long, K. A., & Weinert, C. (1989). Rural nursing: Developing the theory base. *Scholarly Inquiry for Nursing Practice, 3*(2), 113–127.

Long, K. A., & Weinert, C. (1999). Rural nursing: Developing the theory base. *Research and Theory for Nursing Practice, 13*(3), 257–269.

McNiven, C. (1999). North is that direction. *Canadian Social Trends*, pp. 8–11. Statistics Canada—Catalogue No. 11–008. Retrieved July 23, 2004, from http://estat.statcan.ca/content/english/articles/pop-a.shtml

Miles, M. B., & Huberman, A. M. (1994). *Qualitative data analysis* (2nd ed.). Thousand Oaks, CA: Sage.

Morse, J. M., & Field, P. A. (1995). *Qualitative research methods for health professions* (2nd ed.). Thousand Oaks, CA: Sage.

Nichols, E. (1989). Response to 'Rural nursing: Developing the theory base'. *Scholarly Inquiry for Nursing Practice, 3*, 129–132.

Nichols, E. (1999). Response to 'Rural nursing: Developing the theory base.' 1989. *Scholarly Inquiry for Nursing Practice, 13*, 271–274.

Rossman, G. B., & Rallis, S. F. (2003). *Learning in the field* (2nd ed.). Thousand Oaks, CA: Sage.

Statistics Canada. (2004). Retrieved May 27, 2004, from http://www.statcan.ca/start.html

Thomlinson, E., McDonagh, M. K., Reimer, M., Crooks, K., & Lees, M. (2002). Health beliefs of rural Canadians: Implications for practice [Abstract]. *Charting the course for rural health in the 21st century*, 18.

Chapter 4

THE RURAL NURSING THEORY: A LITERATURE REVIEW

Deana L. Molinari and Ruiling Guo

THE RURAL NURSING THEORY (RNT) began when Kathleen Long and Clarann Weinert (1989) attempted to describe rural nursing as a unique health care domain (Jackman, Myrick, & Yonge, 2012). The outcome was a contextual theory interpreting qualitative and quantitative data collected by Montana State University students during the 1970s and 1980s. The conceptual framework provided a formula for examining rural community health status and testing intervention effectiveness with the hope of reducing disparities among populations (Bushy, 2000). The theory is based on the common nurse principles: person, nurse, environment, and health.

Nursing theory aims to describe, predict, and explain the phenomenon of nursing (Chinn & Jacobs, 1978). Researchers create and test theory to move science beyond intuition when evaluating health interventions (Croyle, 2005). Theories also help practitioners decide what is known and what needs to be known for better outcomes (Parsons, 1949). The number of times researchers use a theory and the strategies by which theory is tested are measures of the theory's usefulness. The more a theory is tested, the more logic and knowledge expands (Chinn & Jacobs, 1978).

When interventional studies fail to use theoretical foundations, a logical connection with other studies cannot be drawn. Research studies without theoretical foundations reduce science to the equivalent of inductive vignettes or anecdotes (Bushy, 2000). Generalizability becomes impossible and bias is supported. Theoretical foundations also control design error. When a researcher tests an intervention based on incomplete or unsupportive theoretical framework, the study can be negated. For example, employing a psychosocial stress theory to support a physiological intervention is a major error. The potential for logical errors continue throughout the research planning and implementation processes.

Dissemination of results is described in the context of theory in order to clarify the researcher's actions.

Theories serve to standardize research designs and account for diversity. Diversity of thought and environment are inherent in rural samples. Theory controls this type of diversity by unifying construct definitions and logical explanations. Failure to understand a study's conceptual foundation prevents the reader's growth. Therefore, understanding the development and use of a theory is foundational to scientific advancement.

Middle range theories analyze particular situations with a limited number of variables. For example, a contextual framework like the RNT argues that time, space, and place are crucial to the nature of activities. In other words, the environment impacts nursing practice. Therefore, a contextual nursing theory answers questions like: What is rural health? Who are rural nurses? How do rural nurses practice? Who are rural patients? How do residents define health and prefer health care? What are the environmental parameters? Researchers describe nurse and resident behaviors developed from experiences, principles, ideas, and feelings.

According to Bushy (2004a, 2004b), rural life is different from urban life; therefore, context prevents mirrored practices. Rural nurses function as generalists with specialty knowledge in crisis assessment and management (Long, 1999; Long & Weinert, 1991). Even the definition of rural "generalist" is distinct, due to facility and workforce size and cultural traditions (Molinari & Bushy, 2011). Nurses in small communities care for patients from birth to the end of life who suffer from a wide range of health issues. Rural nurses are also expected to know all community health resources and practice public health principles (Bennett, 2009). These facts are included in the RNT but are not the theory itself.

The RNT consists of concepts, definitions, and propositions based on assumptions derived from qualitative and quantitative data (Nichols, 1989). The organization of interrelated concepts gives a systematic view of rural life for practice (Lee & Winters, 2004). The basic concepts are the theory's components and they map the ideas' parameters. Models then depict the processes that occur among the concepts, and frameworks indicate how the behaviors occur.

The RNT's middle range model describes the "provision of health care by professional nurses to persons living in sparsely populated areas" (Long & Weiner, 1989, p. 3). The core ideas of "work and health beliefs, isolation and distance, self-reliance, lack of anonymity, outsider/insider, and old-timers/newcomers" (p. 7) are key to understanding rural health needs. The statement "rural dwellers define health as primarily the ability to work, and to be productive" is frequently discussed in rural nursing.

Dynamic theories change over time. A recent RNT alteration synthesized one of the core statements into the term "functionality." The concept is defined as "performing or able to perform a regular function" and it "contributes to the development or maintenance of a larger whole" (Bennet, 2009, p. 110). Descriptions of the concept include being ambulatory, able to work, feeling good—not just surviving, caring for family, and being self-determining. Functionality relies on the interplay

TABLE 4.1 Rural Nursing Theory Concepts

Concept	Rural Dimensions of Nursing Concepts

Person	Genetic and biological variations
	   – Diversity
	Human relationships
	   – Familiarity among residents
	   – Rural culture
	Values/perceptions
	Caregiving support systems
	   – Caregiving by known persons
	Spiritual relationships
	   – Health and caregiving beliefs
	   – Duties and responsibilities (friends, country)
	   – Newcomer/oldtimer
	   – Insider/Outsider

Environment	Physical/social/cultural
	   Distance and space
	   Sparse population
	   Geographic terrain
	Values formation and orientation
	Time orientation
	Belief systems and manifestations
	   – Lifestyle orientation to natural environment
	   – Occupations/recreation

Health	Definitions of health and illness
	   – Functionality
	Major beliefs
	   – Spiritual emphasis
	   – Cultural variations
	Worldview
	Healing practices
	Health and illness behaviors
	   – Symptom–action–timeline process (SATL)
	Health care systems
	   – Informal and formal supports

The professional nurse	Nursing—Definition and roles
	   – Interprofessional role diffusion
	Interrelationships
	   – Lack of anonymity
	   – Client familiarity
	Community expectation and responsibilities
	   – Generalist role with specialist skills
	   – Role diffusion
	   – Multiple community roles
	Nurse–client interactions
	   – Caring concepts and practices
	   – Provider culture

between mental, physical, and spiritual well-being and is measured by individual actions. When any one of these measures is lacking, health declines. This is also said of community health (see Table 4.1).

Researchers test a theory's concepts, models, and frameworks. Theory usefulness is measured with a variety of strategies. A qualitative literature analysis was conducted to detect the frequency of theory testing found in easy-to-access databases and synthesized theory applications.

METHODOLOGY

A literature search for "rural nursing theory" and "rural health" was conducted in online databases. The databases we searched included PubMed, Web of Science, Cumulative Index to Nursing and Allied Health Literature (CINHAL), Cochrane Library, PsycINFO, Psychology and Behavioral Sciences Collection, Dissertations and Theses, Abstracting and Indexing (A&I) Database, Education Research Complete, SciVerse Scopus, and Google Scholar. The searches focused on publications of the last 15 years. Therefore, the selection criteria for considering studies were journal articles, dissertations and theses, books, and conference proceedings related to RNT. References from the documents were also searched.

Databases

A brief introduction to each database searched is provided.

- *PubMed* is a comprehensive medical database sponsored by the National Library of Medicine. It comprises more than 21 million article citations for biomedical literature from MEDLINE and life science journals, including nursing. Publications include case reports, randomized controlled trials, clinical guidelines, and reviews.
- The *Web of Science* is an online database developed by the Information Scientific Institute and Thomson Reuters. It includes Science Citation Index and Social Sciences Citation Index. So far it covers over 12,000 journals in the sciences and social sciences. The database includes nursing-related journal articles for worldwide access.
- *CINAHL* is considered the authoritative and premier resource for nursing and allied health. It contains journals, book reviews, and conference proceedings dating back to 1981.
- The *Cochrane Library* is an online collection of evidence-based medicine and clinical practice literature. It comprises seven databases. They are Cochrane Database of Systematic Reviews (CDSR),

Database of Abstracts of Reviews of Effectiveness (DARE), Cochrane Central Register of Control Trials (CENTRAL), Cochrane Database of Methodology Reviews (CDMR), Cochrane Methodology Register (CMR), Health Technology Assessment Database (HTA), and NHS Economic Evaluation Database (NHS EED). Bringing together seven databases allows users to look at the effectiveness of different health care treatments and interventions.

- *PsycINFO* contains about 3 million citations and summaries of scholarly journal articles, book chapters, and dissertations in psychological aspects of topics like bioethics, sociology, education, pharmacology, physiology, and medicine. The journal coverage spans from 1840s to present. It includes more than 2,400 journals in about 30 languages.

- *Psychology and Behavioral Sciences Collection* is another comprehensive database, covering topics in emotional and behavioral characteristics, psychiatry and psychology, mental processes, anthropology, and observational and experimental methods. This database offers about 400 journals related to psychology.

- *Dissertations and Theses, A&I* provides access to 2.3 million index and abstract records for the United States, Canada, and some other international dissertations and master's theses. It covers a variety of disciplines, including nursing.

- *Education Research Complete* is a definitive resource for education research. Indexing and abstracts from more than 2,100 journals include all levels of education from early childhood to higher education, and all educational specialties, such as multilingual education, health education, and testing. The search engine also includes full text for nearly 500 books and monographs.

- *SciVerse Scopus* is the world's largest abstract and citation database of peer-reviewed literature. The indexing contains 46 million records, nearly 19,500 titles from 5,000 publishers, and 4.6 million conference papers.

- *Google Scholar* is an online search engine for articles, theses, books, abstracts, and court opinions from academic publishers, professional societies, online repositories, universities, and other websites across many disciplines and sources. Selection criteria included the words "rural nursing theory" and "rural health."

Articles and book chapters discussing rural nursing and rural health care were chosen. Article data were then placed in a matrix with fields listing theories, citation, dates, sample size, research design, outcome concepts, and study location. A synthesis of findings for frequency and diversity was conducted.

RESULTS

In all, 215 articles met inclusion criteria. Of those, 24 articles addressed the RNT as the main topic. In total, 101 publications focused upon rural residents' health issues. Out of these, 25 publications targeted the rural environment and 60 explored professional rural nurse concepts. Although the proportion of rural articles identified was miniscule when compared with urban sites, publication frequency increased with each passing decade (see Table 4.2).

Many articles employing rural samples were not theory based and therefore were not included in the review. In all, 40 articles and chapters used aspects of the RNT theory to support the research effort. Several other theories and models were mentioned, including: (1) Caplan's theory of crisis, (2) social judgment theory, (3) local clinical scientist model, (4) place-based model, (5) central place theory, (6) effort recovery model, (7) biopsychosocial model, (8) international classification of functioning, (9) disability and health, (10) belonging, (11) social capital, (12) translational environmental research, (13) locus of control, (14) health belief, (15) resource scarcity (Long, 2000), and (16) health literacy. Research topics included, development of the RNT (Long & Weinert, 1989), workforce analysis (Molinari, Jaiswal, & Hollinger-Forrest, 2011; Molinari, Monserud, & Hudzinski, 2008), and health issues (Magilvy & Congdon, 2000).

The most frequently mentioned research design was Grounded Theory (Seright, 2011). The majority of articles were descriptive. Literature reviews, interviews, surveys, and focus groups were methods used to gather data. Ethnography, phenomenology, content analysis (Shookner, Scott, & Vollman, 2008), and general descriptive designs were also employed. Few articles studied intervention outcomes and only one randomized trial was identified.

Studies mentioned the following locations: Arizona, Montana, Mississippi, New England, Northwest United States, rural Canada, Texas; 30 unidentified rural sites, and the Western United States. Most studies did not mention a location. One way of providing confidentiality is by not

TABLE 4.2 Number of Database Articles Meeting Inclusion Criteria, By Decade

Year	Articles Published
1980–1989	3
1990–1999	48
2000–2009	130
2010–2012	34
Total	**215**

providing location clues. The practice hampered analyzing the theory's geographical scope.

The review framework addressed articles employing a theory addressing rural as either a concept or a location. Overall, 24 articles addressed the RNT as the main topic. The authors wrote about the concepts, theory development, theory testing, and methodological issues. Researchers explored the impact of gender and of other theories, on the RNT. Theoretical implications on practice were examined.

One of the four main concepts of RNT is "person." The database searches uncovered 55 different rural health resident issues. The most frequently published topic was mental health (13). Other topics included: Diverse samples living with specific health conditions, perceptions and beliefs, managing distance, and needed supports. Researchers deliberated on specific population and gender issues (Sellers et al., 1999). Journals published articles about farmers, families, elders, Hispanics/Blacks/single women, mothers, adolescents, special needs children, and caregivers. Little was found about male or veteran populations. Sub concepts identified included rural residents' health definitions, independence impacts on health care, choice of provider, access, and the time elapsing from the first symptom identification until the time of care seeking (Moran, 2005; Winters et al., 2010).

The second main concept of RNT is "environment." Some articles explicitly focused on care delivery locations like the hospital, home, and long-term care. Researchers commonly addressed the distance and time needed to reach providers. Implicitly, all articles explored "rural" environments. The authors also examined: community assessment, the importance of location (Poland, Lehoux, Holmes, & Andrews, 2005), rural routes, rural definitions (Pitblado, 2005), market position, and competition. Isolation impacted many studies (Conger & Plager, 2008).

The third concept addressed by RNT is the professional "nurse." In total, 60 articles addressed provider perceptions, values, needs, education, peer relationships, practice issues, social capital, leadership, lifestyle, organizational culture, employment choice factors, autonomy, role definition, connectedness, efficacy, leadership, case management, and litigation (Crooks, 2004). The most frequently discussed item explored nurses' preparation for practice (Molinari, 2011). Of the 25 different nurse topics found in the literature, recruitment and retention were the most frequently mentioned.

The purpose of all research studies was to examine some aspect of "health," the fourth concept in the RNT (Niemoller, Ide, & Nichols, 2000). Rural studies addressed improving health, the definition of health, perceptions of independence, autonomy, and help seeking. The most frequently found studies explored mental health treatment issues. Less frequent studies were devoted to health promotion and disease prevention. Cultural, sports, and activity influences on health were also examined.

Some researchers explored personal characteristics or conditions influencing health: Values, culture, roles, coherence, resilience, behaviors, inequities, perceptions, literacy, care giving, generational care, chronic illness, uncertainty, balance, and homelessness. Specific tests and treatments, health care delivery models, peer group interventions, assessments, and the delivery of psychology and mental health care fill the literature databases. Rural conditions or situations influenced individuals' health, including hypertension, AIDS, pregnancy, obesity, cardiac issues, mental illness, pain, and sexuality. Not all publications focused on adverse issues. Although fewer in number, some articles spoke to concept strengths like independence, exercise, and lifestyle.

DISCUSSION

The literature review identified several issues. Search engine limitations inhibit finding rural studies and synthesizing them. Many research design issues were noted. The infrequency of RNT testing inhibits study results generalizations.

Although PubMed and Web of Science databases identified a few articles related to RNT, the search engines did not provide many results. Some of the most important journals are not included in databases with worldwide access. For instance, the *Online Journal of Rural Nursing and Health Care*, the official journal of the Rural Nursing Organization, publishes extensive information about rural nursing practice. PubMed did not include the journal until 2010. The *Journal of Rural Health* covers many rural health topics and is the official publication of the National Rural Health Association, and yet the journal was not selected by Web of Science for indexing. These restrictions inhibit synthesis studies. Few systematic reviews or meta-analyses were found in any database. Other rural and remote health organizations' journals were not included in the databases. In addition, databases hosted by individual journals were difficult to use. Therefore, this study's publication frequency information lists fewer articles than actually were published. The inability to access studies is a major problem for both researchers and program developers.

Google Scholar was added to the search strategy to identify articles addressing RNT applications. More articles were found with earlier publication dates than were with recent dates, which is a relevance issue. *Google Scholar* allows metadata searching on the Internet while the other online databases require restricted searching fields for titles, authors, abstracts, and subject headings. Database improvements allowing sophisticated search options are needed when studying specific health conditions of specific sample characteristics. For instance, comparison studies require many database search options. Without search capabilities, many research questions cannot be answered. Researchers wishing to test RNT need to compare disease treatments with rural and urban behaviors, issues, and characteristics. Policy and funding issues for specific treatment also require sophisticated search strategies.

Only 19% of the articles studied mentioned RNT's conceptual components. Researchers need to identify the reasons for the infrequent application. Since a majority of articles failed to identify any conceptual framework, suppositions for infrequent use cannot be narrowed from generalities such as researcher's lack of knowledge, a research reporting culture, or a lack of the theory's appropriateness.

The assertion that the RNT does not fit all rural populations cannot be analyzed. The common practice of not including sample locations in reports prevents a detailed analysis of this claim. Limited access to rural nursing literature slows discovery and research application.

Rural Definitions

Research purposes and topics alter over time. Rural definitions have changed since 1989. Initial rural nursing research analyzed qualitative data from small, isolated communities. During the 1990s, the purpose of research shifted from describing conditions to comparing treatment outcomes. Around the globe, the importance of synthesizing multiple studies using new designs grew. Basing new treatments on research studies influences funding opportunities. Large populations for clinical trials are desired for this research design.

One common rural care characteristic is "small." There are small hospitals, small populations, and few providers. Smaller samples hampered small clinical trials, so qualitative designs retained popularity and may have influenced the number of published rural studies.

The traditional definition of *rural* relates to space and distance. "Being rural means being a long way from anywhere and pretty close to nowhere" (Scharff, 1998, p. 21). Economic conditions caused populations to grow and shrink. The fluctuations challenged the rural definition.

Cloke (2003) proposed that "rurality" should be understood as a socially and culturally constructed phenomenon rather than as a location. The idea of space has been replaced by a romanticism of rural as an ideal place to live rather than a fixed location. Populations moved from urban communities into the countryside. Rural began to include manufacturing as well as forestry and agriculture. Leisure and tourism industries changed the view of rural to a preferred location with new social, moral, cultural, ideals. The mobile population increased the number of urban values transferred to countryside locations.

Cloke's definition could alter the RNT's of a rural nurse. Traditionally a rural nurse is one who cares for people in locations with sparse populations. Place and distance are commonly mentioned in rural and frontier studies but differing rural perceptions are rarely mentioned. The RNT is associated with an agrarian definition and yet rural realities have altered. Modifying the rural definition to include cultural and social norms should influence researchers' topics as well as policy makers' funding decisions. Sparsely populated areas today host most high-risk occupations. No longer do rural communities consist of stable generations inheriting the family business. Tourism can double the size of some communities. Large agricultural corporations eliminated small towns. Still other communities find retirement population growth influences public service tax support, thus reducing the number of young families.

Ross (2008) contends there is no one definition of *rural* and that many definitions can occur at once. Traditional descriptions are usually narrow and represent agrarian perceptions. Dichotomous definitions limit research to polar comparisons while typologies place characteristics on a continuum. Rural can be described in terms of size, density, locality, culture, ways of knowing, and so on. Indices using multiple variables can compare health care differences. Definitions including occupations like tourism, mining, fishing as well as size, urban proximity, and population stability may enable researchers to focus on causal relationships. For instance, how do populations in stable, small, isolated communities manage self-care when compared with fluctuating populations in small, isolated communities?

Communities

National phenomena impact rural communities. National policies, economics, and technologies impact all citizens (Hartley, 2005). "Because nursing is a social phenomenon shaped by the society in which it is practiced, an understanding of rural persons along with their self-defined needs and preferences is essential to the development of a theory base for professional practice" (Bushy, 2000, p. 34). The Institute of Medicine (IOM) (2004) indicated smaller, poorer, and more isolated communities experience more difficulty ensuring high-quality health services. The IOM posits that small, isolated communities experience higher health risks and disparities. The lack of rural comparison research constrains innovative interventions. Size and distance may not be as strongly connected to health care as cultural values, self-care, and accountability are. More sophisticated studies are needed.

Rural nursing investigators need a sound understanding of community sampling. Studies sponsored by large urban centers may introduce design bias and yet the nature of research funding predisposes awarding funds to large urban organizations. A standard employment of RNT could control for bias. The RNT posits that community outsiders are not trusted as much as longtime residents, so data collection may be impacted by familiarity with the data collectors (McNeely &

Shreffler, 1998). Community membership can also impact data analysis. Researchers may miss logical reasons for findings they lack a community identity.

Other reasons for supporting rural nurse researchers are written into the theory. Driving forces behind a local economy influence a sample's health care beliefs and perceptions, thus impacting habits and care access. For instance, the loss of a local business can impact a community's view of prosperity. Families may reduce health expenses when concerned about the ripple effects of a business closure.

Larger and more reliable rural samples can be collected using technologies to reach participants from many communities. Studies that include various community types can control for rural diversity and may lead to new rural definitions.

Research is influenced by national initiatives such as health reform. Accountable care organizations and medical homes are expected to produce a new concept called the regional health care center. As the new organizations grow in popularity, residents may adjust expectations of provider access and travel distance. Reforms may also modify the concept of "place." Telemedicine technologies can also revise travel expectations and what constitutes "care." Future collaborative care coordination functions could modify preferences for familiar providers and modify people's self-care expectations.

Competition among urban and rural providers for political power is common. Health care depends on political power and funding; therefore, standardization of definitions and conceptual frameworks need universal understanding. The funding shifts from acute care treatments to community health prevention need more interprofessional, collaborative, and comparative research designs. Health reform is expected to encourage regional studies that could increase impact research about providers. Small samples support qualitative designs while large samples support outcome studies. Outcome studies are preferred for influencing policies and yet small samples so prevalent in rural domains can produce influential data. Gary Donaldson suggests research designs promoting qualitative analysis of quantitative variables can provide a new type of data. A focus on comparative intervention effectiveness or the analysis of treatment response diversities requires fewer participants and more variables per individual to understand that some individuals respond and others do not (Donaldson, 2012).

The RNT's concept of nurse can be expanded. Few studies have focused on the economics of health care, except in terms of access, work setting, and resources. Little was presented about the value of nurse generalists. The review indicated that most researchers studied small community deficiencies. By focusing on a sparse population definition of rural nursing, many cultural and social aspects of "rural" are ignored. The strengths of collaboration, teamwork, cultural diversity, innovations, survival strengths, family, governance, and networking are currently ignored in research (Bunce, 2003; Cloke, 2003).

CONCLUSION

Theories provide a genealogy of researchers' logic and make predictions for the future. Theories are based on populations and behavior principles. The database searches conducted about the RNT indicate a pressing need for more testing. Fast paced health care delivery reforms require a deeper understanding of rural perceptions and practices (Molinari et al., 2011; Molinari, Jaiswal, & Peterson, 2011). This study found researchers describing basic rural health and nursing practice concepts whereas nursing science requires theoretically based treatment outcome studies. There is much for rural researchers to accomplish before improving rural health.

Research requires further theoretical development as economics, policy, health reform, and research designs change over time. Improved patient care will involve standardized definitions and complex research designs. Synthesis studies necessitate theory, design, and analysis commonalities. Rural evidence-based practice will need to compare rural studies based on mid-range contextual theories. Quality patient care also calls for improved database technologies. Testing the RNT appears imperative to understand patients, nurses, the environment, and health interventions.

REFERENCES

Bennett, A. (2009). *Project genesis: Community assessment of rural southeastern Arizona border community*. Dissertation, University of Arizona.

Bunce, M. (2003). Reproducing rural idylls. In P. Cloke (Ed.), *Country visions* (pp. 14–30). Harlow, Essex, UK: Pearson.

Bushy, A. (2000). *Orientation to nursing in the rural community*. Thousand Oaks, CA. Sage.

Bushy, A. (2004a). Creating nursing research opportunities in rural healthcare facilities. *Journal of Nursing Care Quality, 19*(2), 162–168.

Bushy, A. (2004b). *Rural nursing: Practice and issues*. American Nurses Association Continuing Education Program module. American Nurses Association, 51. Retrieved, November 24, 2004, from http://www.nursingworld.org/mods/mod700/rural.pdf

Chinn, P. L., & Jacobs, M. K. (1978). A model for theory development in nursing. *Advances in Nursing Science, 1*(1), 1–12.

Cloke, P. (2003). Knowing ruralities. In P. Cloke (Ed.), *Country visions* (pp. 1–13). Harlow: Pearson.

Conger, M. M., & Plager, K. A. (2008). Advanced practice nursing practice in rural areas: Connectedness versus disconnectedness. *Online Journal of Rural Nursing and Health Care, 8*(1), 24–38. Retrieved January 24, 2009 from http://rno.org

Crooks, K. (2004). Is rural nursing a specialty? *Online Journal of Rural Nursing and Health Care, 4*(1). Retrieved July 25, 2004 from http://www.rno.org/journal/issues/Vol-4/issue-1/crooks_column.htm

Croyle, R. T. (2005). *Theory at a glance: Application to health promotion and health behavior* (2nd ed.). Washington, DC: U.S. Department of Health and Human Services, National Institutes of Health.

Donaldson, G. (2012). *Advanced Quantitative Approaches in Nursing Science: Dyadic and Latent/Growth Mixture Modeling*. Communicating Nursing Research Conference, Western Institute of Nursing Keynote Address, Portland, Oregon, April 20, 2012.

Hartley, D. (2005). Rural health research: Building capacity and influencing policy in the United States and Canada. *Canadian Journal of Nursing Research, 37*(1), 7–13.

Jackman, D., Myrick, F., & Yonge, O. (2012). Putting the (r)ural in preceptorship. *Nurse Research Practice,* 528580. doi: 10.1155/2012/528580. Retrieved June 17, 2012, from http://www.ncbi.nlm.nih.gov/pmc/articles/PMC3368593/?tool=pubmed

Lee, H. J., & Winters, C. A. (2004). Testing rural nurse theory: Perceptions and needs of service providers. *Online Journal of Rural Nursing and Health Care, 4*(1). 51–63.

Long, C. (2000). Rural communities feel sting of nursing shortage. *The Daily Camera*. Retrieved October 10, 2011, from http://www.broomfieldnews.com/news/statewest/09lnurs.html

Long, K. A. (1999). Reflections on "Rural nursing: Developing the theory base." *Scholarly Inquiry Nursing Practice, 13*(3), 275–279.

Long, K. A., & Weinert, C. (1989). Rural nursing: Developing the theory base. *Scholarly Inquiry for Nursing Practice, 3,* 113–127.

Long, K. A., & Weinert, C. (1991). *Rural nursing: developing the theory base (NLN Publication No. 21-2408,* pp. 389–406). New York, NY: National League of Nursing.

Long, K. A., & Weinert, C. (2006). Rural nursing: Developing the theory base. In H. J. Lee, & C. A. Winters (Eds.), *Rural nursing: Concepts, theory and practice* (2nd ed., pp. 3–16). New York, NY: Springer Publishing.

Magilvy, J. K., & Congdon, J. G. (2000). The crisis nature of health care transitions for rural older adults. *Public Health Nursing, 17*(5), 336–345.

McNeely, A. G., & Shreffler, M. J. (1998). Familiarity. In H. J. Lee (Ed.) *Conceptual basis for rural nursing* (pp. 89–101). New York, NY: Springer Publishing.

Molinari, D. L. (2011). Rural nurse transition-to-practice programs. In D. L. Molinari, & A. Bushy (Eds.), *Rural nurse transition to practice* (pp. 23–34). New York, NY: Springer Publishing.

Molinari, D. L., & Bushy, A. (2011). Editor. *Rural nurse: Transition to practice.* New York, NY: Springer Publishing.

Molinari, D. L., Jaiswal, A., & Hollinger-Forrest, T. (2011). Rural nurse: Lifestyle preferences and educational perceptions. *Online Journal of Rural Nursing and Health Care, 2*. Retrieved January 30, 2012, from http://www.google.com/url?sa=t&rct=j&q=&esrc=s&source=web&cd=8&ved=0CFkQFjAH&url=http%3A%2F%2Frnojournal.binghamton.edu%2Findex.php%2FRNO%2Farticle%2Fdownload%2F27%2F19&ei=rdrgT-6vF4qW2QXrvqjgCw&usg=AFQjCNFzMZC3DG3LgkV0UeyTQlBSVUxryg

Molinari, D. L., Jaiswal, A., & Peterson, T. (2011). Rural nurse perceptions of organizational culture and the intent to move. In D. L. Molinari, & A. Bushy (Eds.), *Rural nurse transition to practice* (pp. 61–70). New York, NY: Springer Publishing.

Molinari, D. L., Monserud, M., & Hudzinski, D. (2008). A new type of rural nurse residency. *The Journal of Continuing Education in Nursing, 39*(1), 42–46.

Moran, C. A. (2005). *Replication study of rural nursing theory: A Missouri perspective.* Unpublished master's thesis, Central Missouri State University.

Nichols, E. (1989). Response to "Rural nursing, developing the theory base". *Scholarly Inquiry in Nursing Practice, 13*(3), 271–274.

Niemoller, J. K., Ide, B. A., & Nichols, E. G. (2000). Issues in studying health-related hardiness and use of services among older rural adults. *Texas Journal of Rural Health, 18*, 35–43.

Parsons, T. (1949). *The structure of social action.* Glencoe, Illinois: Free Press.

Pitblado, J. R. (2005). So, what do we mean by "rural", "remote" and "northern"? *Canadian Journal of Nursing Research, 37*(1), 163–168.

Poland, B., Lehoux, P., Holmes, D., & Andrews, G. (2005). How place matters: Unpacking technology and power in health and social care. *Health & Social Care in the Community, 13*, 170–180.

Ross, J. (2008). *Rural nursing: Aspects of practice.* Dunedin, New Zealand: Rural Health Opportunities.

Scharff, J. E. (1998). The distinctive nature and scope of rural nursing practice: Philosophical bases. In H. J. Lee, & C. A. Winters (Eds.), *Rural nursing: Concepts, theory and practice* (2nd ed., pp. 179–196). New York, NY: Springer.

Sellers, S. C., Poduska, M. D., Propp, L. H., & White, S. E. (1999). The health care meanings, values, and practices of Anglo-American males in the rural Midwest. *Journal of Transcultural Nursing, 10,* 320–330.

Seright, T. J. (2011). Clinical decision-making of rural novice nurses. *Rural Remote Health, 11*(3). Retrieved January 16, 2012, from http://www.rrh.org.au/articles/subviewnew.asp?ArticleID=1726

Shookner, M., Scott, C. M., & Vollman, A. R. (2008). Creating supportive environments for health: Social network analysis. In A. R. Vollman, E. T. Anderson, & J. McFarlane (Eds.), *Canadian community as partner: Theory & multidisciplinary practice* (2nd ed.). Philadelphia, PA: Lippincott Williams & Wilkins.

Winters, C., Thomlinson, E. H., O'Lynn, C., Lee, H. J., McDonagh, M. K., Edge, D. S., & Reimer, M. A. (2010). Exploring rural nursing theory across borders. In C. A. Winters, & H. J. Lee (Eds.). *Rural nursing: Concepts, theory and practice* (3rd ed., pp. 41–54). New York, NY: Springer Publishing.

Chapter 5

HEALTH NEEDS AND PERCEPTIONS OF RURAL PERSONS

Ronda L. Bales, Charlene A. Winters, and Helen J. Lee

HEALTH PRACTICES OF RURAL DWELLERS are known to be influenced by their perceptions of health and illness. Long and Weinert (1989) remarked on the individuality of health perceptions among rural dwellers and noted that those assumptions regarding concepts of health cannot be generalized among rural populations. Understanding the health perceptions, needs, and behaviors of an individual, family, or community can be instrumental in health promotion planning. This chapter addresses the health needs, perceptions, and behaviors of six individuals living in one community in rural Montana.

INTRODUCTION TO THE COMMUNITY

The echoed phrase 'closer to heaven than I may ever get' is a vivid reference to the vast and beautiful wilderness known as Montana City, with its elevation of nearly 7500 feet above sea level.[1] The community is nestled in the midst of mountain peaks and lies just east of the northeast entrance to a national park (Glidden, 1982). The location of Montana City is one of its unique attributes, and access to and from the community varies from summer to winter. Although travel in and out of Montana City during the summer may be slow because of the winding mountain roads, it is not limited. The winter months, however, bring additional challenges beyond distance to the members of this community that other rural Montanans may not face. When the snow begins to fly in October, residents are faced with isolation in terms of travel outside their community. From October to May, when the snow typically melts, the only passable route by automobile is 55 miles on a narrow, winding highway through a national park with an additional 55 miles to expanded health care services

(National Geographic Road Atlas, 2000). Passage via this route is dependent on snowplows to keep the roads passable. An alternative route out of Montana City is available. This route allows for travel to towns and cities in Montana and a neighboring state, about 100 and 120 miles, respectively (Glidden; *National Geographic Road Atlas*). There is a catch, however; this route includes a stretch of road over a pass approximately 10 miles long that is left unplowed during the winter (Fahlberg, 1983). Therefore, access to and from Montana City via this route during the winter months is limited to those with snowmobiles. Thus, one can visualize that winter brings challenges to these rural dwellers that affect access not only to health care but also to all dimensions of life outside the community.

METHODS

RONDA L. BALES: My purpose in this study was to explore the health needs and perceptions of rural persons living in Montana City, Montana. I chose descriptive qualitative research methods for this research project because they provide an opportunity "to try to understand how people make sense of their worlds" (Rossman & Rallis, 1998, p. 8). In this case, it allowed me an opportunity to understand how, when, where, and why the residents of Montana City seek health care and the factors that influence health care behaviors, access, and usage.

After obtaining informed consent, I conducted semi-structured interviews with members of the community. Initially, I identified participants through a key informant who owned a cabin located within the community. I approached the remaining participants directly and asked about their interest in participation in the study.

Sample

The convenience sample consisted of five women and one man, aged 37 to 76 years. The participants had lived in the community from 3 to 30 years.

Montana City met the definition of remote rural described by Koehler (1998): "A community with a population of 2,500 or less located forty miles or further from a city with a population of 50,000 or greater. Remote rural communities do not have a hospital or medical assistance facility" (pp. 238–239).

Data Collection and Analysis

I collected data by using a semi-structured interview guide. Questions were open-ended and intended to elicit information regarding the individuals' health perceptions and needs. Interviews were audiotaped and transcribed. Field notes were kept to document observations and impressions about the community and persons interviewed. I analyzed the transcribed interviews and field notes for emergent themes.

FINDINGS: MONTANA CITY

The population of this community varies drastically in accordance with the change of seasons. The participants of the study estimated the year-round population to be 70 to 100 persons and stated that it tripled during the summer. All participants identified themselves as "year-round" residents of the community.

I identified two main groups within the sample: (a) those who had lived in the community for a number of years, and (b) those who had recently moved there. A comparison was provided by one participant, who gave a description of the long-time members of the community.

If you live here long enough, you can tell who lives here by how they dress and the snowmobiles they drive; the clothes they wear are patched up with duct tape. They have the old style stuff, but then maybe that's a sign of the culture too. I just think that some of that goes with it, that you choose to live that way because you want to. It is not important, material things are not important here. I am really speaking generally, because there are people moving in who have a lot more money to spend and they have the nicer homes. So you see, we are seeing a change in our culture here.

Health Care

Health care resources within the community of Montana City were limited. There was no clinic, hospital, or other formal health care. However, emergency medical services (EMS) was available. The EMS network composed of volunteers from the community who were mainly trained at the first responder level and one member who was prepared to practice at the emergency medical technician (EMT) level at the time I conducted the interviews. There was a dedicated ambulance for the national park, located at the entrance, and the park ranger stationed there was an EMT. The EMS process was explained by a participant.

> If someone calls 911, they call me or someone on the roster. Then I go and appraise the situation and call for the ambulance if it is needed. See, we do have an ambulance available, but it is at the gate [to the national park]. But the park administration doesn't think the community should rely solely on the Park for its EMS services. So that is why they call someone on the list first, and then if we need it, we call for the ambulance.
>
> The park ambulance is equipped for advanced life support and can travel to a clinic located in Maryville, approximately 55

miles through the national park. If transport to a hospital was necessary, a second ambulance from Littlewood had to meet the park ambulance and transport the patient. Medical flight services are typically not available to the community because the location presents a dangerous situation for helicopters.

All participants interviewed identified a retired doctor who lived in the community as a health care resource. Participants indicated they had accessed him at one time or another and that he helped them make judgments about whether or not it was necessary to obtain further or immediate care for a health-related issue. The identified retired physician had lived in Montana City for 5 years at the time I conducted the study. I contacted and interviewed this individual, not as a participant of the study, but rather to gain insight into the health care needs of the community in general. The retired physician indicated that he was available for emergencies and did what he could "on the spot," but that he did not encourage members of the community to use him as their regular health care provider. He also stated that he made the decisions about what he would treat and how far he would go in treating patients before sending them to a medical facility because he had very limited resources and equipment available to him in Montana City. He commented that he had very little besides his "five senses" with which to provide care.

Health Status

Two participants described themselves as having major medical illnesses. Several other participants made reference to the fact that there were a number of people in the community who had suffered major illnesses. According to the retired physician, the illnesses suffered by members of the community included heart failure, stroke, cancer, leukemia, pulmonary hypertension, and pheochromocytoma. Furthermore, he had the impression that the incidence of serious illness in the community was higher in comparison with other communities of similar size. Several interviewed participants also indicated that there appeared to be a high rate of smoking and alcohol consumption within the community. As one participant stated,

> There is a high rate of alcohol consumption and drugs too here, even for a small community. And that is a big factor in health issues here. And smoking, that is another issue, everybody smokes. I am sure for the percentage of smokers in a community we are way off the top end.

Data such as average income, poverty rates, and unemployment percentages were not available for Montana City. Therefore, I could not draw any conclusions about these data for the community.

Themes

Six major themes emerged from the analysis of the data. They included self-reliance, hardiness, conscientious consumer, informed risk, community support, and inadequate insurance. Two themes (self-reliance and hardiness) were reported previously in rural nursing literature (Chafey, Sullivan, & Shannon, 1998; Wirtz, Lee, & Running, 1998). Four themes (conscientious consumer, informed risk, community support, and inadequate insurance) were new.

Self-Reliance

Self-reliance has been defined as "the capacity to provide for one's own need" (Agich, 1993, as cited in Chafey et al., 1998, p. 159). All participants expressed that they take care of themselves first. However, varying degrees of self-reliance were described. Two participants, a married couple who moved into the community to retire, expressed self-reliance but also stated they probably accessed formal health care more quickly than long-time residents of the community. Factors that may have influenced their self-reliance included good health insurance, easy access to health care prior to moving to Montana City, and one participant's diagnosis of pulmonary hypertension. They explained,

> We are a little different because we retired here from a very different background and there are several other couples like that. So you are seeing some different things in the rural areas than maybe before because our experience is to take advantage of good medical care where we were and so we sort of expect or do the same thing here, although it is a bit harder, but I think we would be much more apt to take advantage of it than people who have lived here for 50 years. They have had to do things on their own and are very resourceful and they take care of things on their own. But we are spoiled the other way and so it is a little [different].

Another participant, who also moved into the community to retire, stated, "It has to be pretty bad [to seek health care]. I usually wait it out or take care of it myself." Then he described a contrast between himself and long-time residents of the community.

> I think that a lot of people here, because they have lived here all their life and haven't had access to immediate care, wait it out. The locals definitely try to treat themselves first and do wait it out when they probably should leave right away and get there before it is too bad. So, in a way, I guess we are probably

different from some of the people who have lived here a long time.

Another example of self-reliance was reported by a participant when she described how she and her husband planned for surgery.

> We chose May because we knew we wanted to come home after his surgery so he could recuperate up here. Since we live on Montana Pass and there was still snow that meant we still had to get him to the house, and that had to be by snowmobile. The doctor said not to sit on the snowmobile, but that he could stand on our pull sled. So, I drove the snowmobile and he stood up on the pull sled and I took him home.

Hardiness

The participants demonstrated several characteristics of hardiness identified by Wirtz et al. (1998). Those included adaptability, positive attitude, and endurance. The following excerpt from the interview with the participant who was suffering from pulmonary hypertension demonstrates adaptability and a positive attitude.

> I suppose I am concerned [about my health], but I happen to know this is a progressive disease and it's just going to progress and so we will just deal with it as it comes. I think by nature I am an up person and so you just do it.

Another participant, who suffered from a major medical condition causing her severe pain, demonstrated adaptability and endurance. She commented, "I just worked . . . I just go until I drop." "Our thing is we go until I scream [because of pain] and if I scream, I go in."

An older participant, recovering from surgery, also demonstrated endurance while caring for her terminally ill husband.

> I was in the hospital with my new shoulder when they called me at the hospital and told me that I had to either have him out of the hospital by the tenth of June or come up with $118 a day. I can't afford $118 a day. They said I couldn't take him home with [my] shoulder and I said, "well, I am going to. I don't have $118 a day." My grandson came and stayed with me for four days and that really helped until I learned how to handle him, getting him in and out of bed and I had to lift. I felt more comfortable when I had him [my husband] at home, though I didn't sleep much, but I knew he was taken care of and that is where he wanted to be.

Conscientious Consumer

The theme of conscientious consumer was a new one, identified in this study. Many participants made reference to making decisions about where to seek care depending on the type of illness or injury involved and the time of year. "In the summer you can go to Conway or Robertson or Littlewood, or Bowman or Lackwood. We have those options depending on how important it is." Another participant, a little over 8 months pregnant at the time of the interview, made a statement about selecting a health care provider and making arrangements for the birth of her child.

> I chose the Littlewood clinic but Conway would actually be a little closer but they have sometimes a little bit more weather concerns, whereas the road to Littlewood is always open. I chose it [Littlewood] after comparing it with Lackwood and other places.

Another participant demonstrated the concept of conscientious consumer by his explanation of his decisions about emergency care.

> That [miles to emergency care] depends on what type of emergency. If right now I cut my finger off working with the saw over there, I would head for Conway. If I was having chest pains, if I was able to make a conscious decision, I would be heading to Lackwood. Now they do have the clinic in Maryville and they are very good there. They have a really good doctor, but he is in the process of leaving. And it depends on who comes in there. If I like the doctor, I would go there for some things. If I don't like him, I wouldn't go back for anything. And in a few months if I cut my finger I would be heading to the clinic in Maryville and then on to Lackwood because the road to Conway will be closing. And it really does depend on what is going on. I would base my decision on where to go on the situation and the problem.

Informed Risk

Informed risk was a second new theme that emerged from the analysis. Informed risk was evidenced by the two participants with major health problems. One participant, who had pulmonary hypertension, explained that she was aware of the health risks associated with where she lived, but chose to remain in Montana City because of other benefits it provided that she valued. In other words, the risk was worth it to her because she was where she wanted to be.

> There are times when I wonder if I will be here in the morning and sometime I probably won't, but there is no future in worrying about it. I probably shouldn't be at this altitude, but what we have up here, what we enjoy [is here], and so we [are] loath to give that up.

She further explained that she was aware of the implications of living in Montana City.

> I am aware [of the risks and concerns] because the doctors keep telling me that I probably shouldn't be at this altitude, but obviously I'm still here so that must tell you something about my attitude. It would probably be more convenient closer to the hospital and yet I don't really want to live having to be close to the hospital when friends and activities are all up here. It's more fun to be up here and have to deal with whatever happens because I shouldn't be here.

The husband of the above participant was also involved in the research project and stated,

> Well, there were a lot of concerns when this [diagnosis of pulmonary hypertension] first happened. The doctors in Denver were very concerned about us coming back here without what they considered any backup. All the patients they have treated have been with [in] twenty minutes of the hospital and a backup. See, with primary pulmonary hypertension, the literature has showed that within 20 minutes of the prostacyclin infusion being stopped, there are severe, rebound reactions, including death in some cases. The infusion must be continuous, and if something happens, say the pump is dropped and it pulls on the catheter, or if she falls and it somehow stops, or even if the catheter gets clogged, but if the infusion is stopped for any reason, you must start another IV. . . . We are aware of what the doctors think and we know what it might mean to live here because of the altitude or problems with the catheter.

He further explained and defined informed risk in the following statement:

> The altitude here is a problem and the doctors really think we should move. This altitude is not good for [my wife] and the pulmonary hypertension can be worse because of it, but we know that and like I said, maybe one day we will have to move to Lackwood or whatever, but right now this where we want to be.

Another participant who also suffered from a major disease process stated,

> As far as being this far away, we have talked about it, my surgeon and I talked about it. I mean jeepers, if it is time to go in [to the hospital]; it is time to go in. And if it is too late, it is too late. I don't have a concern about that at all, at all.

She further explained by stating,

> I would never move just for medical care, just simply because I love it here. I mean how can you not go out here [outside her home] and think, "oh cool." It is a heart song and it is a peace of heart for me to be here and that is a lot of help. It really is. I can go out there and look at the mountains and get something out of that and that makes the difference.

Another participant stated, "Those of us who have been here for years, we just try to take care of ourselves without having to get any medical attention. Sometimes that is ok. We realize the risk we are taking."

Community Support

Another theme that emerged was community support. Each of the individuals made statements that the community pulls together when someone needs help. The hardy individual described previously who cared for her husband stated,

> There is a lot of people here I could have called. That is one thing about Montana City. If you ever need help, even if you are a stranger to them, you get help. That is one thing about up here. It is a great community.

Another participant shared her perception of support.

> The people in the community are great. Every time I am having a bad day all we have to do is make a phone call or stand out on the street and they are here, taking care of my boys and my business. It is incredible. It really is. They had a benefit auction for us one time when I was in the hospital. And those times too, the boys get spoiled rotten by the whole community.

Inadequate Insurance

All participants had insurance. Five stated that insurance was a concern for them. Four commented it was expensive, had high deductibles, or was inadequate. One participant stated,

> Yes, we have health insurance. It is very expensive and we pay it all ourselves. That has been a real burden. And a lot of people up here do not have health insurance, at all. I don't know if any business has health insurance and benefits, or even provides part of it. So that is a very difficult thing here. When you don't make a lot of money and the health insurance keeps going up all the time. A major part of our income goes to health insurance. That is a real burden.

Another longtime resident of the community stated she had health insurance, "but it doesn't leave me much to live on. I live on about $250 a month after that." Two retired participants brought medical insurance with them from their jobs. One stated, "We are different than a lot of people here in the community in that we brought our insurance here with us. A lot of people here do not have insurance, or do not have adequate insurance."

All participants stated their health insurance coverage did not affect how they accessed care. When I asked a longtime member of the community if her health insurance affected how she sought care, she stated,

> No, I don't think so. I know it does for a lot of people here, if they don't have health insurance, which a lot of them don't, I think it affects them as a choice of going to the doctor, or the hospital, or not seeking care.

Participants estimated that one-half to three-quarters of the members of the Montana City community did not have insurance.

DISCUSSION

The themes that emerged provided valuable information for comparison to previously identified concepts in the rural nursing literature. The primary characteristics of self-reliance included "self-reliance as learned, decisional choice, and independence" (Chafey et al., 1998, p. 162). Self-reliance as learned was demonstrated by several participants and was clearly more evident in those who had lived in the community for a long period of time. The individuals who had more recently moved into the community considered themselves self-reliant, stating that they try to take care of things themselves first. They also acknowledged that those who had grown up in the community or had lived there a long time did more for themselves than they did.

Self-reliance as a decisional choice was not as clear in the data from the Montana City participants. Participants implied they made many choices on a daily basis, but never indicated that was of great importance to them. They all mentioned a sense of security provided by knowing a retired doctor lived in the community who was willing to provide information as they engaged in the decision-making process.

Hardiness is another theme that emerged. As previously discussed, the data from Montana City participants showed evidence of adaptability, positive attitude, and endurance, characteristics of hardiness (Wirtz et al., 1998). All participants expressed in some manner that one must "adjust to what life had to offer" (p. 262). Two long-time residents demonstrated learned experience, an additional characteristic of hardiness, by making statements such as "the way it had always been" or "that's all we have ever known." Overall, the Montana City residents demonstrated hardiness congruent with hardiness previously described in the rural nursing literature.

Four of the themes I identified were new themes or variations of existing themes. Conscientious consumer was a theme that I identified in the Montana City data, and it appeared to be similar to concepts previously discussed in the nursing literature. Distance played a role in where the Montana City participants accessed care for a particular injury or illness. Mileage, time, and perception are attributes of distance (Henson, Sadler, & Walton, 1998). Mileage and time are congruent with the attributes of conscientious consumer as the participants weighed these two factors when determining where to seek care for a particular health problem. For the Montana City participants, weather was a key factor that the conscientious consumers had to consider in their decision-making process.

The theme of conscientious consumer also paralleled health resources concepts (Ballantyne, 1998). Ballantyne stated, "If the client is motivated to seek health care beyond the immediate boundaries of the community, factors such as transportation, distance, inclement weather, and finances become important issues" (p. 182).

Informed risk was a new theme or perhaps a variation of an existing theme. Informed risk was not specifically found in the nursing literature. Informed risk means that individuals are aware of the risks or consequences of their decisions, but desire for quality of life outweighs the risks presented. The participants acknowledged that there may be some risks in living where they did, but they also were weighing their options when making these decisions.

Community support has been discussed in the nursing literature in a variety of ways. The concept of community support may be related to previously presented concepts, e.g., informal networks (Grossman & McNerney, 1998) and familiarity (McNeely & Shreffler, 1998). Community support was clearly demonstrated by "rallying," "benefit auctions," and "helping take care of my business and my kids."

Inadequate insurance had an impact on a number of participants. Inadequate insurance was not a concept in itself, but I identified it as a potential modifying factor for health care usage in the community.

Although I did not identify a concept that paralleled inadequate insurance in the nursing literature, it is an issue related to resource accessibility and health care access that warrants further investigation.

IMPLICATIONS FOR NURSING PRACTICE

Informed risk affects the way health care practitioners relate to their clients. It is important that the practitioner confirm that it is truly informed risk and that individuals are able to make informed decisions. For example, it was important for the individual with pulmonary hypertension to understand the risk of being further than 20 minutes away from an appropriate medical facility and the risk she was taking with the prostacyclin infusion. It was also important for her to understand physiologically the impact altitude may have on the progression of her disease. Once practitioners are clear that their client is truly informed, then it is important to respect their decisions. Furthermore, once the decision has been made by the individual to remain in a particular environment or situation, the practitioner should provide the appropriate information and education, teach the client and family necessary skills, and assist them in identifying available resources. Even if a practitioner disagrees with a client's informed decision, the individual's choice should be respected.

Health care practitioners should be aware of modifying factors such as time and distance that affect access to care and the health care decision-making process of conscientious consumers. The participant who was 8 months pregnant at the time of the interview provides an example.

> When they [practitioners in general] tell you "well leave your house when your contractions are five minutes part," well that could make for a child born in Gateway. They [rural doctors in Littlewood] do realize that even if you are racing it is a good two-hour drive and at night you cannot go that fast.

In this example, inaccurate perceptions on the part of providers caring for pregnant clients may result in babies being born in the back seat of an automobile in the middle of nowhere. Therefore, it is imperative for providers to understand conscientious consumers when making decisions relative to health care. Discussing what-if scenarios with rural clients, particularly in relation to distance, time, and weather, will help them be the best and wisest conscientious consumers.

Self-reliance and hardiness both have an impact on when, why, and how rural individuals will seek care. As with informed risk, health care providers should work with individuals in an attempt to provide the necessary information, skills, and available resources, although allowing persons to be self-reliant.

Understanding the presence or lack of community support for clients in rural communities gives the practitioner insight into the availability of resources. For example, individuals who have been hospitalized and want to return home rather than stay on a transitional care unit may be able to do so with strong community support.

Inadequate insurance affected participants' use of health care. High deductibles, out-of-pocket expenses, distance, and availability of services also influenced health care decision making for these isolated rural residents. The combination of these issues warrants thorough investigation to fully understand health care access.

As indicated by Long and Weinert (1989), "continued research can provide a more solid base for the nursing theory that is required to guide practice and the delivery of health care to rural populations" (p. 126). Thus, previously identified concepts as well as newly emerging concepts or themes warrant further investigation to help health care practitioners provide the highest quality care to rural individuals.

NOTE

1. The names of all communities in this chapter were changed to maintain anonymity of participants.

REFERENCES

Ballantyne, J. (1998). Health resources and the rural client. In H. J. Lee (Ed.), *Conceptual basis for rural nursing* (pp. 178–188). New York, NY: Springer Publishing.

Chafey, K., Sullivan, T., & Shannon, A. (1998). Self-reliance: Characterization of their own autonomy by elderly rural women. In H. J. Lee (Ed.), *Conceptual basis for rural nursing* (pp. 156–177). New York, NY: Springer Publishing.

Fahlberg, L. (1983). *Nine months of winter*. Montana City: Pilot Peak.

Glidden, R. (1982). *Exploring the Montana high country: History of the Montana City area* (2nd ed.). Montana City: Ralph Glidden.

Grossman, L. L., & McNerney, S. (1998). Informal networks. In H. J. Lee (Ed.), *Conceptual basis for rural nursing* (pp. 200–208). New York, NY: Springer Publishing.

Henson, D., Sadler, T., & Walton, S. (1998). Distance. In H. J. Lee (Ed.), *Conceptual basis for rural nursing* (pp. 51–60). New York, NY: Springer Publishing.

Koehler, V. (1998). The substantive theory of protecting independence. In H. J. Lee (Ed.), *Conceptual basis for rural nursing* (pp. 236–256). New York, NY: Springer Publishing.

Long, K. A., & Weinert, C. (1989). Rural nursing: Developing the theory base. *Scholarly Inquiry for Nursing Practice: An International Journal, 3*, 113–127.

McNeely, A. G., & Shreffier, M. J. (1998). Familiarity. In H. J. Lee (Ed.), *Conceptual basis for rural nursing* (pp. 89–101). New York, NY: Springer Publishing.

National Geographic Road Atlas. (2000). *Canada*. MapQuest.com, Inc.

Rossman, G. B., & Rallis, S. F. (1998). *Learning in the field: An introduction to qualitative research*. Thousand Oaks, CA: Sage.

Wirtz, E. F., Lee, H. J., & Running, A. (1998). The lived experience of hardiness in rural men and women. In H. J. Lee (Ed.), *Conceptual basis for rural nursing* (pp. 257–274). New York, NY: Springer Publishing.

Chapter 6

ASSESSING RESILIENCE IN OLDER FRONTIER WOMEN

Gail M. Wagnild and Linda M. Torma

How Do We Help Aging adults recognize and perhaps strengthen their resilience? While there is much written that describes resilience and resilient individuals, there is less information on how one might evaluate individual resilience. Wagnild and Collins (2009) presented a framework for assessing resilience that included the Resilience Scale™ (Wagnild & Young, 1993) and open-ended questions that provide individuals with opportunities to reflect on and perhaps rediscover their resilience. This strength-based approach encourages individuals to focus on their capabilities and is an important step in helping individuals develop a personal strategy to strengthen resilience. Resilience may facilitate adaptation to changes and challenges that often accompany aging, and this adaptation perhaps will lead to less depression and anxiety, more effective coping, and a more satisfying life. In this chapter, we report on a preliminary study applying this assessment approach with 25 older women.

REVIEW OF LITERATURE

Resilience is frequently defined as the ability to adapt or "bounce back" following adversity; it connotes inner strength, competence, optimism, flexibility, and the ability to cope effectively when faced with life's challenges (Hardy, Concato, & Gill, 2004; Wagnild & Young, 1990). Several studies have reported associations between resilience and positive characteristics among aging adults, including forgiveness (Broyles, 2005), morale (March, 2004; Wagnild & Young, 1993), purpose in life, sense of coherence, self-transcendence (Nygren et al., 2005), and self-efficacy (Caltabiano & Caltabiano, 2006). Resilience has also been inversely associated with depression (Torma, 2010; Wagnild & Young, 1993; Wagnild, 2009a, 2012), perceived stress (March, 2005), anxiety (Humphreys, 2003), and fibromyalgia (FM) impact (Torma, 2010).

Successful or healthy aging has often been defined as physical and mental health that continues into old age, as well as continued social involvement and meaningful activities (Hartman-Stein & Potkanowicz, 2003; Rowe & Kahn, 1997, 1998; Ruuskanen & Ruoppila, 1995; Unger, Johnson, & Marks, 1997). Recently, Harris (2008) has challenged this definition and suggested that rather than striving for successful aging, we should be striving for resilience and resilient responses to life's inevitable difficulties. Aging is a dynamic process, often accompanied by significant adversity, due to the cumulative and synergistic effects of lifestyle behaviors, disease, genetics, and age-related changes (Miller, 2008). The biomedical definition of health as absence of disease inadequately describes the experience of health in persons 65 years of age and older—nearly 90% of Medicare beneficiaries have at least one chronic condition (Hoffman, Rice, & Sung, 1996), and 60% have two or more (Wolff, Starfield, & Anderson, 2002). A person's subjective assessment of his/her ability to function psychologically and physically despite this adversity is a much more accurate measure of health in this population (Bryant, Beck, & Fairclough, 2000; Bryant, Corbett, & Kutner, 2001; Wilson & Cleary, 1995).

Aging adults with health problems cannot realistically regain or maintain robust health and independent functioning often associated with a more typical definition of successful aging (Holstein & Minkler, 2003). Many aging adults can strengthen their resilience, however, leading to a meaningful, satisfying, and successful old age, despite declines in health.

BACKGROUND

The percentage of persons over 65 years of age is expected to grow to an unprecedented 19.6% of the United States population by 2030 (Centers for Disease Control and Prevention [CDC], 2003). Currently, older adults constitute approximately 12.2% of the population. In states with substantial frontier populations (six or fewer persons per square mile), the percentage of elders is higher. There are 10 U.S. states in which 30% to 75% of the land area is considered frontier. The proportion of elders in these frontier communities is growing and is projected to double by 2025 (U.S. Census Bureau, 2000). Approximately 15% of the frontier population is 65 years and older; in the three communities reported in this study, 18% to 25% are 65 years and older (Montana County Profiles, 2004).

The majority of elders who survive into old age are women. Approximately 57% of persons 65 years and older are women, and of those 85 and older, 69% are women. With aging comes a higher incidence of chronic illness and a greater need for health care (Wolff et al., 2002). Increasing resilience may help older adults adapt to changes and challenges associated with aging.

Resilience

Resilience is the ability to adapt to, learn, and grow stronger from challenges and adversity, leading to lives that are rich, rewarding, and meaningful. Wagnild and Young (1990) identified five interrelated characteristics that constitute resilience and thus enable an individual to adapt and age in a meaningful and satisfying way. These characteristics are: (1) perseverance—the act of persistence despite adversity or discouragement; (2) equanimity—a balanced perspective of life viewed as "sitting loose" and accepting life as it comes; (3) meaningfulness—recognition of life purpose and a reason for which to live; (4) self-reliance—belief in one's strengths and capabilities that often comes from experience and wisdom; (5) existential aloneness—the realization that each life is unique and that while some experiences can be shared, others must be faced alone. Existential aloneness conveys not only a sense of uniqueness but perhaps freedom as well.

The process of strengthening resilience in adulthood consists of challenge, support, and success. When confronted with adversity or challenge, a woman who finds a way to meet the challenge and adapt successfully will likely increase her resilience. When she meets subsequent challenges, self-confidence and new problem-solving skills will enable her to adapt successfully again, thus increasing resilience. The process of developing resilience may start early in life with challenges that are successfully met, leading to a greater repertoire of effective problem-solving approaches (Rutter, 1985).

According to Richardson (2002), when individuals are confronted by either planned or unplanned life events, they can choose to reintegrate resiliently, resulting in growth, self-knowledge, and understanding. This leads to an increase in resilience. They can also choose to return to homeostasis, referred to as the "comfort zone." Finally they can choose to reintegrate with loss, meaning that they may resort to destructive behaviors and substance abuse as a response to life's challenges.

Resilience and Healthy Aging

Resilient women are able to adapt successfully to stress and adversity (Hardy et al., 2004; Wagnild & Young, 1990). Resilience is frequently associated with optimism, flexibility, inner strength, and effective coping. According to Rutter (1985), resilience is not a fixed personality trait. Rather resilience changes as life's demands and circumstances change.

Researchers have focused on resilience and aging only in the last 25 to 30 years with most early research on resilience focusing on children (Garmezy, 1993; Rutter, 1985, 1987, 1993; Werner, 1984; 1992). Wagnild and Young (1990) published one of the first studies on resilience among older women. Their study emphasized strengths and capabilities rather than decline, decrepitude, and disability prevalent in literature up until that time.

The relationship between resilience and healthy aging has been supported in several studies. For instance, resilience is inversely associated with depression (Humphreys, 2003; Wagnild & Young, 1993; Wagnild, 2009a, 2009b, 2012), anxiety (Humphreys, 2003), and perceived stress (March, 2004) and directly related to purpose in life, sense of coherence, self-transcendence, mental health (Nygren et al., 2005; Wells, 2010), morale (March, 2004; Wagnild & Young, 1993), and forgiveness (Broyles, 2005). In several studies with women, resilience is associated with self-reported health status and health-promoting lifestyle practices (Wagnild, 2009a, 2009b; Wells, 2010). In a recent report on 467 urban older women whose average age was 72.3 years (standard deviation [SD] = 7.9), those who were more resilient were significantly more likely to report healthier lifestyles including diet, exercise, stress management, interpersonal support, health responsibility, and self-actualization. More resilient women also reported better overall health and less depression (Wagnild, 2012). This finding was also reported in a recent study that examined resilience as a moderator of the relationship between pain and physical function in older persons who had been living with fibromyalgia (FM) for an average of 23 years ($N = 224$, average age = 62 years). Levels of resilience were moderately high in this sample despite moderately high levels of pain and functional limitations. Resilience was also positively correlated with age, income, and education, and negatively correlated with depressive symptoms, overall FM impact, and FM pain (Torma, 2010). Resilience did not moderate the effect of pain on physical function as hypothesized, but was instead an independent predictor of physical function in this sample. These findings highlight the important role resilience plays in healthy aging.

RESEARCH METHOD

Design

A descriptive exploratory research design was used for this study. A valid and reliable instrument was used to measure resilience, and open-ended questions specific to the five characteristics of resilience were asked of each participant (Morse, 1991). In addition, each participant was asked about specific challenges she was facing and how she was meeting these challenges. Open-ended questions complemented quantitative measures obtained using the Resilience Scale (RS) (Wagnild & Young, 1993).

Sample

The purposive sample comprised 25 older women who were living independently in their own homes in frontier communities. Inclusion criteria were: being 65 years of age or older; being able to read, speak, and write English; and having no known history of cognitive impairment.

Procedures

The study was conducted with the approval of the Institutional Review Board at Montana State University. The researchers invited women to participate who were at Senior Centers, through the Area Agency on Aging, and using a snowball or networking sampling method. The study was explained to women who were interested in participating. Each woman was asked for her consent to participate and to have the assessment audiotaped. The average assessment took 1 hour, with a range of 45 minutes to 2 hours. All were conducted in the women's homes.

Instruments

The RS measured the degree of individual resilience (Wagnild & Young, 1993). The scale covers two factors: personal competence and acceptance of self and life. The RS has been positively correlated with optimism, stress management, self-esteem, and life satisfaction and negatively with depression and helplessness. Items are scored on a 7-point scale from $1 =$ disagree to $7 =$ agree. Two sub-scales derived from factor analysis measure acceptance of self and life (8 items) and personal competence (17 items). Possible scores range from 25 to 175, with higher scores reflecting higher resilience. Scores of 146 to 175 are considered moderate to high, scores from 121 to 145 fall within the mid-range, and scores 120 and lower are at the low end of the scale. Cronbach's alpha reliability for the RS in the current study was .93.

The health-promoting lifestyle profile (HPLP) (Walker, Sechrist, & Pender, 1987) was used to measure health-promoting lifestyles. The HPLP is a 48-item 4-point summated rating scale with "never" coded as 1, "infrequently" coded as 2, "frequently" coded as 3, and "routinely" coded as 4. The HPLP investigates the following six sub-scales, derived through item analysis: (1) self-actualization, (2) health responsibility, (3) exercise, (4) nutrition, (5) interpersonal support, and (6) stress management. Duffy (1993) reported a Cronbach's alpha internal consistency reliability of .92 for the 48-item HPLP with reliability of sub-scales ranging from .65 to .85. Cronbach's alpha reliability measures for the HPLP in the current study were $.91 =$ total HPLP; $.91 =$ self-actualization; $.87 =$ health responsibility; $.65 =$ exercise; $.71 =$ nutrition; $.80 =$ interpersonal support; and $.74 =$ stress management. These scores are comparable to those reported in previous studies.

Self-reported health status was measured by asking respondents to rate their current health on a 5-point scale as compared to others their age (poor, fair, good, very good, and excellent). This self-report method has been used extensively, corresponds to objective health indicators, and is an acceptable indicator of physical health status (Idler & Benyamini, 1997).

FINDINGS

Demographic Profile

The participants were 25 Caucasian women whose ages ranged from 66 to 85 years (mean age = 75.7 years). Of these, 11 participants were married and living with their spouses and 12 women were widowed; one was divorced and one had never married. Only one participant had fewer than 12 years of education, 11 had completed high school, and 13 had education beyond high school. Nine women reported an annual income of less than $25,000 and eight did not report their income level.

The mean length of time that participants had lived in their community was 45.6 years and ranged from 6 to 73 years. In all, 21 participants reported that they had lived in their communities 25 years or more. Overall, 15 participants resided in a small town, with the remaining 10 participants residing within 2 to 20 miles of the nearest small town. In all, 23 rated their health as good to excellent, with only two reporting their health as fair. All participants reported that they were able to perform activities of daily living without assistance with the exception of one participant who experienced some episodes of urinary incontinence. Most performed instrumental activities of daily living without assistance, with the exception of one participant who needed assistance with housework.

RS and HPLP Scores

The average RS score was 147.1, which is similar to scores obtained on the RS in prior studies with healthy samples of middle-aged and older adults (Broyles, 2005; March, 2004; Nygren et al., 2005; Wagnild, 2003, 2012; Wagnild & Young, 1993) and indicated a moderate-to-high level of resilience. There were nonsignificant relationships between the RS and age, education, and income. The correlation between RS and self-reported health was .53 ($p < .02$).

The average score on the HPLP was 142.2. The maximum score possible on the HPLP is 192, suggesting moderate–to-high scores within this sample. There were nonsignificant relationships between the HPLP and age, education, years lived in the community, and income. There were significant relationships between the HPLP and self-reported health status ($r = .47, p < .04$). The RS and HPLP were related to each other (.52, $p < .03$).

Interview Results Within the Resilience Model

Resilience is the ability to adapt successfully to adversity and challenge. Successful adaptation leads to personal growth and self-confidence, which in turn strengthens resilience. According to the model, as resilience develops and strengthens, the probability of adapting successfully to new challenges increases also.

Each participant was asked to describe challenges in her life and responses she used to respond to difficult events. Responses were organized within five essential characteristics of resilience: Perseverance, Meaningfulness, Self-Reliance, Equanimity, and Existential Aloneness. Further, each participant was asked to describe how she responded to both minor and major life challenges and the effects of childhood on later adaptation to adversity.

Perseverance: The Ability to Keep Going Despite Setbacks

Every participant reported that she had been confronted with many challenges; every woman described that meeting challenges required that she put one foot in front of the other and keep going. One woman lost her husband of 45 years to cancer after caring for him throughout his 5-year illness. She admitted that for at least a year after his death, she did not even bother to vacuum or dust because "what was the point?" Gradually she adapted to the loss but it was not easy. She said, "I just made myself make my bed one day, make it the next, and kept on going."

Another participant living with cancer and struggling with the loss of loved ones said, "My sister was murdered two years ago and I've lost two husbands. And that is the hardest. Losing somebody. But my children have seen me get going again. I always get going again. I've been told I have grit!"

A third participant described a friend who was not resilient and aging poorly and said that she stayed in bed with depression most days. She said, "You have to fight all of your life not to be depressed. Sure I could find a lot to get blue about, too. Because life is kind of depressing. Hard."

Meaningfulness: A Sense of Purpose in Life

The study participants reported that staying involved in life, having a sense of community maintaining interests, and developing new ones were essential to a healthy old age. Many believed that disengaging from the usual activities of life led to a premature death.

One woman said,

> You have to do something! My husband said that ranchers retired to town and in three years they walk themselves to death. They're used to getting up in the morning even if they don't feel good because they have animals to take care of. I think we all have to get up. I think it makes you live longer.

According to the participants, having a purpose in life kept them mentally challenged and permitted them an opportunity to contribute to the well-being of the communities in which they lived. The majority of the women in the study were extensively involved in volunteer work in their communities, which was an important source of productivity for the women and gave them a sense of accomplishment. Many of them had lived in their communities for several decades and were well known.

Self-Reliance: Depending on One's Own Resources, Judgment, and Capabilities

Each woman discussed the process of becoming self-sufficient, or "managing on her own and doing without." There are few if any health care resources in many frontier communities, and these women described how they managed nonetheless. In relation to exercising to stay fit, one woman described her resourcefulness while snowbound.

> There's many a trip I've made around the room here. When the walls get to closing in on me, I just make figure eights and walk in my own home. And you can sit in your chair and move your arms and your legs if you have to. There's a lot of things you can make up as you go just to keep moving.

Another woman described how she drove on 1200 miles of icy roads and frequent blizzard conditions to take her husband to a regional health care center for specialized care. She said,

> It was really scary. I thought my husband might die any moment; he was in a lot of pain. And I also knew that we could slide off a mountain pass and never be found. I just kept saying, "one more mile; just one more mile."

But she succeeded and her journey strengthened her self-reliance.

A 76-year-old woman whose husband was terminally ill had to learn to manage their finances for the first time even though her spouse had done so for more than 50 years. She successfully met the challenge.

Equanimity: A Balanced Perspective of Life

Most of the participants were from farming and ranching communities and they had first-hand experience with adversities that many who live in more urban communities do not experience. Because they lived "off the land," drought, hailstorms, early and late frost, poor cattle/grain prices, and the daily uncertainties of farming and ranching led to an attitude of "sitting loose" and "taking what comes." When a crop failed, they learned to start planning for the next season.

Each of the participants reported that a positive attitude was a vital component of health. Many felt that being optimistic, not worrying, focusing on the good parts of life, and having a zest for living were essential to good health. One woman advised, "You don't brood on yourself. You should have a good attitude towards life. Be cheerful. Don't be down in the dumps all the time. Have something to look forward to."

Several participants reported believing that worrying, complaining, and being negative would lead to illness. When asked how they recognized others who were not aging in a healthy way, the most frequent response concerned attitude and outlook on life. One woman expressed it this way:

> You can tell someone is aging well by engaging in a conversation with them. They are outgoing, not gripers and complainers, they are doers. It's more than physical. They may look the age but mentally they are in their 50s.

Another participant, describing someone who responded to life's uncertainties in a positive way said,

> Their attitude. They'd have a sense of humor; they'd have a smile on their face. They'd have themselves taken care of, you know, not be sloppy, and I guess that's about it. They get out and in amongst people. Do things.

Existential Aloneness: Recognition of One's Unique Path and the Acceptance of One's Life

The women in this study lived in frontier communities, often far from town and even from neighbors. Many were children of early pioneers and homesteaders. Yet they did not complain of loneliness.

One woman had been widowed twice. She lived alone. During our interview together, she looked around her home and described changes she had made to the house. She said, "I've been living the way everyone else wanted me to live and I've finally reached a point where I'm going to do what works for me." Accordingly, her bedroom was open to the living room and she had a walk-in pantry as big as most kitchens because she liked "putting up food." She had gotten rid of her guest room because she didn't want houseguests anymore.

Another woman expressed her aloneness this way: "I don't mind being alone. I have so much to do. And I like being able to do exactly what I want, when I want, how I want. No one tells me what to do."

Success and Support

The women's responses to adversity described many creative and successful approaches to relatively minor challenges (e.g., exercising) and to major challenges (e.g., dealing with spouse's terminal illness). These women were also asked about support in their lives that helped them deal with difficulties. While all identified close family members and friends, their sense of community was a source of strength and meaning to each of them as well. Because most had lived in their communities for several decades, they expressed a feeling of connection and affection for their communities. These older women also stated that they continued to contribute to their communities and were recognized by others as a source of valuable information, guidance, and wisdom.

Contribution of Early Life to Resilience

When participants were asked to talk about their childhood and how it influenced their current life in terms of health and resilience, each had much to say. These women saw a good start in life as laying the foundation for a lifestyle that helped them to stay resilient throughout their lives. Many reported the importance of having childhood chores and work, which gave them a reason to get up in the morning. Chores also led to self-reliance and "stick-to-itiveness."

One participant said,

> Ranch kids have a different outlook on life than the kids that are raised on the asphalt. I mean they have their animals and they have to take care of them. And if you have something in a pen, you gotta feed 'em. When you're a kid, you don't always feel like getting up early in the morning but you just have to keep doing it or the livestock will die. And kids in town, well I say that they don't have that close association with any other living thing. Maybe they got a dog or a cat or a lizard or something, which is good for them, but they don't have that responsibility that kids do that are raised on a ranch.

Each discussed the simplicity of her early life. Most had been raised with very little in terms of material possessions and had learned to be content in their relatively humble circumstances. As farm and ranch kids, they had quickly learned that there were lean and fat years and you "take what comes." This most certainly influenced their equanimity and self-determination to not give up.

Comparison of Quantitative and Qualitative Data

As part of the data analysis, each study participant's individual interview data were compared to her quantitative data; there was consistency between the women's perceptions of health and resilience as described in the interview data and the way they rated themselves on the instruments. A resilient woman continues despite hardship and bounces back from adversity; resilence was a characteristic the participants exemplified. As expected, scores obtained on the RS were moderately high. One would also expect that persons aging well, as these women described themselves, would participate in health-promoting behaviors. Again, scores on the HPLP were moderately high, supporting reports of self-responsibility for health in this sample. Every woman in her interview knew about diet, exercise, stress management, and the need for adequate amounts of sleep. Each had learned from television, reading, and conversations with family and friends. These women were not highly educated and did not have access to specialized health care and information. Even so, they were motivated to obtain information that promoted healthy aging.

CONCLUSION AND IMPLICATIONS

Role Models for Resilient Aging

The elderly frontier women in this study were resilient and healthy, as indicated by their reported independence, moderate-to-high scores in resilience, self-reported health, and health-promoting behaviors. Consistent with Richardson's (2002) position that individuals choose to reintegrate resiliently, return to homeostasis, or reintegrate with loss, these women provided examples within each of the five characteristics of resilience that demonstrated their choices to grow in resilience. They told us that individuals must have a reason to get up in the morning (purposeful life), learn to take what comes (equanimity), never quit trying (perseverance), get comfortable with being alone (existential aloneness), and learn to do what needs to be done (self-reliance). Each woman in this study described the importance of community involvement, identified as a protective factor in older adults' psychological well-being by Greenfield and Marks (2004). These findings are similar to those in a qualitative study by Kinsel (2005), who identified social connectedness and a head-on approach to challenge as factors contributing to resilience.

The women in this study provided many examples of resilient behaviors. Like everyone, they suffered setbacks and losses but they got up again and kept going. More than once did we hear the following expression from these ranching and farming women: "When you fall off a horse, you just get back on again." These women knew literally that falling off a horse and getting back on meant not only being able to continue your journey, but also overcoming the fear of getting back on a horse that has thrown you. Ranchers and farmers know that a horse that throws you once may try to throw you again, and this can be intimidating. Dusting yourself off, gathering the reins and stepping into the stirrup again means facing fear head-on. Achieving success increases resilience.

Future Research and Practice

Research is needed that will develop and test interventions to strengthen resilience among middle-aged and older women. There are many studies that describe the importance of having resilience, but fewer studies describe how to strengthen resilience within this population. Using the resilience model as a guide, a resilience-centered approach would motivate and engage women by focusing on strengths and building personal capacity. This would include working with women to identify what is meaningful in their lives, especially in the midst of loss, illness, and other challenges and encouraging them to give of themselves to others. It means providing support to women who are facing difficulties to develop their self-reliance and encouraging perseverance one step at a time. A resilience-centered intervention would include exploring aloneness or "coming home to yourself" (Northrup, 2006). And finally, strengthening resilience would work toward achieving balance in life and learning to "sit loose" in the saddle of life.

Do early childhood experiences have an effect on later resilience? For instance, Werner, in her 30-year longitudinal study of 698 infants born in 1955, identified protective factors that strengthened resilience that included strong bonds with adults and involvement in a community group such as a church (1992). The women in this study identified childhood factors they believed had an effect on current resilience such as responsibility resulting in self-reliance and the uncertainty of farming/ranching leading to equanimity and perseverance. They identified their parents as role models and described their involvement in their communities even as children. Their responses and childhood memories were consistent with observations made by Garmezy (1993), Rutter (1985), and Werner (1984) that when children experience a nurturing environment, are given responsibility, experience self-efficacy, and develop a positive outlook in addition to other qualities, they grow into resilient adults.

It is important for health care providers to assess risk along with strengths in order to promote health and physical function in older adults. This research was designed to inform the development of methods to assess resilience in older frontier women and to plan interventions designed to strengthen this important protective factor. Increasing resilience will reduce the risk of disability and will promote health and quality of life for a growing number of older adults living in rural and frontier settings.

ACKNOWLEDGMENTS

This research was funded by a grant from Friends Research Institute, Inc, Baltimore, MD, and a block grant from Montana State University College of Nursing, Bozeman, MT. We would like to thank Vonna Koehler, RN, PhD, ARNP, for help in conducting the interviews.

REFERENCES

Broyles, L. C. (2005). *Resilience: Its Relationships to Forgiveness in Older Adults.* Unpublished doctoral dissertation, University of Tennessee, Knoxville.

Bryant, L. L., Beck, A., & Fairclough, D. L. (2000). Factors that contribute to positive perceived health in an older population. *Journal of Aging & Health, 12*(2), 169–192.

Bryant, L. L., Corbett, K. K., & Kutner, J. S. (2001). In their own words: A model of healthy aging [comment]. *Social Science & Medicine, 53*(7), 927–941.

Caltabiano, M. L., & Caltabiano, N. J. (2006). *Resilience and health outcomes in the elderly.* Proceedings of the 39th Annual Conference of the Australian Association of Gerontology., November 22–24, 2006. Sydney, NSW, Australia. Available at: http://eprints.jcu.edu.au/4271/

Centers for Disease Control and Prevention. (2003). Trends in aging: United States and worldwide. *MMWR - Morbidity & Mortality Weekly Report, 52*(6), 101–106.

Duffy, M. E. (1993). Determinants of health-promoting lifestyles in older persons. *Image: Journal of Nursing Scholarship, 25*(1), 23–28.

Garmezy, N. (1993). Children in poverty: Resilience despite risk. *Psychiatry, 56*(1), 127–136.

Greenfield, E. A., & Marks, N. F. (2004). Formal volunteering as a protective factor for older adults' psychological well-being. *The Journals of Gerontology. Series B, Psychological Sciences and Social Sciences, 59*(5), S258–S264.

Hardy, S. E., Concato, J., & Gill, T. M. (2004). Resilience of community-dwelling older persons. *Journal of the American Geriatrics Society, 52*(2), 257–262.

Harris, P. B. (2008). Another wrinkle in the debate about successful aging: The undervalued concept of resilience and the lived experience of dementia. *International Journal of Aging & Human Development, 67*(1), 43–61.

Hartman-Stein, P. E., & Potkanowicz, E. S. (2003). Behavioral determinants of healthy aging: Good news for the Baby Boomer generation. *Online Journal on Issues in Nursing, 8*(2), 6.

Hoffman, C., Rice, D., & Sung, H. Y. (1996). Persons with chronic conditions. Their prevalence and costs. *Journal of the American Medical Association, 276*(18), 1473–1479.

Holstein, M. B., & Minkler, M. (2003). Self, society, and the "new gerontology" *The Gerontologist, 43*(6), 787–796.

Humphreys, J. (2003). Research in sheltered battered women. *Issues in Mental Health Nursing, 24,* 137–152.

Idler, E. L., & Benyamini, Y. (1997). Self-rated health and mortality: A review of twenty-seven community studies. *Journal of Health and Social Behavior, 38*(1), 21–37.

Kinsel, B. (2005). Resilience as adaptation in older women. *Journal of Women and Aging, 17*(3), 23–39.

March, M. (2004). *Well being of older Australians: The interplay of life adversity and resilience in late life development.* Unpublished doctoral dissertation, Charles Sturt University, Australia.

Miller, C. A. (2008). *Nursing wellness in older adults* (5th ed.). Philadelphia, PA: Lippincott.

Montana County Health Profiles (2004). Retrieved May 25, 2012, from http://www.dphs.mt.gov/PHSD/health-profiles/health-profiles-2004.shtml.

Morse, J. M. (1991). Approaches to qualitative–quantitative methodological triangulation. *Nursing Research, 40*(1), 120–123.

Northrup, C. (2006). *The wisdom of menopause.* New York, NY: Bantam Dell.

Nygren, B., Aléx, L., Jonsén, E., Gustafson, Y., Norberg, A., & Lundman, B. (2005). Sense of coherence, purpose in life and self-transcendence in relation to perceived physical and mental health among the oldest old. *Aging and Mental Health, 9*(4), 354–362.

Richardson, G. E. (2002). The metatheory of resilience and resiliency. *Journal of Clinical Psychology, 58*(3), 307–321.

Rowe, J. W., & Kahn, R. L. (1997). Successful aging. *The Gerontologist, 37*(4), 433–440.

Rowe, J. W., & Kahn, R. L. (1998). *Successful aging.* New York, NY: Random House.

Rutter, M. (1985). Resilience in the face of adversity: Protective factors and resistance to psychiatric disorder. *British Journal of Psychiatry, 147,* 598–611.

Rutter, M. (1987). Psychosocial resilience and protective mechanisms. *American Journal of Orthopsychiatry, 57*(3), 316–331.

Rutter, M. (1993). Resilience: Some conceptual considerations. *Journal of Adolescent Health, 14*(8), 626–631, 690–696.

Ruuskanen, J. M., & Ruoppila, I. (1995). Physical activity and psychological well-being among people aged 65 to 84 years. *Age and Ageing, 24*(4), 292–296.

Torma, L. M. (2010). *Fibromyalgia pain and physical function: The influence of resilience.* Doctoral dissertation, Oregon Health & Science University. Portland, OR. Available at: http://drl.ohsu.edu/cdm/ref/collection/etd/id/809

Unger, J. B., Johnson, C. A., & Marks, G. (1997). Functional decline in the elderly: Evidence for direct and stress-buffering protective effects of social interactions and physical activity. *Annals of Behavioral Medicine, 19*(2), 152–160.

U.S. Census Bureau. Index of census 2000/states. Retrieved January 7, 2008, from http://www.census.gov/census2000/states.

Wagnild, G. (2003). Resilience and successful aging: Comparison among low and high income older adults. *Journal of Gerontological Nursing, 29*(12), 42–49.

Wagnild, G. (2009a). A review of the resilience scale. *Journal of Nursing Measurement, 17*(2), 105–113.

Wagnild, G. (2009b). *The resilience scale user's guide for the US English version of the resilience scale and the 14-item resilience scale (RS-14)*. Worden, MT: The Resilience Center.

Wagnild, G. (2012). [Resilience and health-promoting behaviors among healthy middle-aged and older adults]. Unpublished data.

Wagnild, G. M., & Collins, J. A. (2009). Assessing resilience. *Journal of Psychosocial Nursing and Mental Health Services, 47*(12), 28–33.

Wagnild, G., & Young, H. (1990). Resilience among older women. *Image: Journal of Nursing Scholarship, 22*, 252–255.

Wagnild, G. M., & Young, H. M. (1993). Development and psychometric evaluation of the resilience scale. *Journal of Nursing Measurement, 1*(2), 165–178.

Walker, S. N., Sechrist, K. R., & Pender, N. J. (1987). The health-promoting lifestyle profile: Development and psychometric characteristics. *Nursing Research, 36*(2), 76–81.

Wells, M. (2010). Resilience in older adults living in rural, suburban, and urban areas. *Online Journal of Rural Nursing & Health Care*, May 25, 2012. Available at: http://findarticles.com/p/articles/mi_m0555/is_2_10/ai_n56708887/

Werner, E. E. (1984). Resilient children. *Young Child, 40*, 68–72.

Werner, E. E. (1992). The children of Kauai: Resiliency and recovery in adolescence and adulthood. *Journal of Adolescent Health, 13*, 262–268.

Wilson, I. B., & Cleary, P. D. (1995). Linking clinical variables with health-related quality of life. *Journal of the American Medical Association, 273*(1), 59–65.

Wolff, J. L., Starfield, B., & Anderson, G. (2002). Prevalence, expenditures, and complications of multiple chronic conditions in the elderly. *Archives of Internal Medicine, 162*(20), 2269–2276.

Chapter 7

RURAL AND REMOTE WOMEN AND RESILIENCE: GROUNDED THEORY AND PHOTOVOICE VARIATIONS ON A THEME: AN UPDATE

Beverly D. Leipert

RURAL SETTINGS IN CANADA ARE increasingly becoming aging feminized communities. In some rural communities, seniors presently comprise up to 40% of the population (Statistics Canada, 2001), and it is anticipated that by 2021 one in four seniors will reside in a rural setting (Health Canada, 2002). Not only are farmers and other rural people aging in place in rural settings, retirees and older individuals seeking a quieter, slower pace of life are also relocating to rural locations, as younger populations leave for cities for education and employment (Keating, 2008). Older and middle-aged women form the backbone of rural communities and provide significant friend, family, and community support (Keating, Leipert, & George, 2008; Leipert & Smith, 2008; Sutherns, McPhedran, & Haworth-Brockman, 2004). As women tend to live longer than men and often experience greater chronic conditions, isolation, and poverty (Canadian Institute for Health Information, 2006; Clark & Leipert, 2007; Leipert et al., 2012; McPherson & Wister, 2008; Ministry of Industry, 2006), attention to the health and resilience of older women is an especially important aspect of rural health care.

In this chapter, I explore the resilience of women in rural and remote Canada as perceived and depicted in two research studies conducted with rural women in northern British Columbia (NBC study) and southwest Ontario (SWO study). The majority of the participants in these studies were women who were middle-aged (40 years plus) and older.

PURPOSES OF THE STUDIES

The purpose of the NBC study was to examine how women perceive and maintain their health within geographical, social, economic, and other contexts within NBC, Canada. The purpose of the SWO study was to explore the nature of pictorial and descriptive data about social and health promotion needs and resources provided by older rural women in SWO using the photovoice method. The resilience of rural women emerged as a theme in both studies.

METHODS

Both studies were guided by a feminist theoretical approach. Feminist inquiry considers not only women's individual voices and experiences, but also larger sociopolitical, economic, and cultural structures that influence women's lives (MacDonald, 2001). The NBC study also used a grounded theory method to identify and describe complex and hidden processes (Morse, 2001) related to rural and northern women's health. The SWO study used a unique method called photovoice, which was developed specifically for research with rural women (Wang, Burris, & Ping, 1996). Using this method, cameras were provided to participants so that they could take pictures of social and health promotion needs and resources in their rural communities (Leipert et al., 2012). The women also recorded perspectives in log books and participated in two focus groups to discuss the pictorial and narrative data and their perspectives.

Setting

The NBC study included both urban and rural settings in NBC. Northern rural settings are characterized as rural, rural remote, and rural isolated. Rural communities have a population of less than 1,000 people with less than 400 people per square kilometer (Statistics Canada, 1993). Rural remote communities are 80 to 400 kilometers or 1 to 4 hours, travel in good weather to a major regional hospital (Canadian Association of Emergency Physicians, Rural Committee, 1997). Rural isolated communities are more than 400 kilometers or 4 hours, travel in good weather to a major regional hospital (Rennie, Baird-Crooks, Remus, & Engel, 2000). In the north, both urban and rural settings are considered remote and isolated because of their distant location from health care and other resources.

The SWO study was conducted in four counties in SWO. These counties are considered rural because they are "outside of urban centres with 10,000 or more population" (du Plessis, Beshiri, & Bollman, 2002, p. 1). Although distances are less and the number of people are greater in SWO compared to NBC, SWO is still considered rural because farmland covers 75% of the land area (Turner & Gutmanis, 2005) and major amounts of agricultural products are grown there (Caldwell, Brown, Thomson, & Auld, 2006).

Sample

In the NBC study, the sample was constructed using theoretical sampling (Glaser, 1978) and consisted of 25 women who had lived in northern settings for a minimum of 2 years. The women were aged 21 to 86 years (the majority within 41–60 years), had less than Grade 9 to university education, and had incomes ranging from less than $10,000 ($n = 2$) to over $60,000 ($n = 5$). The women reported Aboriginal, Métis, South Asian, British, Swiss, and Canadian cultural backgrounds. The majority of the women were married or living common law, employed full-time or part-time, and in good health. Two-thirds ($n = 17$) of the study participants resided in rural and remote settings (farms, ranches) as well as in villages of less than 100 residents and in small towns, whereas the remaining one-third ($n = 8$) of the participants resided in Prince George, population 75,000, the only city in the north.

In the SWO study, purposeful snowball sampling (Patton, 2002) was used to create a sample of 31 women who ranged in age from 55 to 89 years, had less than Grade 9 to a university degree, and had incomes ranging from less than $10,000 ($n = 1$) to over $50,000 ($n = 3$) (not all participants answered all of the sociodemographic questions). The women claimed Aboriginal, Mennonite, Dutch, Belgian, and Canadian cultural backgrounds. The majority of the women were widowed ($n = 18$), lived in towns of 250 to 7500 residents ($n = 14$) or on farms ($n = 4$), and reported good ($n = 11$) or excellent ($n = 8$) health.

Data Collection

Prior to data collection in the NBC study, ethical approval was obtained from the University of Alberta Health Research Ethics Board and University of Northern British Columbia Ethics Review Board. Narrative data were then collected through semi-structured interviews using open-ended questions; observational data were also collected during travels to interviews on farms and ranches and in northern communities as well as from written documents such as maps, tourist guides, community histories, and newspapers (Leipert, 2006). Each participant was interviewed 3 times; the first interview was in person and the second and third interviews were predominantly by telephone. The first and second interviews were taped and transcribed, then imported into the NVivo (Version 1) computer program for analysis. Pseudonyms selected by each woman were used in transcribing to protect participants' identities. Notes taken during third interviews and memos containing researcher reflections subsequent to interviews were also collected.

Prior to data collection in the SWO study, ethical approval was obtained from the University of Western Ontario Health Research Ethics Board. The 31 participants consisted of five groups in four rural communities. Each group participated in two group interview sessions; both group sessions were audiotaped. In the first group session, the research was explained and cameras were demonstrated and provided to the women, along with log books for recording perspectives (Leipert et al., 2012). Participants were invited to photograph images and record reflections in log books about social and health promotion needs and resources for older rural women in rural settings. After 2 weeks, the cameras and log books were retrieved and the films were developed. At the second group session, the photos were returned to the women, and they were invited to select two images: one that best represented a social and health promotion need and one that best represented a social and health promotion resource. Participants were asked for titles for each of these pictures and discussion ensued as to the meaning of the pictures and their importance regarding social and health promotion needs and resources of rural older women. The second interview session concluded with participants completing a brief sociodemographic questionnaire.

Data Analysis

In the NBC study, analysis was conducted concurrently with data collection and followed the grounded theory constant comparative method (Glaser, 1978, 1992). With the assistance of the NVivo (1999) computer program, I reviewed interview transcripts line by line and coded them for categories and themes. Participants clarified, elaborated upon, and verified emerging categories, subcategories, and relationships in second and third interviews. A fourth interview was conducted with three participants for verification of the theory that emerged in the study (Leipert, 2006). Analysis and data collection ceased when no new information or insight was forthcoming about the categories and their relationships and when the theory seemed to be elaborate in complexity and clear in its articulation of the central problem and the process used to address it (Glaser, 1978).

In the SWO study, data were analyzed using a rigorous three-phase process. In the first phase, the second group interview participants: (1) identified key data by selecting their photos, (2) contextualized data by explaining the meaning of their photos, and (3) codified data by identifying issues, concepts, themes, and theories (Wang & Burris, 1997). These audiotaped data were transcribed and, in the second phase, were analyzed by a minimum of two researchers using NVivo to determine themes related to rural social and health promotion needs and resources (Leipert et al., 2012). As a result of this analysis, themes related to rural women and resilience also emerged. In the third phase, a three-stage analysis process (Oliffe, Bottorff, Kelly, & Halpin, 2008) was used. In the first stage, preview, the researchers viewed participants' photographs alongside the narratives about each picture to understand intended representations and to situate the participants within the context of their photographs. In the second stage, cross-photo comparison, the researchers developed themes that were reflected in the entire photograph collection. We reviewed the total data set of 575 usable pictures taken by the participants. The final stage, theorizing, allowed the researchers to develop abstract understandings by linking the themes to the feminist theoretical approach of the study. As resilience began to emerge as an important theme in the original analysis, the photos were reanalyzed using this rigorous three-stage process to determine more consistently and accurately findings regarding rural women and resilience.

Limitations

A limitation of the NBC study is the exclusion of non-English-speaking women; for both the NBC and SWO studies, representation of various groups of women, such as very remote women, lesbian women, and women, who live in extreme poverty, were limited. In addition, the grounded theory and photovoice methods used in the two research studies differed to some degree. Nonetheless, data analysis in both studies revealed rich information regarding the resilience of rural women in two diverse locations in Canada.

FINDINGS

The NBC Study

The findings and theory that emerged regarding resilience in the NBC study have been elaborated elsewhere (Leipert, 2006). Only some elements of the theory will be summarized here; the main focus in this section of the chapter will be on the findings regarding the nature of the resilience revealed by the women in the NBC study.

The intent of grounded theory is to generate a theory that explains a process of how individuals respond to a main concern or problem (Glaser, 1978). The main problem for the women in this study was vulnerability to health risks, in particular, physical health and safety risks, psychosocial health risks, and risks of inadequate health care. Women responded to these health risks by developing a process of resilience, which included strategies of becoming hardy, making the best of the north, and supplementing the north (Leipert, 2006) (see Figure 7.1).

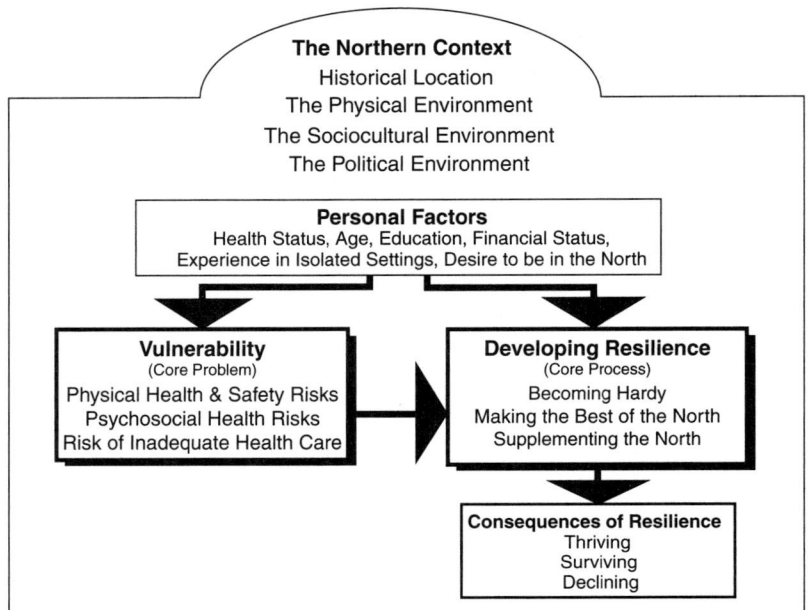

FIGURE 7.1 Developing resilience to manage vulnerability: Northern Canadian Women's Health.

Developing Resilience

In response to vulnerability to health risks, women in the study engaged in a core process of developing resilience. This process involved strategies of becoming hardy, making the best of the north, and supplementing the north.

Becoming Hardy

Becoming hardy for northern women involved taking a positive attitude, following spiritual beliefs, developing fortitude, and establishing self-reliance. Taking a positive attitude helped women put northern challenges into perspective and deal with them, thereby enhancing their commitment to northern life. Spiritual beliefs provided personal comfort, meaning and balance, opportunities for cultural and social connections, and a sense of peace, control, care, and belonging. Spirituality included religious and cultural beliefs, as well as friendships, personal reflection, and communing with nature. Establishing self-reliance increased women's confidence, courage, and skills to tackle new and difficult challenges. Examples of self-reliant strategies included learning to drive, using various strategies to defend oneself against wildlife and threatening humans in isolated settings, and learning to suture wounds if women lived in remote locations.

Women were better able to develop hardiness if they were healthy and motivated to be in the north, could address isolation and other northern context issues, were able to learn about and purchase resources, and had a social support network. Women who were ill, in low income or remote situations, worked outdoors, or traveled on isolated or winter roads were especially challenged in becoming hardy. Adequate personal and social resources were essential. Carmen noted, "You have to have an upbeat attitude. What makes you hardy is the fact that you don't dwell on the fact that you're living where it's cold and remote"; Lilac recommended "having things to amuse you at home in winter"; and Gert valued "the company of women."

Making the Best of the North

Making the best of the north meant that women used and developed available resources and opportunities. These included participating in northern activities, making decisions about health care services, seeking education and information, seeking and providing social support, and working on financial and employment issues.

Women participated in northern activities by (a) enjoying the ready access to outdoor activities, such as camping and hiking; (b) developing indoor interests, such as quilting, painting, and computer use; and (c) volunteering for community groups. Sometimes making the best of the north through participation required a conscious effort. Carmen explained, "When you live in more remote areas, you have to make yourself be positive. It's not something that just happens." For example, Carmen planned trips to Prince George for entertainment and "to do something different."

Study participants made a variety of decisions about health care. They tried to circumvent inadequate care by seeking a second opinion from another physician or by changing their physician. These circumventions were not always possible because of a scarcity of physicians and physician refusals in small communities to provide advice to patients of colleagues. Women also sought the more accessible and sometimes more appropriate services of public health nurses. Public health nurses were valued because they were "approachable" and took a "holistic approach to health" (Rosie), and because they accorded time, education, and respect to women. Other times, women sought health care in another northern community or outside the north. However, women with low incomes and women who were older, ill, or disabled often had to settle for inadequate care provided locally. To supplement the limited health care in the north, and because alternative therapies were believed to be legitimate in their own right, women also made decisions to use alternative health care such as massage and naturopathic options. Health needs, age, cultural and educational backgrounds, economic circumstances, available time, and their knowledge about care accessibility and quality influenced women's decisions about health care.

Women also developed resilience by seeking education and information from nurses, physicians, universities, community colleges, and distance education programs. Education and information helped to change attitudes, enhanced job and career opportunities, increased knowledge and abilities regarding health and health care, and enriched quality of life. Factors that affected women's ability to access educational resources included women's geographic location; their access to finances for tuition and travel; time for study and travel; and access to technology, such as electricity, telephones, computers, roads, and automobiles.

Social support provided women with instrumental (practical), emotional, affirmational, and informational resources (House & Kahn, 1985). Marie explained, "When people in the north go out of town shopping, they always ask their friends, 'Is there anything you want me to pick up for you?'" Signe noted that it was important "to find somebody to talk to, to ease the loneliness of the long dreary winters." Frequently, northern residents had left extended family to seek employment in the north. Thus, friends often took the place of family. In addition, social support, especially by women, helped women who were new to a community become insiders and thus better able to secure friends, information, support, employment, and other resources.

Financial and work issues included limited employment options for women, lack of child care, male attitudes about what women can and should do, inadequate remuneration, lack of respect, sexual harassment at work, and reluctance of communities to employ women who were new to the community. The boom and bust nature of northern resource-based economies compromised job prospects for men, with resultant financial implications for their female partners. Study participants addressed these limitations by engaging in diverse full-time and part-time employment in both the public and private sector. Part-time work decreased risks by decreasing travel in dangerous climates and terrains and helped women maintain control and make the most of their talents, interests, and opportunities. However, part-time employment also decreased women's incomes.

Nevertheless, women in the study illustrated that through resourcefullness, assertiveness, and effective decision making, part-time and full-time work sometimes improved their financial and employment situations. For example, Casey capitalized on her computer and ranching resources and developed part-time employment "helping a friend do a seed catalogue, babysitting, baking, I [have] eggs and we have hay...." Rumi developed assertiveness skills to deal with harassment at her restaurant job, and other women made decisions to work part-time, change jobs, or do volunteer work to address employment situations. With adequate incomes, women were better able to access health resources both near and far.

Supplementing the North

Supplementing the north involved being political (personally and for the community) and leaving the north, temporarily or permanently. Supplementing the north included adding to, as well as changing, what presently existed in the north, thereby enriching northern resources and minimizing vulnerability.

The main mode of political action used was that of advocacy, speaking out for themselves and others. Leah advised, "It's important to learn to advocate for yourself with your doctor," and Casey believed that "being your own advocate will take you far." Women engaged in community advocacy to increase awareness about and access to resources. Community advocacy activities included participating in Take Back the Night walks, subscribing to and writing for a regional publication that focused on northern women's interests, and serving as a member of a community committee that met with the premier of the province about local health matters. Participation in this research was also seen as a political act. Eileen explained, "Women up here feel disempowered, under, and invisible ... this research will help women become more visible to themselves and that's part of becoming more empowered." Women needed time and finances, as well as commitment, courage, assertiveness, and tact to be successful as political activists in and for northern communities.

Leaving the north temporarily was a strategy that every participant used to decrease exposure to vulnerabilities and to supplement resources. Obtaining health care in southern locations increased the quality, timeliness, and appropriateness of care, and for women who required special or more diverse care, increased their ability to obtain any care at all. Goods and services obtained from southern locations increased women's quality of life by increasing choices and decreasing costs of living in the north. Women who were able to travel to vacations and events outside the north brought back expertise and experiences that enriched their lives and the lives of other northerners. Women who were poor, ill, or very geographically isolated often had greater need to leave the north; however, their ability to leave was also compromised by their needs and circumstances.

Leaving the north permanently was a resilient strategy because it required courage and self-assertion to leave friends and family and an established life in the north. Leaving permanently was a strategy that was considered especially salient for single women and for women who wanted enriched education, employment, and sociocultural options. Eileen, a single mother, was considering leaving because she felt that people in her community "look at single moms as having made mistakes, not quite fitting in, as being peripheral." Marie, a single retired woman, was looking forward to leaving the "redneck rough crude" north to lead "the quality of life I want to lead." Leah, a young single woman, was moving south where "all my friends are" and where she could access desired education. Although leaving permanently may increase women's resources and quality of life, their leaving would mean that the north would lose vital resources—women with an informed vision of how northern women's health could and should be advanced.

Women's location within the northern context, the degree of vulnerability they experienced, and personal factors (age, health and financial status, and cultural background) affected the degree to which women could develop and use resilient strategies. Although older women and women who were isolated, ill, or poor experienced greater vulnerability to health risks and a greater need for resilience, their ability to be resilient was compromised by their situations. Thus, those with the greatest needs were often the least able to address their needs.

The SWO Study

Similar to the NBC study, rural older women in the SWO study also experienced vulnerability risks. Physical health and safety risks were associated with poor climate, especially in winter; broken sidewalks and limited rails along walking trails, which contributed to unsafe sites for physical exercise; and spraying and other farming practices. For Aboriginal women, the increased use of alcohol and other drugs on their reserve contributed to physical health risks not only for the users, but also for women who lived close by. Although most of the women were retired, and thus not employed, one woman in her 80s still actively farmed and, although

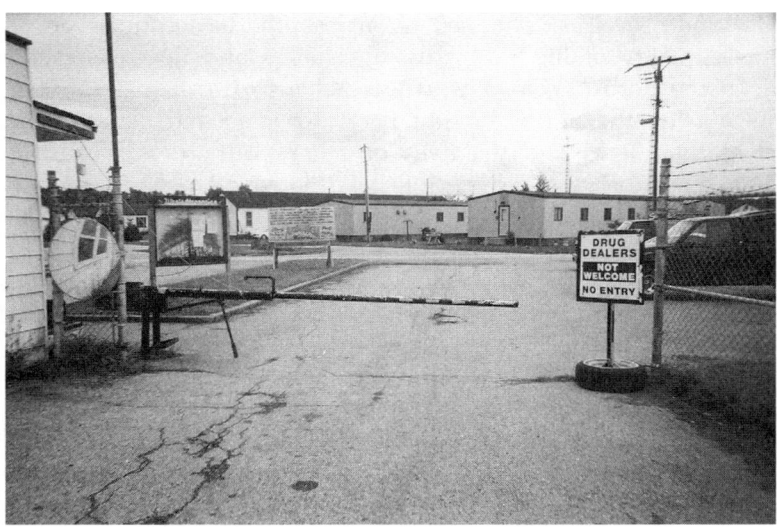

Drug dealers not welcome.

she did not comment on employment risks to her health, working around farm machinery could pose a risk to her physical health.

Psychosocial health risks were perhaps a larger concern for women in the SWO study. Although they were not as geographically isolated from each other compared to the NBC participants, nonetheless for this group of older rural women isolation was an issue. Isolation from friends and family due to limited transportation or the inability to drive any longer lack of access to family members such as spouses who were deceased or in distant long-term care facilities, limited abilities to travel in winter, and not having access to exercise resources in winter, such as an indoor pool, contributed to feelings of loneliness and depression. Histories of abuse and neglect experienced by Mennonite and Aboriginal women and the frequent closure of rural churches contributed to mental health and spiritual concerns. The following quotes illustrate these issues:

> All our children ... were raised there.... We went ... across the road to the church all the time. I don't know what I'll do when they close [the church].... We bought [our home here] because we figured the church would be there ... you could walk [across the road] to church in your old age but you can't do that I guess ...
>
> I got married ... had eight children.... This was not [a] very good ... marriage ... my husband left ... I was always scared of him, all the time.... Until we finally came across the border [from Mexico] into the United States [on our way to Canada] ... I finally felt better ... I didn't have to watch all the time.

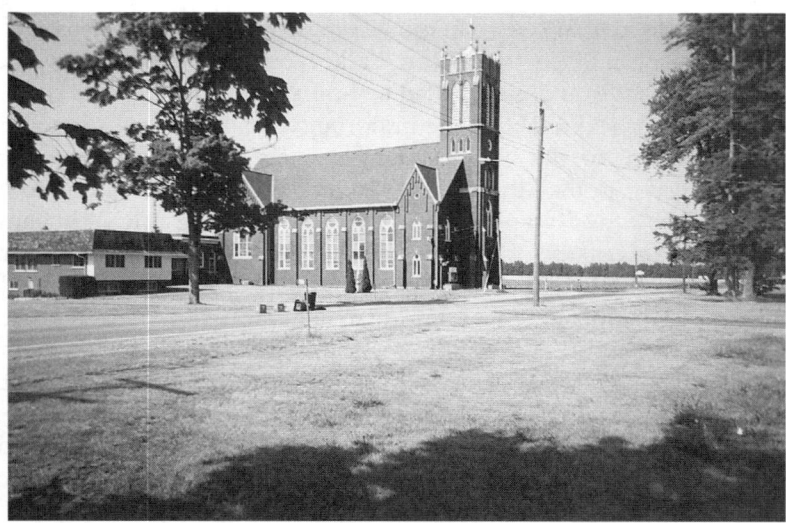

A rural church.

> Residential schools ... caused a significant loss in native cultural/identity. This can be seen in areas such as language, parenting skills, family and community values and roles, loss of living in ancestral land base, day to day living values and belief systems. [The] inflict[ion] of physical, psychological, emotional and sexual abuse ... resulted in ... generations of mental health issues ... post-traumatic stress disorders ... all of these factors have affected me during my childhood, youth, adult life and as a senior.

The older rural women in this study also experienced risks of inadequate health care. Closure of pharmacies in rural communities, lack of access to hospitals that were close by, and poor or distant long-term care facilities were major areas of concern. The following quote illustrates this latter issue:

> This is the nursing home where my husband lived. The reason we chose [it] is because it was close to where we lived.... [When it closed] we had to take the first one that came up ... 23 km away [from home].

Developing Resilience

Becoming Hardy

The older rural women in this study also developed hardiness as they took a positive attitude and followed spiritual beliefs, as exhibited in the numerous comments ("I go to church every Sunday ... I feel it helps me when I pray. I feel if there are any problems in your family, you know, it's like a support to you ... that's my opinion.") and pictures of rural churches, and bibles (especially in the pictures taken by the Mennonite women); developed fortitude; and established self-reliance.

One woman spoke about the importance that taking a nursing aide course had been for her in her younger years and the challenges she endured in order to take this course, "Well I had always wanted to be a nurse from the time I was twelve years old.... [Being a RNA] changed my life.... It gives me more incentive of living now [in my senior years]." The fortitude and self-reliance that this woman exhibited resulted in a sense of accomplishment and pride in her ability to care for others and to complete an education program, especially when almost overwhelmed with childbearing, child care, and farming responsibilities. Another woman, aged 83, revealed elements of fortitude and self-reliance in her narratives of active farming and tractor driving activities, "I used to work nights all the time.... I loved to come home ... jump on the tractor ... go out to the fields ... think ... I can watch the birds ... the trees ... the sand blow, how relaxing to get away from the stressful night's work".

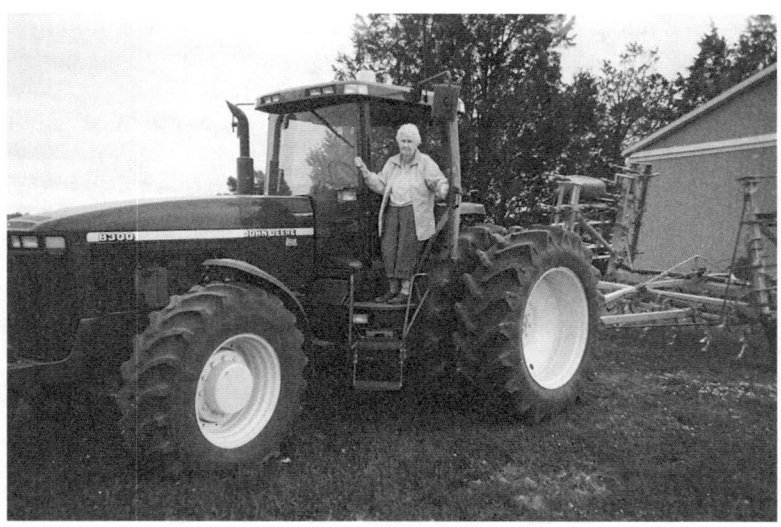

The love of John Deeres.

The hardiness of one of the Aboriginal women was revealed in the poetry she wrote in which she addressed past injustices and hopes for the future:

Our hopes and dreams became a war zone ...

May our Nation

give us peace in heart

As we come together from a broken promise

We speak with one voice through the wisdom

Given to us by our ancestors

many moons back.

Arise, and come together our First nation

Together we'll heal from

a broken promise

Let our drums beat

coming together lock

Step of the way: stamping

our feet, good spirits coming together.

These activities helped the women contribute to their families and communities in the past and in the present, and gave them a sense of accomplishment, pride, independence, and agency.

Of all of the above attributes of hardiness, perhaps the most important attributes for participants in this study were their attitudes toward themselves and their past and present lives. The women in this study frequently spoke about the importance of accepting some of life's situations, not engaging in self-pity, and enjoying what you have without constantly striving to have more and better, as these quotes exemplify:

> I am happy. I have a good life. We are going through hard times but, hey, that's life. But I am not unhappy because of circumstance. I'm glad we came to Canada.

> I think everyone here has been a role model in some way to family or friends and yet there may be a reluctance to claim that, to say that you've done that, even though you have been a role model ... none of us really see ourselves as a leader ... [but] as a mother or a daughter or anything you are a leader no matter how you look at it.

These attitudes provided peace of mind as well as the ability to be inspired and objective when considering issues and ways to address them. The many challenging situations with which the participants in this study engaged throughout the course of their lives, and the many ways they needed to develop resilience in the past to address difficult circumstances, no doubt provided rich experience that formed the basis for these hardy attitudes. For example, participants had experienced extreme poverty, societal discrimination, oppression and abuse by spouses, issues related to adapting to a new country, having to learn a new language (English), raising an often large family in challenging circumstances, and making new friends in a new land. Thus, life experiences and fortitude developed over the years in stressful and challenging circumstances may assist in the development of resilience for a satisfying older age in rural contexts.

Making the Best of the Rural Context

Several women in the study were proud of their ability to drive, even if this was only during the good weather and road conditions in the summer. For women who were older, who lived alone, and who lived in an area where resources were decreasing or nonexistent, being able to drive afforded them access to resources in other communities and social support from friends and families. A participant summarized the perspectives of most of the women in the study when she stated, "Without wheels, we're stuck. We can't go anywhere ... there's no bus stopping where I live.... When stores are closing ... and no new stores come in ... makes you feel like there's something missing.... Like you can't get what you would get, say, in a larger community."

Examples of titles that participants gave to pictures related to their vehicle included "My Best Companion" and "Freedom." Women with sufficient funds were able to purchase electric carts that helped them get around in town situations, although these were of limited use in more rural and unpaved contexts.

Participants enjoyed the outdoors, especially in the summer. The planting and tending of gardens was a major theme in the women's development and enactment of resilience. Titles of their photographs, such as "Peace/Happiness" and "My Sanctuary," illustrate the importance of gardens to these women, as do their comments: "My garden is like my haven ... my peace of mind.... It's the best way to relax, sit out there and read.... Look at the flowers in the morning.... It's just beautiful"; and "My little garden creates a feeling of peace and enjoyment which of course, makes me happy and healthy."

In addition, participants enjoyed physical activities such as swimming in the neighborhood or their own outdoor pools, lawn bowling, biking, and walking. These activities helped them stay physically healthy, facilitated mental health as they interacted with grandchildren, neighbors, and friends, and helped participants support future generations, as this participant remarked:

> I believe in setting a good example [for my grandchildren] for their physical health ... The other day my daughters were talking to me and they said, "Our parents have taught us to be physical [and] they're still in their 70's ... and we have all followed suit" ... I do feel good that they have all ... said to me that I have been a good example.

Participants also believed that it was important for one's mental health to keep busy in the winter months, when it was more difficult and risky for older people to be physically active outdoors. Some of the resilient activities in winter included meeting with friends for card and board games, quilting baking gatherings, and indoor exercise classes.

In addition, pets, such as birds, dogs, and cats, provided companionship and meaning to their lives, and helped participants be resilient in the face of isolation and loneliness brought about through the loss of a spouse or the enforced isolation of being housebound in winter. Titles of pictures of pets revealed how important they were to participants, for example, "Joy," "Happiness," and "The Loves of My Life."

Participants were also able to be resilient in the face of adversity and health challenges because of their contributions from and to their communities. For women who lived alone, helpful neighbors who could be relied on to do chores, such as check smoke detectors and pick up groceries in

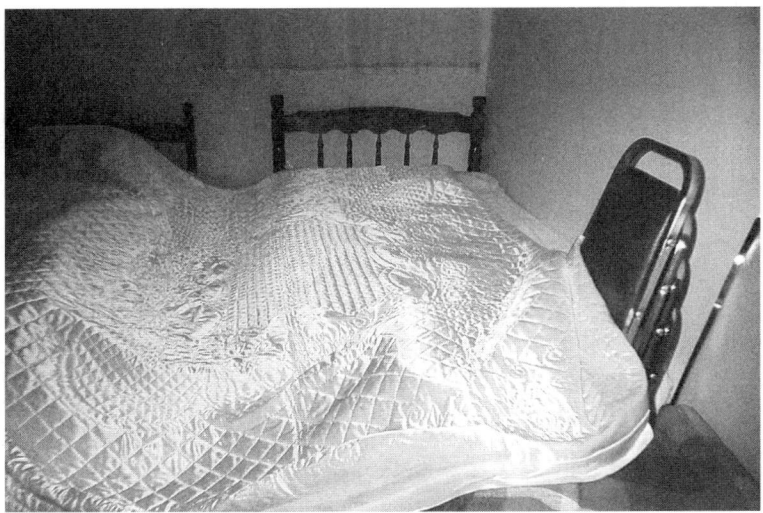
Made out of love.

winter, were essential and very much appreciated: "My neighbor... [helped] change the battery on the smoke alarm.... Women that live alone need to have good friends and neighbors... we get so we depend on them".

Home delivery of prescription drugs by pharmacies and access to local or home visiting health care resources such as nurses, massage therapists, and housekeeping services were also very welcome. Because participants were assisted in these and other ways to be resilient and independent, and because they could see the need for and the value of their contributions, participants were able and eager to give back to their rural communities. Thus, they contributed in many and several ways, including assisting at church and other community events, volunteering at community agencies such as the Mennonite Central Committee, which provides clothing and other resources to the Mennonite community, and providing services such as transportation to others in the community.

Supplementing the Rural Context

Participants supplemented the resources in their rural communities by traveling to other towns and cities for goods and services. They also provided transportation to others and often carpooled so that they could access distant resources.

Women with sufficient funds valued traveling to warmer climates in winter so as to avoid dealing with winter challenges ("I'm very fortunate that I am in Florida in the wintertime, but not everybody's that fortunate"). Participants who did not have access to funds for travel supplemented their

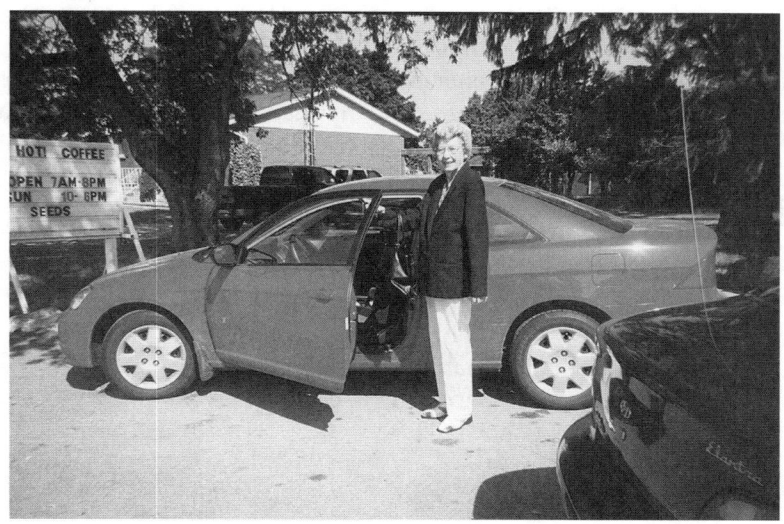

Driving to keep an appointment.

resilience, especially during the isolating winter months, by cultivating enjoyment of local available resources such as seniors centers and by their creation of activities that could be experienced individually or with others, such as quilting, cooking, watching TV, reading, and enjoying pets. In addition, some women who still actively farmed enhanced their safety and peace of mind by learning to use technology, as this 83-year-old participant noted:

> What's helping more is the younger farmers all have cell phones in their tractors. If you get alarmed, you can phone 'em ... or they can phone you.... They've got me educated on how to use one 'cause I'm out driving the tractor.... He [her son] can phone me and say "Are you alright, mother?"

Whether and how participants wanted to, needed to, or could supplement the rural context with resilient approaches depended on several factors. Women who were healthy could physically manage to access distant resources such as health care and shopping. Women who needed health care resources were often compromised in their ability to be resilient and travel, especially in winter, to health care resources that were at a distance. Women with financial and social resources could purchase what they needed, rather than do without or manage with limited or delayed resources available more locally; occasionally, friends, spouses, and children assisted with funds and support. Several women in the study, especially those who were older and more isolated and the First Nations and

Mennonite women, depended on their spiritual beliefs and on each other to help them be resilient so that they could meet needs or develop acceptance of limitations, as these comments indicate: "My church is the most important part of my physical, mental, social and general well-being.... I travel quite a long distance to attend services...." And, "When [I] go to church, I feel him [my husband] in the seat with me ... he's not there but ... he is in spirit..." Another said,

> I believe that to have a healthy sense of well-being, it has to be holistic including social/emotional, physical, cognitive and spiritual. Native people ... embrace their spirituality in a strong and meaningful sense ... usually in a belief system that can be Native Traditional, or Christian belief. In our community most people chose one of these belief systems [for] a sense of identity, belonging, and self-worth.

DISCUSSION AND IMPLICATIONS

Findings from both of these studies revealed that rural women in the NBC study and the SWO study developed resilience in response to a number of factors, such as life experiences, stages in life, resources and needs, and the nature of rural contexts. Although the nature and degree of resilience may have varied according to participant circumstance, geographical location, and other factors, the elements of resilience, of becoming hardy, making the best of the context, and supplementing the context remained relevant for women in both rural settings.

Findings from the two studies reported here included data from 56 rural women between the ages of 21 to 89 years, with the majority aged 41 years and older. Thus, the findings have particular relevance to middle-aged and older rural women, populations about which little is known, but who provide and require the bulk of health and social care in rural settings (Forbes & Hawranik, 2012; Keating, 2008; Leipert et al., 2012). Thus, findings from these studies are significant in articulating how middle-aged and older women may experience vulnerability and develop resilience in the context of limited health care resources and increasing personal and social demands, but also within the context of personal and community strengths. For example, although older rural women may experience more physical and psychosocial health risks and vulnerability to inadequate health care, they may also have enhanced maturity and life experience to develop resilient strategies of hardiness and make the best of and supplement personal and geographical limitations. Study findings may also be useful in suggesting diverse and innovative strategies to facilitate resilience, and in highlighting issues of aging in rural settings to anticipate and prepare for, issues that may benefit from present and future support, programs, and services. For example, realization that resilience is not static, but that it changes and can lead not only to thriving and surviving but also to declining, indicates that personal abilities, needs, and resources, as well as seasonal variations and other circumstances, must constantly be monitored to ensure that aging rural residents stay healthy.

Keating and Eales (2012) note that older rural women are not a homogeneous group, that they experience diversity related to geographical location, physical and psychosocial health issues and connections, and styles of living in their rural communities. Keating and Eales describe rural seniors in terms of four groups: community-active, stoic, marginalized, and frail seniors, and note that each group requires and facilitates good health in various ways. For example, community-active and stoic seniors tend to be in good health, well connected socially, have the resources to age well, and are net contributors to their communities, whereas marginalized and frail seniors have more perilous health, more limited finances and social connections, and higher support needs that are difficult to address in rural settings (Keating & Eales, 2012). In addition, in new retirement communities, such as those in particularly isolated and under-resourced frontier settings, social structures, and existing health care resources may not be sufficient to sustain seniors or to assist them to develop the resilience needed to address vulnerabilities in these harsh settings (Skinner, Hanlon, & Halseth, 2012). Indeed, the "double jeopardy of caring for increasingly vulnerable rural people in increasingly vulnerable rural places" (Skinner et al., p. 463) has serious implications for the ability of rural and remote communities to cope with the needs of rural seniors. Thus, differences in vulnerability and resilience needs and resources for diverse rural seniors in diverse rural contexts must be acknowledged and incorporated to develop effective health promotion, illness and injury prevention, treatment, and rehabilitation resources. In addition, this diversity must be appreciated by health care policy-makers and funders to ensure that rural residents, in whatever rural context in which they live, receive appropriate care and support.

Recent research is revealing rural infrastructure that could provide rich resources for rural women's health, especially for older rural residents. Churches represent some of the last remaining infrastructures in many rural communities, and, as such, could be utilized as locations for health events and programs in addition to spiritual support (Plunkett & Leipert, 2011). As rural communities are aging communities and older residents are more likely to use church facilities (Plunkett & Leipert), these facilities would be familiar, acceptable, and accessible to many older rural women. Although depopulation and diminishing financial resources can affect the utility and viability of churches in some rural communities (Pletsch, Amaratunga, Corneil, Crowe, & Krewski, 2012), nonetheless, in other communities, active and well-supported churches may serve as vital resources for rural women and rural health care providers, such as public health nurses, in which to plan and engage in health-related activities.

Rural sport and recreation facilities, such as skating and curling rinks, are additional rural resources that could be adapted for health-based initiatives in addition to the social support and community sustainability that they already provide (Leipert et al., 2011; Mair, 2009). For example, in Canada more than 60% of the curling clubs are located in communities with fewer than 10,000 people (Canadian Curling Association, 2004), and rural senior women and men often curl weekly or drop in regularly at their local rink to visit, watch a game, or volunteer (Leipert et al., 2011). As "sporting clubs are usually the last organizations to fold in small declining communities, often lasting longer than local shops, pubs and churches" (Tonts, 2005, p. 142), curling rinks can be viable rural community-gathering centers that could be utilized to promote rural seniors' health. These rinks could be used in both summer and winter for community lunches, physical activity, and recreational and leisure groups, as well as for more formal health education meetings. The exploration of sport and recreational facilities as important resources for rural health is a new area of research; more information is needed to determine if and how factors such as lack of finances, an aging membership, rural women's balancing of family and community responsibilities, and volunteer burn-out are affecting rural women's health and their sport participation.

Successful aging and rural women's health have been characterized as including the ability to plan ahead, be intellectually curious and in touch with creative abilities, do physical activity, have serenity and spirituality, care for friendships and other social connections, and volunteer and have civic responsibilities (Coward et al., 2006; Glicken, 2006; McPherson & Wister, 2008). Clearly, the photovoice method used in these studies acted not only as an effective research approach, but, as importantly, it assisted women to successfully age by helping them to voice and hear about needs and resources that they could address, individually or collectively. As such, photovoice is obviously a method to consider in rural research with rural women in other locations and age groups to assist them to access knowledge and develop abilities and perspectives that may help them to enrich resilience and age successfully.

This study and others (Forbes & Hawranik, 2012; Keating & Eales, 2012; Leipert et al., 2012; Skinner et al., 2012; Sutherns et al., 2004) indicate that more feminist qualitative research is needed in isolated settings, particularly regarding the health issues and resilience of women who may be more vulnerable to health risks, such as older rural women, and women who were not well represented in this study, such as those in very remote settings and disabled women. Additional qualitative and quantitative research could expand and test components of the theory revealed in the NBC study with women in other rural and remote settings. Additional research that explores aspects of resilience, such as factors that facilitate and hinder rural women's resilience, would provide important information for rural health care practice and policy.

REFERENCES

Caldwell, W., Brown, C., Thomson, S., & Auld, G. (2006). *The urbanite's guide to the countryside*. Guelph, ON: University of Guelph.

Canadian Association of Emergency Physicians, Rural Committee. (1997). *Recommendations for the management of rural, remote, and isolated emergency health care facilities in Canada*. Ottawa, ON: Author.

Canadian Curling Association [CCA]. (2004). *Survey of Canadian curling facilities*. Retrieved May 14, 2012 from http://www.curling.ca/start-curling/profile-of-the-canadian-curler

Canadian Institute for Health Information [CIHI]. (2006). *How healthy are rural Canadians? An assessment of their health status and health determinants*. Ottawa, ON: CIHI.

Clark, K., & Leipert, B. (2007). Strengthening and sustaining social supports for rural elders. *Online Journal of Rural Nursing and Health Care*, 7(1), 13–26.

Coward, R., Davis, L., Gold, C., Smiciklas-Wright, H., Thorndyke, L, & Vondracek, F. (Eds.). (2006). *Rural women's health: Mental, behavioral, and physical issues*. New York, NY: Springer Publishing.

du Plessis, V., Beshiri, R., & Bollman, R. (2002). Definitions of rural. *Rural and Small Town Canada Analysis Bulletin*, 3(3), 1–16. Statistics Canada, Catalogue 21-006- XIE.

Forbes, D., & Hawranik, P. (2012). Looming dementia care crisis: Are Canadian rural and remote settings ready? J. Kulig, & A. Williams (Eds.), *Health in rural Canada* (pp. 447–461). Vancouver, BC: UBC Press.

Glaser, B. (1978). *Theoretical sensitivity*. Mill Valley, CA: Sociology Press.

Glaser, B. (1992). *Basics of grounded theory analysis: Emergence vs. forcing*. Mill Valley, CA: Sociology Press.

Glicken, M. (2006). *Learning from resilient people: Lessons we can apply to counseling and psychotherapy*. London: Sage.

Health Canada. (2002). *Canada's aging population*. Ottawa, ON: Minister of Public Works and Government Services Canada.

House, J., & Kahn, R. (1985). Measure and concepts of social support. In S. Cohen, & S. Syme (Eds.), *Social support and health* (pp. 83–108). Orlando, FL: Academic Press.

Keating, N. (2008). *Rural ageing: A good place to grow old?* Bristol, UK: The Policy Press.

Keating, N., & Eales, J. (2012). Diversity among older adults in rural Canada: Health in context. In J. Kulig, & A. Williams (Eds.), *Health in rural Canada* (pp. 427–446). Vancouver, BC: UBC Press.

Leipert, B. (2006). Rural and remote women developing resilience to manage vulnerability. In H. Lee, & C. Winters (Eds.), *Rural nursing: Concepts, theory, and practice* (pp. 79–95). New York, NY: Springer Publishing.

Leipert, B., & George, J. (2008). Determinants of rural women's health: A qualitative study in southwest Ontario. *The Journal of Rural Health, 24*(2), 210–218.

Leipert, B., Landry, T., McWilliam, C., Kelley, M., Forbes, D., Wakewich, P. et al. (2012). Rural women's health promotion needs and resources: A photovoice perspective. In J. Kulig, & A. Williams (Eds.), *Health in rural Canada* (pp. 481–502). Vancouver, BC: UBC Press.

Leipert, B., Plunkett, R., Meagher-Stewart, D., Scruby, L., Mair, H., & Wamsley, K. (2011). I couldn't imagine my life without it! Curling and health promotion: A photovoice study. *The Canadian Journal of Nursing Research, 43*(1), 60–78.

Leipert, B., & Smith, J. (2008). Using photovoice to explore older rural women's health promotion needs and resources. In P. Armstrong (Ed.), *Women's health: Intersections of policy, research, and practice* (pp. 135–150). Toronto: Women's Press.

MacDonald, M. (2001). Finding a critical perspective in grounded theory. In R. Schreiber, & P. Stern (Eds.), *Using grounded theory in nursing* (pp. 113–157). New York, NY: Springer Publishing.

Mair, H. (2009). Club life: Third place and shared leisure in rural Canada. *Leisure Sciences, 31*(5), 450–465.

McPherson, B., & Wister, A. (2008). *Aging as a social process: Canadian perspectives.* Don Mills, ON: Oxford University Press.

Ministry of Industry. (2006). *Women in Canada: A gender-based statistical report.* Ottawa, ON: Statistics Canada.

Morse, J. (2001). Situating grounded theory within qualitative inquiry. In R. Schreiber, & P. Stern (Eds.), *Using grounded theory in nursing* (pp. 159–175). New York, NY: Springer.

NVIVO. (1999). *Version 1. QRS NUD*IST VIVO.* Melbourne, Australia: Qualitative Solutions and Research Pty, Ltd.

Oliffe, J., Bottorff, J., Kelly, M., & Halpin, M. (2008). Analyzing participant produced photographs from an ethnographic study of fatherhood and smoking. *Research in Nursing & Health.* Retrieved June 18, 2008 from, at www.interscience.wiley.com

Patton, M. (2002). *Qualitative research and evaluation methods* (3rd ed.). London, UK: Sage.

Pletsch, V., Amaratunga, C., Corneil, W., Crowe, S., & Krewski, D. (2012). Reflections on the socio-economic and psycho-social impacts of BSE on rural and farm families in Canada. In J. Kulig, & A. Williams (Eds.), *Health in rural Canada* (pp. 352–370). Vancouver, BC: UBC Press.

Plunkett, R., & Leipert, B. (2011). Women's health promotion in the rural church: A Canadian perspective. *Journal of Religion and Health* [Epub ahead of print]. DOI 10.1007/s10943-011-9535-z

Rennie, D., Baird-Crooks, K., Remus, G., & Engel, J. (2000). Rural nursing in Canada. In A. Bushy (Ed.), *Orientation to nursing in the rural community* (pp. 217–231). London, ON: Sage.

Skinner, M., Hanlon, N., & Halseth, G. (2012). Health and social care issues in aging resource communities. In J. Kulig, & A. Williams (Eds.), *Health in rural Canada* (pp. 462–480). Vancouver, BC: UBC Press.

Statistics Canada. (1993). *Census of agriculture: Selected data for Saskatchewan rural municipalities*. Ottawa, ON: Government of Canada.

Statistics Canada. (2001). *Urban and rural population counts for provinces and territories*. Ottawa, ON: Minister of Industry.

Sutherns, R., McPhedran, M., & Haworth-Brockman, M. (2004). *Rural, remote, and northern women's health: Policy and research directions*. Winnipeg, Manitoba: Centres of Excellence for Women's Health.

Tonts, M. (2005). Competitive sport and social capital in rural Australia. *Journal of Rural Studies, 21*, 137–149.

Turner, L., & Gutmanis, I. (2005). *Rural health matters: A look at farming in southwest Ontario: Part 2*. London, ON: Southwest Region Health Information Partnership.

Wang, C., & Burris, M. (1997). Photovoice: Concept, methodology, and use for participatory needs assessment. *Health Education and Behavior, 24*, 369–387.

Wang, C., Burris, M., & Ping, X. (1996). Chinese village women as visual anthropologists: A participatory approach to reaching policy makers. *Social Science and Medicine, 42*, 1391–1400.

Chapter 8

PALLIATIVE CARE AT THE END OF LIFE: A RURAL FAMILY PERSPECTIVE

Dorothy M. "Dale" Mayer and
Rebecca Murphy

AMERICANS ARE LIVING LONGER AND as a result of this longevity individuals often live many years with some type of chronic illness. Chronic medical conditions are frequently associated with distressing symptoms, yet the incurable nature of chronic and debilitating illnesses result in need for ongoing treatments that will not be curative in nature. The alleviation of symptoms without curing the underlying medical condition is what we know as palliative care. Palliative care seeks to prevent, reduce, or soothe the symptoms of disease or disorder without effecting a cure (Field & Cassel, 1997). Fundamental elements of palliative care include management of a person's physical, psychosocial, spiritual, and practical needs along with ongoing communication between the providers of care and the patient and family. Ideally, palliative care should begin at the time a serious illness is diagnosed and continue to the end stages of an illness. Palliative care is particularly beneficial during the dying process and through family bereavement. Due to the ongoing nature of life-threatening or debilitating chronic illnesses, there is a need for coordination of palliative care across all care settings.

In recent years, strides have been made in raising awareness that palliative care is not, and should not be, limited to end-of-life care. Palliative care has been identified as a national priority by several professional groups, including the American Academy of Hospice and Palliative Medicine (AAHPM), the Center to Advance Palliative Care (CAPC), the Hospice and Palliative Nurses Association (HPNA), and the National Hospice and Palliative Care Organization (NHPCO). In an effort to standardize palliative care, the National Consensus Project (NCP) (2009) was formed with members from the above organizations. While these national organizations have reached consensus on the elements of palliative care, access to palliative care services remains challenging, especially in rural areas. The purpose of this chapter is to connect the "real-world" practice setting of rural palliative care with the existing palliative care literature. A case study will be presented to illustrate both the challenges and opportunities that health care providers encounter when providing palliative care services in rural settings.

CASE STUDY

Abe and Cindy (not their real names) are a retired couple who have been married for 52 years, and together they spent most of their adult life ranching and raising five children. Life was hard but they managed well because they had each other and they worked together to overcome the inevitable obstacles that arose over the course of many years on the ranch. When they were in their mid-70s Abe and Cindy decided it was time to move to town because, as Abe said, *"We're not as healthy as we used to be."* Moving to a town of 1,000 residents provided easier access to services like grocery stores and drug stores. Health care resources in town were limited to a small clinic staffed by one physician, one registered nurse (RN), and one home health aide, all of whom lived locally and were employed by a clinic/home health agency affiliated with a hospital located 60 miles away.

At age 80, Abe had a stroke; after spending several weeks in a rehabilitation facility, with Cindy's help, Abe was able to return home. When Abe developed a pressure ulcer on his coccyx, additional help was needed and Nancy, the local home health RN, began making home visits to provide dressing changes and assess healing. Laura, a home health aide, was scheduled 3 times a week to help with activities of daily living (ADL), including bathing and dressing. After this stroke, Abe and Cindy began talking with each other and their children about their desire to stay in their own home, and their children were supportive of this decision.

Over the next few years, Abe developed signs of memory loss which developed into dementia. As Abe's mobility lessened, Dr. Smith, the local physician, began to make house calls, and neighbors and fellow church members began to check in on Abe and Cindy on a regular basis. When Abe's condition had declined to the point he had lost a significant amount of weight and required full-time care, Dr. Smith mentioned it was time to consider adding hospice services.

In many ways the transition to hospice, with its focus on symptom management and comfort, was difficult for Cindy. The previous years of

(Continued)

maintaining or improving Abe's functional status made it hard for Cindy to let go of the rehabilitation philosophy; she was accustomed to getting Abe up every day, making sure he ate, feeding him when needed, and ensuring passive range of motion exercises were done at least twice a day. Cindy told her friends that she would see to it Abe was not going to die. Dr. Smith and Nancy began to gently counsel Cindy that it was time to change the approach to Abe's care and focus on his comfort.

One of the things that eased the transition to a more palliative focus was the fact that the home health agency that had been providing care for Abe over the past several years also provided hospice services. This allowed Nancy and Laura to remain involved and assist Cindy with the transition to hospice care. The addition of hospice made more services available to Abe and Cindy. There was increased availability of nursing and aide services to assist with Abe's ADLs, visits from a social worker/counselor, chaplain visits for spiritual support, and access to music, massage, and pet therapies. Due to the long distance involved, and difficult road conditions during the winter months, these services were not always easily provided. The hospice interdisciplinary team met weekly to help coordinate Abe's care, and often Nancy and Laura attended these team meetings via conference call rather than in person.

Initially, Cindy was resistant to having anyone else involved in her husband's care; after all she had been his primary caregiver and advocate for so many years that she found it hard to accept additional assistance. Family and friends agreed Cindy should meet with the counselor to discuss the slow decline in Abe's health and his approaching death. Initially, Cindy refused because she thought it was pointless to talk to someone about problems when you should be working your way through them. After all, this was how Cindy and Abe got through many tough years on the ranch. When Cindy finally met with the social worker, she discovered it was not the waste of time she was expecting. Due to long distances between the hospice office and their home, there were days when the social worker was not able to come out to the house. Weekly telephone conversations were scheduled to discuss what was going on with Abe's health, and how Cindy was feeling about these changes. These conversations, even by phone, were supportive and helpful for Cindy.

Abe's physical care and symptom management needs increased as he got closer to death. Since supplies at the local pharmacy were limited, it was important to anticipate and order medications that might be needed to control potential symptoms, for example, pain or agitation. Nancy and Laura, as the local care providers, attempted to increase

(Continued)

> their availability for Abe's care, but they had responsibilities to other clients. Hospice provided additional nursing staff members; however, they were often described by Cindy and other family members as the *"outside nurses."* Due to the lack of a preexisting relationship, these additional hospice nurses were not able to develop strong connections with Cindy and Abe, thus reinforcing their status as *"outsiders."*
>
> Nancy and Laura, as employees of the home care/hospice agency located 60 miles away, work very independently. Their work is both physically and emotionally challenging, while also rewarding due to the nature of the long-term relationships they develop with clients. These professionals were Abe's primary caregivers and, since they were well known in town, everyone recognized their car and knew when clients were receiving services. One day while Nancy was visiting Abe, another patient and her husband were driving by and stopped when they noticed *"the nurse's"* car in the driveway. These neighbors knocked on the door and waited to have Nancy listen to this woman's lungs, when she was having trouble breathing.
>
> After many months of decline in his physical and mental condition Abe eventually died at home with Cindy and all their children present. Dr. Smith, Nancy, and Laura, along with other members of the interdisciplinary hospice team, all contributed to supporting this family. Neighbors, friends, and members of the local church were supportive, which bodes well for continued family support. Cindy continues to talk to the social worker, who also serves as the bereavement coordinator for hospice, on a regular basis since Abe's death.

CHALLENGES ASSOCIATED WITH RURAL PALLIATIVE CARE

As illustrated in the case study, there are many challenges associated with providing rural palliative care. Distance and remoteness are real issues, not only for rural residents who are in need of palliative care services, but also for health care providers, who must travel great distances, often in inclement weather, to provide health care services. Abe, Cindy, and their health care providers encountered challenges on a daily basis involving long distances and remote locations. Canadian researchers (Castleden, Crooks, Schuurman, & Hanlon, 2010; Kaasalainen et al., 2011) have documented similar obstacles of great distances and remote locations, two factors that can be negatively influenced by weather during winter months. Health care providers working in rural settings spend more time traveling long distances, in comparison to health care providers working in more urban settings (Kaasalainen et al., 2011).

Initially, Cindy was reluctant to accept that Abe was not going to live forever, and the case study illuminates that the switch from a rehabilitation focus to a palliative focus can be particularly challenging for family members. This challenge has also been reported by Van Vorst and colleagues (2006), who conducted a study in rural Colorado and Kansas that surveyed health care personnel about the care provided to dying patients. In this study, health care providers identified the top three barriers to providing quality care to dying patients as: family member's avoidance of issues of dying (60%), differences in opinion among health care professionals (48%), and patients' avoidance of issues around dying (47%). Additional barriers identified by Van Vorst et al. (2006) included communication difficulties, health care professionals', own discomfort with death, personnel shortages, time constraints, and a lack of knowledge about palliative care.

Milone-Nuzzo, McCorkle, and Ercolano (2010) emphasized the need for a team approach to palliative care. A multi-disciplinary team improves the care provided to patients and their family caregivers and also provides support to all members of the team. Team members should include physicians, nurses, therapists, mental health workers, social workers, pharmacists, and paraprofessionals. In the case study, Dr. Smith, Nancy, and Laura developed a strong relationship with Abe, Cindy, and the rest of the family; however, this preexisting relationship presented a challenge for additional care providers, who were considered *"outsiders"* (Findholt, 2010). Including all members of the interdisciplinary team in weekly palliative care team meetings can build a strong team and facilitate a sense of *"familiarity"* between the team and the family (Lee, Winters, Boland, Raph, & Buehler, 2010), which in turn can assist clients and their families to overcome the perspective that some team members are *"outsiders."*

While multi-disciplinary palliative care teams are the norm in urban settings, developing a palliative care team in rural settings can be especially challenging due to the limited number of professionals available in rural environments. The limited number of interdisciplinary professionals practicing in rural settings means there are often a small number of professionals, perhaps only one physician and one home health registered nurse, available to provide palliative care services to rural residents. Such a shortage of professionals leads to limited or no on-call coverage for health care providers to attend conferences, take a vacation, and so on. Professionals in rural settings frequently report personal and professional role strain (Robinson et al., 2009; Winters & Lee, 2010). An additional challenge reported by Robinson et al. (2009) is that palliative care services account for only a small portion of rural generalists' daily workload, thus making it difficult for rural providers to stay current with best practices associated with palliative care.

A lack of palliative care providers in rural settings may necessitate long distance travel for health care services. Rural residents are generally well accustomed to driving long distances on a regular basis, but travel to more urban centers for health care may be particularly challenging for clients approaching the end of life. Pesut, Robinson, Bottorff, Fyles, and Broughton (2010) conducted a study that examined the experiences of rural cancer patients who traveled to an urban cancer center for palliative care and identified three major themes: "cultures of rural life and care; strategies for commuting; and effects of commuting" (p. 190). Challenges identified by study participants included anxiety related to managing symptoms while on the road and financial hardships associated with travel. Another challenge associated with travel for palliative care services is the necessity for a support person, such as a family member or friend, who is available to handle the logistics of travel while also providing emotional and physical support while away from home.

In addition to health care provider shortages, other resources tend to be more limited in rural settings, especially when compared to more urban centers. When rural residents have a choice between resources available from a distance versus more local resources, rural families often prefer to support local businesses, thus health care providers need knowledge of supplies and medications available locally. Symptom management can be especially challenging in rural settings, and long distances necessitate pre-planning. Health care professionals must be prepared to adequately address symptoms and pain management issues during nonbusiness hours, including holidays and weekends. Kaasalainen and colleagues (2011) surveyed 159 rural and urban nurses who delivered palliative care in community settings. Many of these rural nurses reported the benefits associated with having access to symptom control/response kits, and reported that access to such kits improved quality of care by decreasing the need for clients to travel to more urban settings for symptom management.

The lack of provider education/training is a barrier to providing palliative care in rural settings (Kaasalainen et al., 2011) and it is well documented that there is a need for ongoing continuing educational opportunities for health care providers providing palliative care to rural dwellers (Arnaert, Seller, & Wainwright, 2009; Elsey & McIntyre, 1996; Kaasalainen et al., 2011; Robinson, Pesut, & Bottorff, 2010). Another well acknowledged challenge is a need for team development activities to foster strong collegial relationships among palliative care teams, including opportunities for debriefing (Rushton et al., 2006) and meaning-centered interventions (Fillion, Dupuis, Tremblay, De Grâce, & Breitbart, 2006).

Emotional and physical isolation has been reported by homecare nurses providing palliative care to clients and families in rural Canada (Arnaert et al., 2009). Anonymity and privacy are limited when health care professionals live and work in the same community (Lee et al., 2010). All health care providers know the importance of patient confidentiality, but in small rural communities the lines of patient confidentiality are often blurred. In rural settings when there is an immediate need or concern, it is not uncommon for a family to call the nurse directly at home rather than call the main home health agency or hospice phone number, leave a message with the answering service, and have the on-call nurse, who is located 60 miles away, return their call and troubleshoot over the phone. This blurring of health care professionals' personal and professional identities has been reported by others (Lee et al., 2010; MacLeod, Kulig, Stewart, Pitblado, & Knock, 2004).

OPPORTUNITIES ASSOCIATED WITH RURAL PALLIATIVE CARE

Despite the many challenges that health care providers encounter when providing palliative care in rural settings, there also are tremendous opportunities for professional and personal rewards. The preceding case study illustrated several such opportunities, including community embededness and multi-disciplinary team collaboration (Arnaert et al., 2009). As care providers, nurse Nancy, Dr. Smith, and aide Laura were longstanding members of the rural community, they were well accepted by the rural residents, and were clearly part of the social network of the community. Caring for Abe as he was dying was like caring for a family member, and was both rewarding and emotionally draining. Support was shared among these three care providers, and they were also appreciative of support from the hospice interdisciplinary team, even if most of this support came over the phone. Just knowing there was someone on the other end of the phone line provided much-needed emotional support and reduced feelings of emotional and physical isolation (Arnaert et al., 2009).

Connectedness is an important concept in rural settings, and rural residents have reported feeling connected not only to their formal care providers, but also to their informal network of friends and neighbors (Duggleby et al., 2011). In the case presented here, Nancy, Laura, and Dr. Smith had close ties with Abe and Cindy and their family members, and this closeness developed over the many years they provided cared for Abe. In rural settings, support comes from many people, and in a study of rural cancer patients commuting for cancer treatment, participants expressed the many ways their friends and neighbors supported them, including bringing food over, assisting with chores on rural properties, providing transportation, and hosting fundraisers to obtain financial support to help with medical expenses (Pesut et al., 2010).

Technology can be used to overcome some of the challenges of providing palliative care in rural settings. The case study illustrates that health care providers were able to connect with their colleagues on the hospice interdisciplinary team using the telephone to overcome challenges associated with distance. Connecting to other team members by phone allows palliative care providers to feel supported and part of the team. Technology can also be used to provide continuing education—for example, using telehealth networks and videoconferencing systems to allow rural health care providers a means to participate in continuing education opportunities (Arnaert et al., 2009; Robinson et al., 2010).

The palliative care literature contains reports on additional technological innovations, including the development of an Internet-based consultation model (Kuebler & Bruera, 2000) and the evaluation of after-hours phone support (Phillips, Davidson, Newton, & DiGiacomo, 2008) for palliative care services. Kuebler and Bruera described their Internet-based collaborative consultative relationship and identified it as a potential means of support, which allows practitioners to provide holistic palliative interventions to patients. In rural Australia, researchers reported that patients and their caregivers appreciated access to a palliative care after-hours telephone support service (Phillips et al., 2008). These researchers reported that most calls occurred between the hours of 6 p.m. to midnight and attributed this to the isolation many family caregivers experience during nighttime hours.

Rural residents often report a strong sense of community (Kaasalainen et al., 2011; Kulig, Hegney, & Edge, 2010) and have well-developed social networks, which may offset some of the challenges of providing rural palliative care. Kaasalainen and colleagues (2011) reported that rural nurses reported significantly greater self-efficacy in palliative care than more urban nurses, a finding they believe may be related to the close-knit informal networks that exist in rural settings. Teamwork is important and, as Robinson et al. (2010) noted, in rural communities "it is often the spirit of cooperation and collaboration that overcomes resource challenges" (p. 82). The coordination of palliative care services has been reported to be more efficient in rural communities; this may be due in part to the close-knit communities and interpersonal working relationships that exist between health care providers working in rural areas. It is important to pay attention to the unique characteristics inherent in rural communities so that geographic, cultural, and health care needs of rural residents are considered when developing a team of health care professionals to provide rural palliative care. Researchers who study palliative care in rural settings stress the importance of teamwork as an essential element of palliative care programs (Arnaert et al., 2009; Kaasalainen et al., 2011; Kelley, Williams, DeMiglio, & Mettam, 2011; Robinson et al., 2010; Rosenberg & Canning, 2004).

SUMMARY

Providing palliative care services in rural settings places health care providers in a land of challenges and opportunities. While the challenges associated with providing palliative care in rural settings can be daunting, it is important to recognize the opportunities for personal and professional growth, for clients, family members, and health care professionals. Creativity, community connectedness, and interdisciplinary collaboration provide support for rural health care providers working with clients with incurable conditions and their family members. Challenges such as distance and limited resources can be managed by flexibility and pre-planning, along with an openness to consider new models of care delivery. Technological advances need to be considered to overcome the inherent challenges of distance associated with rural settings. Creative and caring approaches are needed to promote rural residents', quality of life during the illness trajectory. Palliative care includes the relief of suffering and care through the dying process, as well as bereavement care and support for surviving family members and friends after death. Providing palliative care in rural settings can be immensely rewarding for rural residents and their families and for the health care providers who overcome challenges on a daily basis by identifying opportunities for compassionate care.

REFERENCES

Arnaert, A., Seller, R., & Wainwright, M. (2009). Homecare nurses' attitudes toward palliative care in a rural community in western Quebec. *Journal of Hospice and Palliative Nursing, 11*(4), 202–208.

Castleden, H., Crooks, V. A., Schuurman, N., & Hanlon, N. (2010). "It's not necessarily the distance on the map...": Using place as an analytic tool to elucidate geographic issues central to rural palliative care. *Health & Place, 16,* 284–290.

Duggleby, W. D., Penz, K., Leipert, B. D., Wilson, D. M., Goodridge, D., & Williams, A. (2011). 'I am part of the community but ...': The changing context of rural living for persons with advanced cancer and their families. *Rural and Remote Health, 11,* 1733–1744.

Elsey, B., & McIntyre, J. (1996). Assessing a support and learning network for palliative care workers in a country area of South Australia. *Australian Journal of Rural Health, 4*(3), 372–380.

Field, M. J., & Cassel, C. K. (1997). *Approaching death: Improving care at the end of life* [Report of the Institute of Medicine Task Force]. Washington, DC: National Academy Press.

Fillion, L., Dupuis, L., Tremblay, I., De Grâce, G. R., & Breitbart, W. (2006). Enhancing meaning in palliative care practice: A meaning-centered intervention to promote job satisfaction. *Palliative and Supportive Care, 4*(4), 333–344.

Findholt, N. (2010). The culture of rural communities: An examination of rural nursing concepts at the community level. In C. A. Winters, & H. J. Lee

(Eds.), *Rural nursing: Concepts, theory and practice* (3rd ed., pp. 373–383). New York, NY: Springer Publishing.

Kaasalainen, S., Brazil, K., Wilson, D. M., Willison, K., Marshall, D., Taniguchi, A. et al. (2011). Palliative care nursing in rural and urban community settings: A comparative analysis. *International Journal of Palliative Nursing, 17*(7), 344–352.

Kelley, M. L., Williams, A., DeMiglio, L., & Mettam, H. (2011). Developing rural palliative care: Validating a conceptual model. *Rural and Remote Health, 11*, 1717–1728.

Kuebler, K. K., & Bruera, E. (2000). Interactive collaborative consultation model in end-of-life care. *Journal of Pain and Symptom Management, 20*(3), 202–209.

Kulig, J. C., Hegney, D., & Edge, D. S. (2010). Community resiliency and rural nursing: Canadian and Australian perspectives. In C. A. Winters, & H. J. Lee (Eds.), *Rural nursing: Concepts, theory and practice* (3rd ed., pp. 385–400). New York, NY: Springer Publishing.

Lee, H. J., Winters, C. A., Boland, R. L., Raph, S. J., & Buehler, J. A. (2010). An analysis of key concepts for rural nursing. In C. A. Winters, & H. J. Lee (Eds.), *Rural nursing: Concepts, theory and practice* (3rd ed., pp. 447–459). New York, NY: Springer Publishing.

MacLeod, M., Kulig, J. C., Stewart, N. J., Pitblado, J. R., & Knock, M. (2004). The nature of nursing practice in rural and remote Canada. *Australian Journal of Rural Health, 6*(2), 72–8.

Milone-Nuzzo, P., McCorkle, R., & Ercolano, E. (2010). Home care. In B. R. Ferrell, & N. Coyle (Eds.), *Oxford textbook of palliative nursing* (3rd ed., pp. 891–904). New York, NY: Oxford University Press.

National Consensus Project for Quality Palliative Care. (2009). *Clinical practice guidelines for quality palliative care* (2nd ed.). Retrieved February 1, 2011 from http://www.nationalconsensusproject.org/Guideline.pdf

Pesut, B., Robinson, C. A., Bottorff, J. L., Fyles, G., & Broughton, S. (2010). On the road again: Patient perspectives on commuting for palliative care. *Palliative and Supportive Care, 8*, 187–195.

Phillips, J. L., Davidson, P. M., Newton, P. J., & Digiacomo, M. (2008). Supporting patients and their caregivers after-hours at the end of life: The role of telephone support. *Journal of Pain and Symptom Management, 36*(1), 11–21.

Robinson, C. A., Pesut, B., & Bottorff, J. L. (2010). Issues in rural palliative care: Views from the countryside. *The Journal of Rural Health, 26*, 78–84.

Robinson, C. A., Pesut, B., Bottorff, J. L., Mowry, A., Broughton, S., & Fyles, G. (2009). Rural palliative care: A comprehensive review. *Journal of Palliative Medicine, 13*(3), 253–258.

Rosenberg, J. P., & Canning, D. F. (2004). Palliative care by nurses in rural and remote practice. *Australian Journal of Rural Health, 12*(4), 166–171.

Rushton, C. H., Reder, E., Hall, B., Comella, K., Sellers, D. E., & Hutton, N. (2006). Interdisciplinary interventions to improve pediatric palliative care and reduce health care professional suffering. *Journal of Palliative Medicine, 9*(4), 922–933.

Van Vorst, R. F., Crane, L. A., Barton, P. L., Kutner, J. S., Kallail, K. J., & Westfall, J. M. (2006). Barriers to quality care for dying patients in rural communities. *The Journal of Rural Health, 22*(3), 248–253.

Winters, C. A., & Lee, H. J. (2010). *Rural nursing: Concepts, theory and practice* (3rd ed.). New York, NY: Springer Publishing.

Chapter 9

PATTERNS OF RESPONSES TO SYMPTOMS IN RURAL RESIDENTS: THE SYMPTOM–ACTION–TIMELINE PROCESS

Janice A. Buehler, Maureen Malone, and Janis M. Majerus-Wegerhoff

HOW PEOPLE IDENTIFY, EVALUATE, AND RESPOND to symptoms is an important determinant of their health and illness behavior (Lenz, 1984). An increasing amount of literature addresses health behaviors of rural people (Lee, 1991; Long, 1993; Long & Weinert, 1989; Moon & Graybird, 1982; Weinert & Long, 1990). However, less information is available on the patterns of responses of rural people to symptom occurrence that signifies actual or potential health problems. In addition, there is a paucity of information on health behaviors of certain rural groups, specifically, women and Plains Indians.

Although actual processes of health-seeking behavior are not delineated in most research on rural health behaviors, some patterns are evident. A survey of health risk prevalence in rural Montana (Moon & Graybird, 1982) revealed that participants believed in self-responsibility for health. Lee (1991) noted that the quality of hardiness may be responsible for some rural dwellers' delay in seeking assistance from the professional health care system when symptoms of illness appear. Rural people were viewed as delaying health care until they were very ill, thus often needing hospitalization at the point care was sought (Long, 1993; Long & Weinert, 1989; Rosenblatt & Moscovice, 1982; Weinert & Long, 1990).

Studies of responses to symptom occurrence not specific to rural people have been conducted by behavioral and social scientists. Mechanic (1960) stated that possible responses to illness include discretionary inaction, the use of medicines, seeking professional care, and using a lay network. Suchman (1966) described individual responses to symptom occurrence as proceeding in this sequential pattern: (a) symptom experience stage, (b) assumption of sick role stage, (c) medical care contact stage, and (d) dependent patient role stage.

Segall and Goldstein (1989) noted that lay persons clearly do routinely self-evaluate and self-treat many of their health problems as a part of daily living and that the nature and extent of these self-care practices are not well understood. They concluded it is not clear whether self-care behavior is equally prevalent among different social groups, whether self-care is used for both health maintenance and the treatment of illness, and whether self-care is used only in response to selected symptomatic conditions.

METHODS

The qualitative method of grounded theory was used in this study (Glaser & Strauss, 1967). Grounded theory provides a means of understanding behavioral patterns from the perspective of the participants. It enables learning about their world and the interacting influences of personal, social, and cultural characteristics without imposing the cultural biases of the interviewer (Chenitz & Swanson, 1986). Grounded theory allows for the direct examination of the world of rural residents in a naturalistic way (Schatzman & Strauss, 1973).

The convenience sample was composed of 16 rural or frontier Montana women, 8 of whom were Native American women living on a federal reservation, and 8 of whom were Caucasian farm or ranch women. Elison (1986) defined *rural* as a population density of more than 6 but less than 100 per square mile and a driving distance to a hospital of at least 30 minutes. *Frontier* is defined as a population density of less than 6 per square mile and driving time to a hospital of either 60 minutes or severe geographic and/or seasonal climatic conditions.

The eight Caucasian farm or ranch women were married and had at least two children. Six of these women were self-employed, actively farming and ranching with their husbands. Two were employed in a small city 60 miles from their homes. Four of these women lived in rural locations and four in frontier locations. Their nearest neighbors lived one-fourth mile to 8 miles away. One informant's nearest neighbor was 5 miles away but did not have a phone. For emergencies, this informant would travel 12 miles to the nearest neighbor with a telephone. The primary means of paying for health services for these women was through private pay and individual health insurance.

Of the eight Native American women, seven were classified as rural and one as frontier. Five of the informants lived on small ranches and three lived in one of two towns each with populations of less than 200

(U.S. Bureau of Census, 1987). Seven of the informants have lived on the reservation all of their lives. Three of the women were unemployed and on Aid to Families with Dependent Children, two considered themselves full-time homemakers, and the remaining three were employed in local towns. Five of the Native American women were married, two were single, and one was divorced. All informants had children, with an average number of 2.3 children per household and a range of 1 to 6 children per household. Five informants lived with extended family members, and three lived with only their children and husbands. All eight women used the Indian Health Service, which provided free health care, as entitled by the treaty.

Face-to-face focused interviews were conducted in the homes of the participants. Open-ended interview questions and probes were used to stimulate free responses (Woods & Catanzaro, 1988). Topics included describing the steps used when someone in the home becomes ill, examples of when self-treatment would be used or when someone would be consulted, signs indicating illness, examples of home remedies, length of time before seeking help, and reasons for deterrence in obtaining care from professional health resources.

The grounded theory data analysis for this study revealed a basic social process (BSP) termed the *symptom–action–timeline* (SATL) *process*.

FINDINGS

Both Native American and Caucasian farm/ranch women used the SATL process to respond to symptoms of actual or potential health problems. The process consists of four stages in which symptoms are identified and actions are taken to move to a desired state of health. The stages are (a) symptom identification, (b) self-care, (c) lay resources, and (d) professional resources. Each stage has a time period (timeline) in which the participant takes actions in response to a symptom, evaluates the effectiveness of the actions in resolving the symptom, and decides whether to go on to the next stage. Time periods during stages are dependent on the intensity, duration, and amount of interference in function caused by the symptom and may be minutes, days, or years. The first stage, symptom identification, is the stimulus leading to the other stages.

Symptom Identification Stage

Symptom identification was preceded by symptom occurrence and included assessment of conditions or signs perceived as being an undesired alteration in the person's usual state of health that required actions to move the person to his or her desired state. Participants identified their desired state as being the way they were before the symptoms occurred. The symptoms had three properties: physical signs and sensations, degree of interference in the ability to function, and intensity and duration. Physical signs included "fever," "vomiting," "pain," "pulling at ears," "broken bones," "hard to breathe," and "losing blood." Interference in function included "not being able to do ordinary things like housework," "I couldn't move my finger," and "unable to eat or play." Intensity and duration of symptoms were the degree and rate of change in symptoms, the onset of new symptoms, and the length of time they persist. Examples included "temperatures over 102 degrees for 3 days" and "a bloody nose that couldn't be stopped after 2 hours." After the symptoms were assessed, they were given meaning, and a decision was made whether to take action. This was dependent on knowledge and past experience with illness, intensity and duration of the symptoms, and degree of interference with normal functioning. A Native American woman stated, "Whenever my girl pulls at her ears and is fussy, I know from before that she probably has an ear infection and we should go in [to the clinic].... The first time [she was sick] I waited until she had a fever, and it went so high it really scared me." Participants in both groups stated they noticed most symptoms within minutes to a few hours after occurrence.

Variation noted between Caucasian and Native American women in symptom identification was due to meanings given to symptoms. For example, one of the Native American women, after getting no relief from headaches through use of medications prescribed by a physician, attributed her headaches to supernatural origins and sought care from a medicine man. Both groups of women described lower thresholds of tolerance for duration and intensity of symptoms in their children. This resulted in shorter SATL processes for children.

Self-Care Stage

The second stage of the SATL process was characterized by the initiation of self-care. *Self-care* involved those activities self-initiated and performed for self or family members in response to symptoms. Examples of self-care listed by respondents ranged from "getting extra rest," "slowing down," "waiting for more symptoms" to more complicated activities such as "soaking my foot three times a day." The timeline described by both groups of women for starting self-care after symptom identification was seconds for intense symptoms to a "couple of days" for minor symptoms.

The self-care stage was also characterized by using self-care tools, those items used by the respondent to resolve symptoms on her own. Both groups listed such items as nonprescription medications, leftover prescription medicine, teas, thermometers, heating pads, disinfectants, and reference books. The majority of the Native American women used traditional self-care tools to treat certain symptoms. These included sage, sweetgrass, and medicine bundles. One Native American woman used a first aid book for reference whereas half the Caucasian ranch women regularly referred to their "family health textbooks." One informant in this group stated, "I looked up symptoms my daughter had, and the book told me what I could do for her at home or if I needed to see a doctor." Another informant added, "Everyone in my family knows how to look up their illnesses in our health book." All of these informants live in the frontier area. Another self-care tool mentioned only by these frontier women was "animal" ointments to treat hand rashes resulting from feeding lambs.

Actions for this stage included initiating self-care; evaluating its effectiveness based on a decrease in the duration, intensity, or the amount of interference in the ability to function; and deciding to seek help if self-care was ineffective. A typical response, for both Native American and Caucasian informants, regarding the decision to seek help was, "I tried taking Tylenol but after two days I still had a fever, so I called my mother for advice."

Lay Resources Stage

In this third stage, the participants involved their informal network of family, friends, and neighbors, that is, their *lay resources*, by describing the symptoms and obtaining assistance to alleviate symptoms. Properties of this stage included symptom validation, asking advice for self-care or self-care tools, receiving physical care, and seeking emotional support—particularly for deciding to go to a physician. Timelines for consulting lay resources after symptom identification ranged from 1 to 3 days for both groups. Both groups had usually initiated a self-care activity before they consulted their lay resources.

Ranch women stated their most frequently used lay resources were their mothers, but they also consulted with neighbors. Two frontier ranch women described how they had become aware of each other having similar joint pain of the great toe. They compared their symptoms over the phone while referring to their health textbooks that guided them to diagnosing themselves as having gout. They then verified these symptoms and information with another lay resource, a neighbor who was a registered nurse (RN). Ranch women also described an organized informal lay network of volunteer farmers and ranchers who acted as first responders to emergencies. They were called for such symptoms as "chest pain," "losing blood," and "broken bones."

Organized volunteer networks of lay resources were not described by Native American women. The majority identified their mothers as their primary source of help. A few consulted only with their husbands, stating that they had no relatives or friends living in the area for them to contact. Participants stated they would usually consult a relative before they would consult a neighbor who was not a relative. The majority of the Native American women also consulted their lay network for advice on the use of traditional healing practices. The following described this use of a lay resource.

> My son (9-months-old) had been fussy for two days; he was not taking his bottle and had cold sweats. Tylenol didn't seem to be helping, so my mother suggested that I take him to my aunt because he might have colic. My aunt massaged him and blew smoke in his ear. He went to sleep and was OK after that.

Actions for this stage included contacting a lay resource; evaluating whether there was a decrease in the symptom's intensity, duration, or interference with function; and deciding whether to take further action. Varying degrees of self-care continued throughout this stage.

Professional Resources Stage

Seeking help from *professional resources* occurred when there was failure to alleviate symptoms through the use of self-care or lay resources, when symptoms intensified, or when new symptoms developed. Professional resources listed by both groups included physicians, RNs, dentists, and chiropractors. Both groups stated they consulted professional help when "nothing else helped," "there wasn't anything I could do," or "for emergencies." Nurses were sometimes consulted for advice about whether symptoms required immediate attention or could wait a while longer. Nurses were frequently used as lay resources in this instance, since they were called at their homes when off duty. Physicians were usually not called at home unless the participant had been under physician care for a specific condition.

Timelines, from the symptom identification stage to the professional resource stage in situations other than emergencies, were 4 to 7 days for rural women and 1 to 2 weeks for frontier women. Timelines for Native American women ranged from 2 to 5 days in both rural and frontier areas.

Timeline variations occurred for children and in emergencies. For children, total timeline durations were much shorter, ranging from less than 1 day to 3 days. Each stage within the timeline process was shorter; lay resources were consulted sooner and often were used only to help transport the child to the professional resource. Barriers to seeking professional care were minimized so that time and distance became less important for children than for adults. In emergencies, individuals tended to bypass self-care and lay resources and go directly to professionals. Barriers were minimized according to the urgency of symptom occurrence.

If symptoms were not alleviated after going to a professional resource, participants either returned to the same professional or went to a different professional. At times, symptoms were simply "tolerated." Several Native American women sought alternative care by contacting a medicine man.

This occurred because they believed physicians had not helped. The medicine man was described by these participants as another type of professional. The most frequently identified barriers to professional resources were distance and transportation. Other barriers mentioned were fear of "bad news," a lack of women doctors, and the time required to see a professional, especially time spent in waiting rooms.

IMPLICATIONS

The SATL process clarifies response patterns rural women display when confronted with symptoms of actual or potential health problems. The process provides a framework for health care professionals that is client centered, and, therefore has powerful implications for intervention and health education; promotes culturally sensitive planning and provision of health services; and adds to the body of literature on rural use of health resources.

The SATL process provides a systematic framework for health care providers to assess patterns of response to symptoms and to develop interventions to facilitate rural residents' responses to their symptoms. For a full understanding of what actions a rural client will use to alleviate a health problem, each stage in the process must be carefully assessed on an individual basis.

CONCLUSION

Findings in this study suggest that rural residents use several indicators to identify and evaluate their symptoms. These indicators can be clarified by using the properties of the symptom identification stage as an assessment guide. It will yield information on what signs and sensations prompted symptom identification, tolerance levels for symptoms, amount of interference caused by symptoms, knowledge levels about symptoms, meanings of symptoms, and the timeline and conditions necessary for taking further actions. With these baseline data, health care providers can determine a client's capability to accurately interpret a symptom and take appropriate actions. Corresponding interventions may be aimed at increasing the client's knowledge of indicators of disease processes and the preferable time period in which to initiate an action.

Through assessment of the self-care stage of a client's SATL, information can be elicited regarding the client's self-care patterns. This includes the conditions under which self-care is activated and the variety of self-care tools that are available and employed by the client. Interventions can be directed at expanding a person's access to more effective self-care tools or adapting health care to the tools already available to the person. Findings in this study suggest that assessment of self-care resources leads to an evaluation of a client's lay resources, since self-care tools are often shared with a network of relatives or neighbors. Knowing whom a rural client most often relies on for symptom validation provides valuable information about functional support systems actively used by rural/frontier people. Interventions with a rural client may be more effective if key people in these networks are included.

Assessment of the professional resource stage provides information about the conditions necessary for an individual to seek professional care, appropriateness of timelines, and barriers that prevent access to care. For example, if clients are seeking professional care for conditions that could be handled at home, interventions can be aimed at making a client's response pattern clear to both the provider and the client by using the SATL process. With this information, the client and provider can identify which response in the process is deficient and mutually determine a more appropriate response.

The multidimensionality of the SATL process increases health professional's awareness of the dimensions and complexities involved in caring for people from diverse cultural and geographical backgrounds. A health care provider can identify cultural views of health and illness by using the SATL process. These beliefs are deeply entwined within traditional customs and culture. By gaining insight into the traditional attitudes that people have toward health and illness, health care providers can become more sensitive to the issues surrounding health care and the cultural health beliefs of the consumer, thereby providing more comprehensive health care.

Finally, the SATL process has important implications for research. Although research studies appear in the literature on self-care, use of lay or informal health resources, and use of formal health services, these studies tend to focus on single health resource utilization. The SATL process begins to explicate how various types of health resources are used in an integrated manner by actual rural/frontier residents. Furthermore, the preponderance of literature on consumer use of health resources focuses on urban rather than rural populations. Further research is needed to validate the use of the SATL process among rural and urban subpopulations.

REFERENCES

Chenitz, W., & Swanson, J. (1986). *From practice to grounded theory.* Menlo Park, CA: Addison-Wesley.

Elison, G. (1986). Frontier areas: Problems for delivery of health care services. *Rural Health Care, 8*(5), 1, 3.

Glaser, B., & Strauss, A. (1967). *Discovery of grounded theory.* Chicago: Aldine.

Lee, H. J. (1991). Relationship of hardiness and current life events to perceived health in rural adults. *Research in Nursing and Health, 14,* 351–359.

Lenz, E. (1984). Information seeking: A component of client decisions and health behavior. *Advances in Nursing Science, 6*(3), 59–72.

Long, K. A. (1993). The concept of health: Rural perspectives. *Nursing Clinics of North America, 28*(1), 123–130.

Long, K. A., & Weinert, C. (1989). Rural nursing: Developing the theory base. *Scholarly Inquiry for Nursing Practice: An International Journal, 3*(2), 113–131.

Mechanic, D. (1960). Illness behavior and medical diagnosis. *Journal of Health Social Behavior, 1,* 86–94.

Moon, R., & Graybird, D. (1982). *High risk prevalence: A report card for Montana.* Helena, Montana: Department of Health and Environmental Sciences.

Rosenblatt, R., & Moscovice, I. (1982). *Rural health care.* New York, NY: Wiley.

Schatzman, L., & Strauss, A. (1973). *Field research.* Englewood Cliffs, NJ: Prentice-Hall.

Segall, A., & Goldstein, J. (1989). Exploring the correlates of self-provided health care behavior. *Social Science Medicine, 29*(2), 153–161.

Suchman, E. (1966). Health orientation and medical care. *American Journal of Public Health, 56*(1), 97–105.

U.S. Bureau of Census. (1987). *Statistical abstract of the United States: 1988* (108th ed.). Washington, DC: U.S. Government Printing Office.

Weinert, C., & Long, K. A. (1990). Rural families and health care: Refining the knowledge base. *The Journal of Marriage and Family Review, 15*(1–2), 57–75.

Woods, N. F., & Catanzaro, M. (1988). *Nursing research: Theory and practice.* St. Louis: Mosby.

Chapter 10

BEYOND THE SYMPTOM–ACTION–TIMELINE PROCESS: EXPLICATING THE HEALTH-NEEDS–ACTION PROCESS

Andrea D. Rasmussen, Chad O'Lynn,
and Charlene A. Winters

IN CHAPTER 9, AN IMPORTANT STUDY by Buehler, Malone, and Majerus is reprinted from the first edition of this book (1998). The Buehler et al. study is important because the authors proposed an initial model detailing how rural dwellers recognize health symptoms and the process rural dwellers go through in relieving those symptoms. As Buehler et al. noted, the significance of such a model is the provision of a framework from which health care providers can better assess an individual's interpretation and response to symptoms and then work with them to more accurately interpret symptoms and choose responses that optimize health outcomes. The model also offers health care providers a framework to better assess all resources available to individuals (such as self-care or lay resources) that might be tapped to resolve health problems and provide emotional support during illness. Buehler et al. recommended additional research to validate the use of their *Symptom–Action–Timeline* (SATL) process model for rural dwellers.

In 2010, O'Lynn examined the SATL process and made several recommendations that would allow the model to be used in other studies. O'Lynn's literature review supported the SATL process; however, he proposed a revised model titled the *Symptom Action Process* (SAP). The SAP model is intended to be more inclusive of the various rural subgroups and their health behaviors and holistic health needs. In addition, O'Lynn theorized that findings from studies using the new SAP model would provide health professionals and policy makers a better understanding of how health needs are manifested and interpreted in rural settings.

In this chapter, we report the findings of a recent literature review designed to examine the level of support for the SATL process (Buehler et al., 1998) and O'Lynn's (2010) SAP model. We specifically address the recommendations proposed by O'Lynn to: (a) expand the definition of symptom to include psychological symptoms; (b) expand the definition of symptom to be more reflective of a health need so that self-care measures to prevent illness or promote health are included; (c) recognize that intentional disregard of a health need is a type of self-care action, especially when mental health needs are involved; (d) embed the model within an environmental context external to the decision tree to account for demographic variables, access to resources, and so on; and (e) design the model to be more circular in nature, allowing for sequential or concurrent health-related actions.

On the basis of the findings from our review of the literature, we recommend the SAP model be expanded and renamed the *Health-Needs–Action Process* (HNAP) model to incorporate all holistic aspects of the above. We further propose additional studies be conducted with rural populations, both domestically and internationally, to explore support for the revised model.

REVIEW OF THE SATL PROCESS AND THE SAP MODEL

The SATL Process

We present a brief review and graphic depiction of the SATL in this section; however, we refer the reader to chapter 9 for more details about the SATL process. The SATL process and SAP model will be compared in a graphic description later in the chapter.

The SATL process encompasses four phases: (a) symptom identification, (b) self-care, (c) lay resources, and (d) professional resources (Figure 10.1). The process is preceded by the occurrence of a symptom, defined as an alteration in the usual state of health that requires action. Unless that symptom is recognized by an individual (symptom identification), the SATL process does not continue. It is important to note that *symptom* was defined as a negative entity (Buehler et al., 1998) and the SATL process as one of resolving a problem.

Symptoms are characterized by three general components: (a) physical signs and sensations, (b) degree of interference with the person's usual or desired level of functioning, and (c) intensity and duration of the symptom (Buehler et al., 1998). These three characteristics, coupled with an individual's prior experience of and knowledge of the symptom, are used in assigning meaning to the symptom. Based on this meaning, an individual will decide whether to take action. According to Buehler et al., self-care is the first action taken after identifying a symptom.

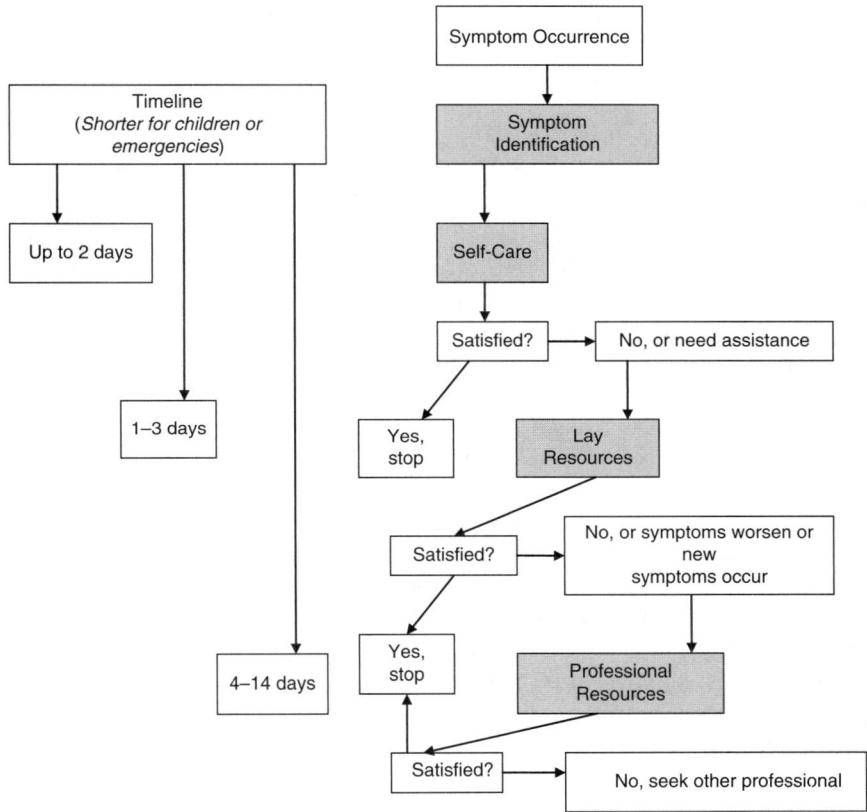

FIGURE 10.1 Symptom–Action–Timeline (SATL) process. (Adapted from Buehler, Malone, & Majerus, 1998)

Self-care refers to the myriad activities initiated by and performed by an individual to relieve a symptom (Buehler et al., 1998). For individuals relying upon others for their health needs (e.g., dependent children and elders), family members or other caretakers would be responsible for initiating activities to address an identified symptom. Self-care activities include applying home remedies, taking over-the-counter medications and herbal preparations, using the Internet and reading reference books to learn more about the symptom and symptom resolution. Self-care activities, as well as all other actions taken in the SATL process, are evaluated by the individual in terms of efficacy, and a decision is made whether to proceed through the SATL process, alter actions, or cease activities.

If self-care activities do not resolve a symptom to the individual's satisfaction, family, friends, and neighbors are consulted. These lay resources are used to provide (a) validation of symptom interpretation, (b) advice and emotional support, and (c) physical care (Buehler et al., 1998). Although not defined by Buehler et al., unlike professional resources, lay resources are not financially reimbursed for their services. If symptoms do not resolve, if symptoms intensify, or additional symptoms occur, professional resources are then sought. If professional resources do not lead to symptom resolution, individuals may seek other professional resources.

The time one takes to navigate the SATL process (Buehler et al., 1998) is influenced by the intensity and duration of a symptom and the degree to which the symptom interferes with usual functioning. Actions are implemented more quickly when a symptom is particularly intense, greatly interferes with usual functioning, or children are involved. If the symptom is interpreted as an emergency, the individual may seek professional care immediately and bypass the early phases of the SATL process. However, if the SATL process is completed in its entirety, the time from symptom identification to self-care can take up to 2 days; from symptom identification to lay resources can take from 1 to 3 days, and from symptom identification to professional resources can take from 4 to 14 days. How individuals progress through the SATL process has great implications for health care providers and researchers. It is important to note that a major limitation to the SATL process is the lack of reference to health prevention and health promotion activities utilized by rural dwellers. This is in contrast to both the SAP model proposed by O'Lynn (2010) and the HNAP model proposed by the authors of the present chapter, which accounts for health promotion and prevention and incorporates a holistic multitherapeutic approach.

SAP Model

In general, the SAP model supports the SATL process as described by Buehler et al. (1998), but with a few revisions. Buehler et al. described a symptom as a physical sign or sensation. SATL is focused on problem solving and does not address activities to prevent illness and promote health. O'Lynn (2010) noted that the SATL definition of symptom was quite narrow and proposed that the concept of *symptom* be replaced with *health need*. A health need can be a biophysical need, as well as a spiritual, emotional, social, and psychological need. A health need is more holistic than a symptom and would provide a broader perspective of rural dwellers' response to perceived health and wellness needs (O'Lynn, 2010). The inclusion of psychological symptoms, such as those typically seen in depressive and anxiety disorders, is vital because mental health services are often unavailable or poorly implemented in rural communities (DeLeon, Wakefield, & Hagglund, 2003; Dobalian, Tsao, & Radcliff, 2003; Haard & Anderson, 2004; Kane & Ennis, 1996; National Institute of Nursing Research, 1995).

Unlike the linear SATL process, the SAP model includes a circular process that allows for multiple actions—self-care, lay resources, and

EXTERNAL CONTEXT AND VARIABLES

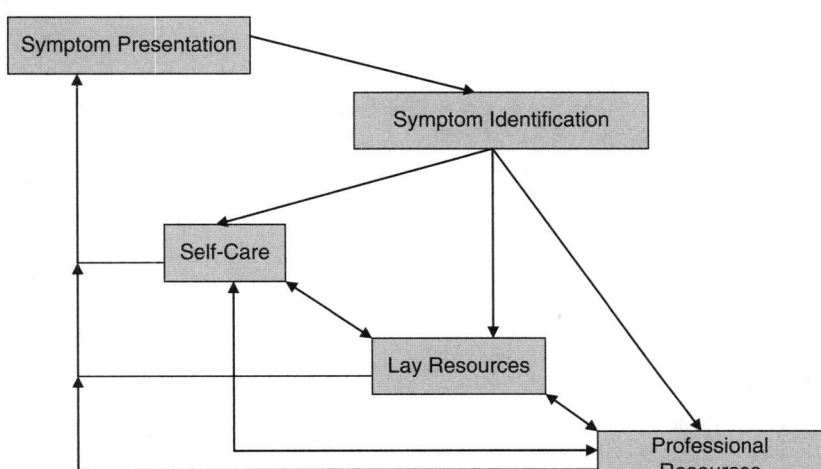

FIGURE 10.2 Symptom–action process (SAP): a revision of the SATL process. (Adapted from O'Lynn, 2010)

professional resources—to be incorporated in a sequential *or* concurrent fashion (Figure 10.2). This approach is different from the more linear SATL process, which details the process of resolving a single symptom or health problem, for example, fever or broken bone. The SAP can be used by individuals for multiple symptoms, an important consideration when responding to chronic illnesses. Chronic conditions, such as diabetes or congestive heart failure, are characterized by the recurrence of multiple symptoms with varying degrees of intensity and duration. Using the more circular SAP model, one can readily explain how an individual might use prayer, hot packs, support from friends, prescription drugs, and physical therapy concurrently to manage an illness or injury, and might vary use of these strategies over time as health needs wax and wane.

The SAP model also recognizes the act of ignoring a health need or symptom as a type of self-care action. This is often seen with rural men (Levant & Habben, 2003; Sellers, Poduska, Propp, & White, 1999) and depressed persons seeking treatment for somatic health needs (such as fatigue, pain, changes in appetite) while ignoring the depressive symptomatology (lack of interest in usual habits, sadness, etc.) that accompanies the somatic issues. Moreover, some cultural beliefs are rooted in traditions that perceive psychological health needs as conditions resulting from spiritual or magical causes or see the needs as a weakness (Garcia, Gilchrist, Vazquez, Leite, & Raymond, 2011), highlighting the need to consider the context external to the decision-making process to understand rural persons' approach to health needs. In addition to culture and tradition, gender, race, ethnicity, educational achievement, socioeconomic status, family and social role, residential location, and barriers to resources, among others, provide the environment in which decisions are made.

On the basis of our review of the literature, we propose renaming the SAP model as the HNAP model. By replacing the term *symptom* with *health need* we believe that the model more accurately reflects a broader spectrum of rural health demands, including psychological and physiological acute and chronic conditions.

METHOD USED FOR LITERATURE REVIEW

Much of the literature pertaining to rural health care focuses on (a) disparities in health for rural dwellers as compared with nonrural dwellers, (b) description of the health of rural dwellers, (c) use of complementary alternative medicine and treatments (CAM), (d) barriers to accessing health care services for rural dwellers, and (e) the experiences and demographics of health care providers in rural areas. None of these broad areas of literature directly addresses the SATL process or SAP model in identifying health needs and actions to resolve them, with the possible exception of access barriers. Buehler et al. (1998) touched on access barriers in that additional effort is made to overcome the barriers if children were involved or symptoms were deemed emergent. Access barriers modulate the SATL process rather than serving as foundational antecedents in determining the components of the process itself. O'Lynn (2010) did not include access barriers in his literature review and as a result barriers to care were not included in this review.

In March 2012, we conducted a search of peer-reviewed resources contained in the Cumulative Index to Nursing and Allied Health Literature (CINAHL), MedLine, Psych Info, PubMed, and Google Scholar, to locate research-based support for the SATL process and SAP model. Resources published from July 2004 through March 2012 were searched, using the keyword of *rural* and its associated keywords of *rural health, rural environment, rural community, frontier,* and *rural populations*. Rural keywords were the primary sorting category to ensure that rural dwellers would be salient in the literature, although use of the SATL process and SAP model may be made in nonrural populations as well. We then combined the rural keywords with other keywords, based on available keyword search options within each database that were suggestive of the SATL process and SAP model, including *self-care, health needs, health behaviors, illness behavior, attitudes and beliefs for self-care, decision-making, self-assessment, alternative therapies, complimentary medicine,* and *home remedies*. We excluded dissertation abstracts because of the difficulty of obtaining full texts of multiple dissertations. The search yielded a total of 583 journal articles.

From the 583 articles, we excluded review articles, case studies, and anecdotal reports, resulting in a new pool of 87 research-based journal articles. We then excluded all articles reporting studies occurring outside the United States, congruent with O'Lynn's (2010) review. This latter exclusion is reasonable because the study by Buehler et al. (1998) occurred in the United States. These steps resulted in 71 articles available for review.

Following a critical review of the 71 articles, we excluded studies that did not address components relevant to the SATL process or the SAP model and studies that focused only on health care providers. The final sample of articles for review included 21 research reports.

FINDINGS FROM THE LITERATURE REVIEW

The 21 studies included in this review were published between July 2004 and March 2012. Participants in these studies represented Arizona, Indiana, Louisiana, Michigan, Montana, New Mexico, North Carolina, North and South Dakota, Pennsylvania, Tennessee, Texas, West Virginia, and Wyoming. All of the studies included rural dwellers, although five studies (24%) included urban participants as a comparison group. The mean age of the rural dwellers in this literature review was 63.12 years. The Buehler et al. (1998) study did not include age ranges, therefore this study was not included in the current review's mean age calculation. Table 10.1 shows the gender and racial or ethnic characteristics of

TABLE 10.1 Participants' Demographic Characteristics from Current Review ($N = 21$ studies)

Characteristic	N	%
Gender		
All female	6	29
Mixed	15	71
All male	0	0
Mean age	63.12 y ($N = 20$)	NA
Race/Ethnicity		
All non-Hispanic White	3	14
Mixed	13	62
All minority	2	10
Unknown	3	14
US States represented	14	28

the participants. Notably absent in the studies were Asian or Pacific Islander participants. Otherwise, non-Hispanic Caucasian, African American, Native American, and Hispanic participants were well represented.

Buehler et al. (1998) and O'Lynn (2010) noted a paucity in the literature of resources that describe the *process* rural individuals undertake in managing symptoms/health needs once they have been identified. We confirmed this paucity in the present literature review. Of the 21 studies reviewed, 13 (62%) minimally supported the tendency to use self-care and lay resources before going to a health professional for nonemergent symptoms experienced by adults (Albert, Musa, Kwoh, Hanlon, & Silverman, 2008; Arcury et al., 2006, 2009; Buehler et al., 1998; Clark et al., 2008; Duran et al., 2005; Garcia et al., 2011; Harju, Wuensch, Kuhl, & Cross, 2006; Ruggiero, Gros, McCauley, De Arellano, & Danielson, 2011; Shreffler-Grant, Weinert, Nichols, & Ide, 2005; Stoller et al., 2011; Vallerand, Fouladbakhsh, & Templin, 2005; Zhang, Jones, Spalding, Young, & Ragain, 2009). However, none of these studies described or tested a comprehensive process of health needs identification and actions.

The majority of the studies we reviewed confirmed the *use of self-care strategies* to treat symptoms (Albert et al., 2008; Arcury et al., 2006, 2009; Brown & May, 2005; Buehler et al., 1998; Callaghan, 2005; Clark et al., 2008; Duran et al., 2005; Easom & Quinn, 2006; Garcia et al., 2011; Harju et al., 2006; Ruggiero et al., 2011; Shreffler-Grant et al., 2005; Stoller et al., 2011; Vallerand et al., 2005; Winters, Cudney, & Sullivan, 2010; Winters, Cudney, Sullivan, & Thuesen, 2006; Zhang et al., 2009). Many of these studies supported the self-care strategies described by Buehler et al. (1998) and O'Lynn (2010), including taking over-the-counter medications, herbal remedies, CAM, and family remedies; referring to health information sources via the Internet, books, and television; and using physical treatments (e.g., heating pads, stretching, massage, or yoga). A number of authors reported the value of prayer and spirituality as self-care strategies (Arcury et al., 2011; Duran et al., 2005; Easom & Quinn, 2006; Harju et al., 2006; Winters et al., 2010). Buehler et al. did not discuss these strategies. In some of the studies that compared rural and nonrural dwellers, researchers noted that rural dwellers were more likely than nonrural dwellers to use self-care strategies to treat symptoms (Garcia et al., 2011; Harju et al., 2006; Ruggiero et al., 2011; Winters et al., 2010).

We also found support for the *use of lay resources* in managing symptoms in the studies reviewed. Primarily, researchers reported the strategies of soliciting the assistance and support of friends and family in managing symptoms and in using formal support groups (Albert et al., 2008; Arcury et al., 2006, 2009, 2011; Buehler et al., 1998; Clark et al., 2008; Duran et al., 2005; Easom & Quinn, 2006; Garcia et al., 2011; Goins, Spencer, & Williams, 2010; Ruggiero et al., 2011; Shreffler-Grant et al., 2005; Stoller et al., 2011; Vallerand et al., 2005; Winters et al., 2006, 2010; Zhang et al., 2009). In addition, in nine (43%) of the studies that we reviewed, the researchers reported the progression to lay resource use after self-care had failed, or the use of lay resources prior to the use of professional resources (Arcury et al., 2006; Brown & May, 2005; Buehler et al., 1998; Clark et al., 2008; Easom & Quinn, 2006; Harju et al., 2006; Shreffler-Grant et al., 2005; Vallerand et al., 2005; Winters et al., 2006).

In terms of gender, women were well represented in the sample of studies we reviewed, including six studies in which women were studied exclusively. In only one study from O'Lynn's review in 2010 (Sellers et al., 1999) did researchers examine men or men's health exclusively; our literature review did not return any studies that focused exclusively on men. This limitation is significant because Sellers et al. noted that although both men and women may rely on self-care and lay resources before utilizing professional resources, men may interpret symptoms very differently and may delay use of professional resources as long as possible (Levant & Habben, 2003; Sabo & Gordon, 1995; Sellers et al., 1999). Consequently, men may incorporate very different time frames for actions.

Generally, the results of the studies support the finding from Buehler et al. (1998) and O'Lynn (2010) that professional resources are utilized after self-care or lay resources are used. Some of the studies we reviewed included the use of complementary or alternative therapies to manage symptoms (Arcury et al., 2006, 2009, 2011; Buehler et al., 1998; Duran et al., 2005; Easom & Quinn, 2006; Harju et al., 2006; Shreffler-Grant et al., 2005; Winters et al., 2010). Complementary therapies included spiritual interventions, as noted earlier, but also included the use of professional resources such as those provided by a masseuse, acupuncturist, naturopath, chiropractor, and herbalist. Other results supported the finding that professional resources are utilized if symptoms persisted (Arcury et al., 2006; Brown & May, 2005; Buehler et al., 1998; Clark et al., 2008; Easom & Quinn, 2006; Harju et al., 2006; Shreffler-Grant et al., 2005; Vallerand et al., 2005; Winters et al., 2006, 2010).

Consistent with O'Lynn's review (2010), none of the researchers of the studies we reviewed provided specific time frames for utilizing resources as described by Buehler et al. (1998). However, research results did support the timeline tenets within the SATL process, particularly those referring to the use of professional resources. The results found that progression to and direct utilization of professional resources was quicker if (a) symptoms involved children (Buehler et al., 1998), (b) symptoms were perceived as emergent or crisis in nature (Arcury et al., 2006; Brown & May, 2005; Buehler et al., 1998; Clark et al., 2008; Easom & Quinn, 2006; Harju et al., 2006; Shreffler-Grant et al., 2005; Vallerand et al., 2005), (c) the individual perceived a need for a prescription to treat the symptom (Buehler et al., 1998; Harju et al., 2006; Winters et al., 2010), or (d) if the symptom would result in the individual missing work (Buehler et al., 1998; Cudney et al., 2006; Harju et al., 2006).

Buehler et al. (1998) reported that if professional resources were not effective in relieving symptoms, participants continued to work with the professional, sought another professional (particularly a provider of alternative therapy), or accepted the symptom's nonresolution. As noted by O'Lynn (2010), we also found in the studies we reviewed that researchers did not address this specific decision point in the same fashion. However, a number of researchers reported the concurrent use of multiple strategies, including complementary or alternative therapies (Albert et al., 2008; Arcury et al., 2006, 2009, 2011; Brown & May, 2005; Buehler et al., 1998; Duran et al., 2005; Easom & Quinn, 2006; Garcia et al., 2011; Simmons, Huddleston-Casas, & Berry, 2007; Stoller et al., 2011; Vallerand et al., 2005; Winters et al., 2006, 2010). A table of characteristic variables pulled from the literature review is displayed in Table 10.2.

TABLE 10.2 Characteristic Variables Found in the Current Literature Review (N = 21 studies)

Characteristic Variables	n	%
Self-care resources utilized	18	86
Lay resources	18	86
Decision-making process	17	81
Rural population only	16	76
Multiple strategies used	15	71
Self and lay care used before professional services	13	62
Health promotion	11	52
Barriers to care	11	52
Lay resources to professional	9	43
Cultural beliefs	8	38
Symptom–action process discussed	7	33
Use of CAM* therapies	7	33
Self-efficacy	5	24
Rural vs. nonrural population	5	24
Prayer/Spirituality self-care	4	19
Direct use of professional services when:		
Children are involved	1	5
Prescription is needed	3	14
Possible loss of employment	3	14

*CAM = complementary alternative medicine.

DISCUSSION

The literature review provides overall support for aspects of the SATL process and the SAP model used by rural dwellers. Although none of the researchers contradicted the model proposed by Buehler et al. (1998) or O'Lynn (2010), no researcher discussed or tested a comprehensive process for health needs identification and action. It should be noted, however, that the number of studies we reviewed was small. Most of the studies were cross-sectional and descriptive in design, limiting the ability to confirm use of the SATL process or SAP model over time. Similar to O'Lynn's review, most of the research we reviewed had small sample sizes and focused primarily on rural dwellers over 50 years of age (mean age = 63.12 years). To be consistent with the O'Lynn's review, we did not include participants residing outside the United States. We recommend studies be conducted with larger samples, younger participants, as well as outside of the United States, to further support the proposed change from the SAP to the HNAP model. With the exception of the Asian or Pacific Islander communities, the literature we reviewed represented racial or ethnic diversity. In addition, the literature represented geographic diversity. We recommend that studies examining rural Alaskan and Hawaiian communities be conducted to provide additional information about the HNAP model. We concur with O'Lynn (2010) that additional studies of men in rural communities should be conducted to further strengthen the HNAP model. Rural health needs of men differ from those of women and would add great value to this model.

A limitation of the SATL process model is Buehler et al.'s (1998) lack of attention to symptoms that are recognized as problematic but ignored. For example, one may recognize a self-limiting symptom such as a strained muscle, but choose no action to relieve the strain. An interesting finding in our review is that stigma and embarrassment influence health pattern behaviors in rural women diagnosed with depression and other mental health issues (Simmons, Huddleston-Casas, & Berry, 2007). Both the SAP and HNAP literature reviews found self-efficacy and health behavior patterns to be similar when comparing rural and nonrural dwellers' compliance with personal health needs management and both SAP and HNAP reviews allow for prevention and management of various health needs, including psychological needs (Garcia et al., 2011; Harju et al., 2006; Simmons et al., 2007; Winters et al., 2010; Harju et al., 2006). Additional research is needed to explore how stigma, embarrassment, and other factors such as lack of anonymity, familiarity, and isolation from lay resources influence individuals' recognition and response to health needs.

The emphasis on the timeline aspect of the SATL process model is problematic, in that it suggests a rather linear progression through phases of symptom identification, and actions are taken while previous strategies may be abandoned because of unsatisfactory outcomes. We concur with O'Lynn (2010) that the literature we reviewed did not support this process and that instead, multiple modes of treatment are utilized singularly or concurrently. Our review also supports O'Lynn in that as rural dwellers become more educated and familiar with interpreting and identifying recurring health symptoms, they may bypass self-care and lay care and go directly to professional resources. This is more prevalent in those suffering from chronic conditions (Albert et al., 2008; Buehler et al., 1998; Easom & Quinn, 2006; Stoller et al., 2011; Winters et al., 2006, 2010). A study done by Stoller et al. described the older rural adult who was managing both new symptoms and chronic diseases as a "bricoleur"—a kind of informal professional do-it-yourself person who blends information gathered from multiple sources. Managing the process of chronic symptoms and new health needs is well identified in the proposed HNAP model.

Buehler et al. (1998) and O'Lynn (2010) noted that time frames for action were influenced by whether or not the symptoms were associated with children or with emergent conditions. Our review agrees with this process. In addition, as noted previously, others have suggested that time frames for action are also influenced by whether or not symptoms required a prescription or caused one to miss work (Buehler et al., 1998; Harju et al., 2006; Winters et al., 2006, 2010). It is reasonable to assume that barriers in accessing health resources for rural dwellers, as described widely in the literature, will influence how quickly or slowly one may adopt actions to address health need symptoms. As such, time frames are descriptive outcomes resulting from the contextual variables.

Perceived barriers such as pain, lack of information, and knowledge were noted in three of the studies we reviewed (Callaghan, 2005; Easom & Quinn, 2006; Vallerand et al., 2005). Lack of information and knowledge (coupled with pain) has been found to be related to health promotion activities. (Easom & Quinn, 2006). Adding to that is psychological well-being and the ability of rural dwellers to self-identify their health needs (Callaghan, 2005; Duran et al., 2005; Garcia et al., 2011; Ruggiero et al., 2011; Simmons et al., 2007; Winters et al., 2010). O'Lynn (2010) recognized the importance of including psychological symptoms in the model and noted that mental health services are often unavailable or poorly implemented in rural communities. The HNAP model allows for psychological symptomatology to be identified and treated alongside of physical symptoms (as would be the case in pain management, depression, and/or anxiety with new onset or chronic disease management). Depression in rural women is a growing public health concern, and many of the women underreport their symptoms due to stigma and/or a lack of knowledge regarding their symptoms (Simmons et al., 2007). Oftentimes with depression, anxiety, and other psychological disorders, symptoms present with somatic symptoms as well, making them difficult to identify. Our review validated that multiple strategies are used (as depicted in the

HNAP model) to address both psychological and physical health needs in rural populations.

RECOMMENDATIONS FOR THE NEW HNAP MODEL

Figure 10.3 shows a graphic depiction of the HNAP model. The action process of the HNAP is embedded in an external context identical to the SAP model. The two models are similar in all facets of identification, decision-making processes, and actions taken by rural dwellers. The only difference between the SAP and the HNAP model is the replacement of the term *symptom* with *health needs* to include physical and psychological health conditions and states. After health needs are identified in the HNAP model, individuals may incorporate various types of actions: (a) self-care, (b) lay resources, and (c) professional resources in a sequential or concurrent fashion. The contexts will influence which action, or combination of actions, is taken. The sloping nature of the action types reflects the propensity to progress from self-care to lay resource use to professional resource use. The double arrows between action types account for fluid movement among aspects of the model and concurrent use of types of actions. More explicit in this model are the arrows leading from the

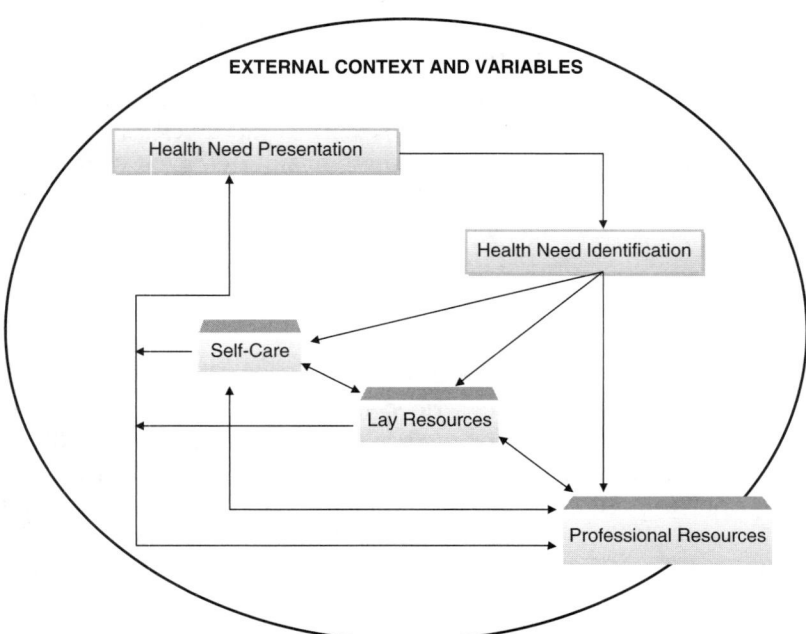

FIGURE 10.3 Health-Needs–Action Process (HNAP) model. (Proposed by Rasmussen, O'Lynn, and Winters, 2012)

action types back to the symptom occurrence aspect of the model. These arrows close the circle of the process and account for symptoms that might recur, new symptoms that develop, or new actions resulting from new information or previous actions taken by an individual.

Both the SATL process model and HNAP model depict a process in which an individual identifies a problem or health need and takes action(s) to address it. As such, these models may describe the behaviors of all individuals, including nonrural dwellers, although how actions are taken may differ across populations. To address the limitations of the newly proposed HNAP model, we recommend that further research be conducted to:

1. Evaluate how well the revised HNAP model is empirically supported. If the revised model is well supported, then it may serve as an ideal framework for comparison studies examining health behaviors across participant demographic variables.
2. Identify responses to health needs in rural men and younger individuals to support the revised HNAP model in these populations.
3. Incorporate studies done both internationally and domestically to support rural populations' health need patterns, behaviors, and treatment processes.
4. Address barriers that prevent rural dwellers from health promotion, prevention, and treatment options, including cultural, physical, and psychological impediments that may interfere with the revised HNAP foundation.
5. Provide insight and support regarding cultural practices, beliefs, and decision-making processes in rural dwellers for overall health promotion, illness prevention, and treatment using a holistic interpretation.

CONCLUSION

Buehler et al. (1998) derived the SATL process model from a grounded theory study in which they described the process that a group of rural Montana women used to respond to health symptoms. O'Lynn (2010) completed a literature review to determine the level of support for the SATL process and proposed changes, resulting in a more circular model called SAP. The current literature review was conducted to determine the level of support for the SATL and SAP models and resulted in the HNAP model. We reviewed 21 research studies located in the CINAHL, MedLine, PsychInfo, PubMed, and Google Scholar databases that focused on the process rural dwellers use to respond to health needs. Those studies provide general support for aspects of the SATL process, the SAP model, and the new HNAP model, although in only seven studies did researchers describe a sequential process of how rural dwellers respond to health symptoms (Albert et al., 2008; Arcury et al., 2009, 2011; Buehler et al., 1998; Stoller et al., 2011; Vallerand et al., 2005; Winters et al., 2010).

We recommend further research with younger participants, rural men, and rural Asian or Pacific Islander participants to determine the support for the revised model. In addition, identifying if cultural, physical, and/or psychological barriers inhibit rural populations (such as rural Asian or Pacific Islander) from health promotion, prevention, and treatment would further support the revised SAP model, now renamed HNAP. Finally, we recommend an examination of studies completed outside the continental U.S. to determine whether the revised model has broad relevance to rural dwellers across the globe.

REFERENCES

Albert, S. M., Musa, D., Kwoh, C. K., Hanlon, J. T., & Silverman, M. (2008). Self-care and professionally guided care in osteoarthritis—Racial differences in a population-based sample. *Journal of Aging and Health*, 20(2), 198–216.

Arcury, T. A., Bell, R. A., Snively, B. M., Smith, S. L., Skelly, A. H., Wetmore, L. K. et al. (2006). Complementary and alternative medicine use as health self-management: Rural older adults with diabetes. *Journal of Gerontology: Social Sciences*, 61B(2), S62–S70.

Arcury, T. A., Grzywacz, J. G., Neiberg, R. H., Lang, W., Nguyen, H. T. et al. (2011). Daily use of complementary and other therapies for symptoms among older adults: Study design and illustrative results. *Journal of Aging and Health*, 23(1), 52–69.

Arcury, T. A., Grzywacz, J. G., Stoller, E. P., Bell, R. A., Altizer, K. P., Chapman, C. et al. (2009). Complementary therapy use and health self-management among rural older adults. *Journal of Gerontology: Social Sciences*, 64B(5), 635–643.

Brown, J. W., & May, B. A. (2005). Rural older Appalachian women's formal patterns of care. *Southern Online Journal of Nursing Research*, 2(6), 1–21.

Buehler, J., Malone, M., & Majerus, J. (1998). Patterns of responses to symptoms in rural residents: The symptom-action-time-line process. In H. Lee (Ed.), *Conceptual basis for rural nursing* (pp. 153–162). New York, NY: Springer Publishing.

Callaghan, D. (2005). Healthy behaviors, self-efficacy, self-care, and basic conditioning factors in older adults. *Journal of Community Health Nursing*, 22(3), 169–178.

Clark, D. O., Frankel, R. M., Morgan, D. L., Ricketts, G., Bair, M. J., Nyland, K. A. et al. (2008). The meaning and significance of self-management among socioeconomically vulnerable older adults. *Journal of Gerontology: Social Sciences, 63B*(5), S312–S319.

DeLeon, P., Wakefield, M., & Hagglund, K. (2003). The behavioral health care needs of rural communities in the 21st century. In B. Stamm (Ed.), *Rural behavioral health care: An interdisciplinary guide* (pp. 23–32). Washington, DC: American Psychological Association.

Dobalian, A., Tsao, J. C., & Radcliff, T. A. (2003). Diagnosed mental and physical health conditions in the United States nursing home population: Differences between urban and rural facilities. *Journal of Rural Health, 19*, 477–483.

Duran, B., Oetzel, J., Lucero, J., Jiang, Y., Novins, D. K., Manson, et al. (2005). Obstacles for rural American Indians seeking alcohol, drug, or mental health treatment. *Journal of Consulting and Clinical Psychology, 73*(5), 819–829.

Easom, L. R., & Quinn, M. E. (2006). Rural elderly caregivers: Exploring folk home remedy use and health promotion activities. *Online Journal of Rural Nursing and Health Care, 6*(1), 32–46.

Garcia, C. M., Gilchrist, L., Vazques, G., Leite, A., & Raymond, N. (2011). Urban and rural immigrant Latino youths and adults' knowledge and beliefs about mental health resources. *Journal of Immigrant Minority Health, 13*, 500–509.

Goins, R. T., Spencer, S. M., & Williams, K. (2010). Lay meanings of health among rural older adults in Appalachia. *The Journal of Rural Health, 27*, 13–20.

Haard, L., & Anderson, E. (2004). Factors related to depression in rural and urban noncustodial, low-income fathers. *Journal of Community Psychology, 32*(1), 103–119.

Harju, B. L., Wuensch, K. L., Kuhl, E. A., & Cross, N. J. (2006). Comparison of rural and urban residents' implicit and explicit attitudes related to seeking medical care. *National Rural Health Association, Fall,* 359–363.

Kane, C. F., & Ennis, J. M. (1996). Health care reform and rural mental health: Severe mental illness. *Community Mental Health Journal, 32*, 445–462.

Levant, R., & Habben, C. (2003). The new psychology of men: Application to rural men. In B. Stamm (Ed.), *Rural behavioral health care: An interdisciplinary guide* (pp. 171–180). Washington, DC: American Psychological Association.

National Institute of Nursing Research. (1995). *Chapter 2: Rural America: Challenges and opportunities*. Retrieved April 9, 2003, from http//ninr.nih.gov/ninr/research/vol7/chapter2.html

O'Lynn, C. (2010). Updating the symptom-action-time-line process. In H. Lee (Ed.), *Conceptual basis for rural nursing* (pp. 163–178). New York, NY: Springer Publishing.

Ruggiero, K. J., Gros, D. F., McCauley, J., de Arellano, M. A., & Danielson, C. K. (2011). Rural adults' use of health-related information online: Data from a 2006 national online health survey. *Telemedicine and e-Health, 17*(5), 329–334.

Sabo, D., & Gordon, D. F. (1995). Rethinking men's health and illness. In D. Sabo & D. F. Gordon (Eds.), *Men's health and illness: Gender, power, and the body* (pp. 1–22). Thousand Oaks, CA: Sage.

Sellers, S. C., Poduska, M. D., Propp, L. H., & White, S. I. (1999). The health care meanings, values, and practices of Anglo-American males in the rural Midwest. *Journal of Transcultural Nursing, 10*, 320–330.

Shreffler-Grant, J., Weinert, C., Nicholls, E., & Ide, B. (2005). Complementary therapy use among older rural adults. *Public Health Nursing, 22*(4), 323–331.

Simmons, L. A., Huddleston-Casas, C., & Berry, A. A. (2007). Low-income rural women and depression: Factors associated with self-reporting. *American Journal of Health Behavior, 31*(6), 657–666.

Stoller, E. P., Grzywacz, J. G., Quandt, S. A., Bell, R. A., Chapman, C., Altizer, K. P., ... Arcury, T. A. (2011). Calling the doctor: A qualitative study of patient-initiated physician consultation among rural older adults. *Journal of Aging and Health, 23*(5), 782–805.

Vallerand, A. H., Fouladbakhsh, J. M., & Templin, T. (2005). Patients' choices for the self-treatment of pain. *Applied Nursing Research, 18*, 90–96.

Winters, C. A., Cudney, S., & Sullivan, T. (2010). Expressions of depression in rural women with chronic illness. *Rural and Remote Health, 10*, 1–14.

Winters, C. A., Cudney, S., Sullivan, T., & Thuesen, A. (2006). The rural context and women's self-management of chronic health conditions. *Chronic Illness, 2*, 273–289.

Zhang, Y., Jones, B., Spalding, M., Young, R., & Ragain, M. (2009). Use of the Internet for health information among primary care patients in rural west Texas. *Southern Medical Journal, 102*(6), 595–601.

Chapter 11

CHRONIC ILLNESS EXPERIENCE OF ISOLATED RURAL WOMEN: USE OF AN ONLINE SUPPORT GROUP INTERVENTION

Charlene A. Winters and
Therese Sullivan

CHRONIC ILLNESS HAS LONG BEEN a major public health problem (Husaine & Moore, 1990; Jensen, 1991; Marks, 2003; Stuifbergen, 1995) affecting more than 133 million Americans in 2005—or nearly one of every two adults (Centers for Disease Control [CDC], 2010; Wu & Green, 2000). Seven of every ten Americans who die each year die of a chronic disease; more than 50% of these deaths can be attributed to cancer, heart disease, and stroke (CDC, 2010; Kung, Hoyert, Xu, & Murphy, 2008). Effective self-management is instrumental to a person's ability to adapt successfully to his or her illness and maintain a quality life. Education; support from family, friends, and health care providers; and the ability to manage uncertainty have long been recognized as important factors in chronic illness self-management (Strauss et al., 1984).

CHRONIC ILLNESS IN AMERICA

Arthritis and other rheumatic conditions, cancer, diabetes, and multiple sclerosis (MS) are common among Americans, affecting more than 75 million people. Recent national figures indicate that arthritis and other rheumatic conditions alone affect nearly 46 million Americans and continue to be the leading causes of disability (Hootman, Bolen, Helmick, & Langmaid, 2006). Cancer continues to be the second leading cause of death in the United States, and more than 11 million people are living with a history of cancer (Ries et al., 2008). Diabetes mellitus (DM) affects 24 million Americans and is the leading cause of new cases of blindness, kidney failure, and lower extremity amputations (CDC, 2011). Just having DM greatly increases a person's risk for heart attack or stroke (Albright, 2008). In 2004, more than 400,000 people living in the United States had multiple sclerosis (MS), and 200 new cases were diagnosed each week (About MS, 2004). MS is most common in the northern states and occurs mostly in women of northern European ancestry aged 20–50 years.

RURAL/URBAN HEALTH DIFFERENCES

Health differences between urban and rural dwellers have long been recognized and can be attributed in part to differences in community demographic, economic, physical, social, and environmental characteristics (recognized by Eberhardt et al., 2001; Ingram & Franco, 2012). The context within which chronic illness occurs has a significant impact on how the chronically ill arrange for services and support. People living in sparsely populated rural areas have few health care providers, hospitals, and other resources (Agency for Healthcare Policy and Research, 1996; Gesler, Hartwell, Ricketts, & Rosenberg, 1992; Health & Human Services [HHS] Rural Task Force, 2002; Meit, 2004; Muskie School, 2003). Living in rural areas with few health care resources may complicate an individual's ability to manage his or her illness. For example, in Montana, a person may need to travel 120 miles one way to a health care specialist (Winters, 1999) or 320 miles round trip to an illness-related support group in many areas public transportation is inadequate or nonexistent.

CHRONIC ILLNESS SELF-MANAGEMENT

Management of chronic illness requires persons to recognize and control symptoms; implement prescribed treatments; adjust to changes in the course of the disease; prevent medical crises; attempt to normalize daily life; fund medical care; and confront emotional, marital, and family problems (Benet, 1996; Hwu, 1995; Robinson, 1993; Strauss et al., 1984; Winters, 1997, 1999). An individual's adaptive behaviors, psychosocial outcomes, and ability to provide self-care are influenced by uncertainty about the meaning of symptoms and treatment outcomes (Mast, 1995; Mishel, 1993; Strauss, et al., 1984; Weiner, 1975). Uncertainty occurs when people lack the information or knowledge needed to understand their illness and is influenced by resources available to assist persons in the interpretation of illness-related events. Resources include relationships individuals have with their health care providers, cognitive ability, and social support (Mast, 1995; Mishel, 1984).

More than one-fifth of America's population lives in rural areas (United States Census Bureau, 2000), yet little is known about how rural persons experience chronic illness (Scott, 2000). Our purpose for this chapter is to describe the chronic illness experiences of isolated rural women living with arthritis, fibromyalgia, cancer, diabetes, and MS.

METHODS

We conducted a secondary analysis of existing data from one cohort of participants in the Women to Women Project (WTW). WTW is a large-scale, multiphase intervention study that provides online peer support and health education via computer and the Internet to isolated rural women living with chronic illness. The overall goal of WTW is to evaluate the impact of participation on psychosocial health. In Phase I of WTW, a purposive sample of 120 chronically ill women from one western American state was randomized into four cohorts of 30 women. Each cohort had 15 women with computers and 15 women without computers. The computer groups participated in an online support group using an asynchronous chat room and structured education sessions spanning a period of 5 months. The groups without computers did not participate in the computer-based activities and continued to use their usual sources of support and information. All participants received a three-ring binder containing a description of the study and articles on a variety of health issues pertinent to women with chronic illness. Each participant completed written questionnaires to measure psychosocial outcomes over a 10-month period (Sullivan, Weinert, & Cudney, 2003; Weinert, 2000). Although WTW addressed psychosocial health, the study we describe in this chapter specifically focused on the experiences of living with chronic illness shared by the women in one computer group. The Montana State University-Bozeman Human Subjects Committee approved this study.

Sample

Eligible participants in WTW were women diagnosed with cancer, DM, rheumatoid diseases, or MS who lived at least 25 miles from an urbanized area (12,500 people or more). All women in WTW were required to read and speak English, have sufficient dexterity to communicate using a computer keyboard, and have a telephone in their home. The women were recruited to participate via word-of-mouth and with the help of voluntary agencies, state agricultural extension services, schools of nursing, parish nurses, nursing students, health professionals, public and professional libraries, newspapers, and public television announcements.

Participants in the study we report on in this chapter came from one computer group ($n = 15$). We chose this cohort because it was the first cohort to complete WTW. We included all women in the computer group in the sample. Fourteen of the women were Caucasian and one was Native American. All the women were from rural areas and lived on farms or in small towns. Eight of the women worked full time outside the home; two were full-time homemakers; five were unemployed. The women reported their primary health problem to be cancer ($n = 2$), MS ($n = 5$), rheumatoid arthritis or fibromyalgia ($n = 5$), and DM ($n = 3$). Mean age was 47.2 years and the average time between illness diagnosis and the beginning of the study was 5.29 years.

Data Collection

We analyzed qualitative and demographic data collected for WTW and made no direct or indirect contact with the participants during this study. The qualitative data consisted of 453 messages posted to the online support group chat room by the women over a 22-week period. The messages were conversations held between group members on topics of their choice. They had been stored verbatim in the end-user database then downloaded by the WTW research assistant for analysis. Although all the women participated in the discussions, the number of messages posted and their lengths varied. The number of postings ranged from 4 to 118 ($m = 57.18$; sd $= 39.30$) and the time spent online ranged from 346 to 3,239 minutes ($m = 1370.23$; sd $= 873.37$), indicating that women were spending time online even if they were not posting.

The quantitative data analyzed for the study consisted of demographic information. The data were collected as part of the screening interview to determine eligibility for participation in WTW. Electronic and printed copies of the data were provided to us by the WTW project manager under the direction of the principal investigator for WTW.

Data Analysis

We checked a printed copy of each chat room conversation for accuracy with the electronic data, and then analyzed the conversations for common themes using methods described by Miles and Huberman (1994). We analyzed chat room conversations specifically by (a) reading each conversation completely to get a sense of the whole, (b) dividing conversations into units denoted by a change in subject matter or activities described, and (c) labeling individual units from each conversation using a word or words that represented the unit topic (descriptive codes) and writing them in the margins of each printed copy. We also wrote theoretic memos (thoughts about the connections between the codes) in the margins. We continued coding until we classified all of the data. After coding by hand on the hard copy, we entered the electronic file of each conversation into QSR

NUD*IST (Version 4), a software program designed to manage qualitative data. We then entered the codes for each conversation and compared them with other coded conversations to identify common themes among them. To confirm and validate findings, we linked all initial codes, theoretic memos, and the emerging themes to primary data sources. We discussed emerging themes until we achieved consensus.

We analyzed quantitative data to provide a description of the participants and to provide context for the qualitative findings. We displayed all data using *Statistical Package for the Social Sciences* (Version 11.5) and analyzed the data using descriptive statistics to determine item frequencies and measures of central tendency.

FINDINGS

It was clear from the qualitative data that the women in the computer group felt positive about the intervention. They were pleased to have access to information about their illness and to other women facing similar challenges. Many expressed feeling a "connection" with group members. Some women referred to the group as their "cyber friends," exchanged phone numbers, and made plans to meet off-line. In addition to talking about their illnesses, the women shared stories about their families, exchanged recipes, described vacations, and told jokes. They offered words of support, prayer, and hope for "better times" for their online peers and their family members. As the computer intervention was nearing conclusion, the women expressed sadness about losing the connection with their newly made friends. They spoke of "going through withdrawal" and having a "hard time" giving up the program. One participant wrote,

> I will miss visiting with you all. There have been times when I felt too crummy to type anything, but I could always read. My last exacerbation would have been 10 times worse if I had not been able to hear your words of wisdom, jokes, and suggestions for better health.

Common Themes

We identified six common themes from analyzing the online support group conversations.

1. Uncertainty/searching for answers
2. Physical and emotional isolation
3. Maintaining balance

4. Others first
5. Vigilance: financial, physical, emotional
6. Ways of coping

Uncertainty/Searching for Answers

The women experienced uncertainty throughout their illness experiences. Before diagnosis, uncertainty was related to not knowing what was happening to them and the inability of their health care providers to provide an immediate explanation of their symptoms. A long diagnostic process was common, requiring trips to more than one health care provider before the correct diagnosis was made. One woman wrote, "I can't even count how many things I went to the doctor for over the years that I am now told are symptoms of this hateful illness." The average time from onset of symptoms to diagnosis was 9.7 years (range = 1–32 years). Frustration and an erosion of trust in their physician's judgment accompanied uncertainty, while women who were quickly diagnosed thought of their health care provider as "good."

Diagnosis did not put an end to the uncertainty. New or changing symptoms were common as were new treatments with unfamiliar outcomes and side effects. Uncertainty prompted a search for information, explanations, and answers. The women read about their illnesses and asked questions of their health care providers. During the intervention, the women asked others in the group if they had similar experiences to their own and were relieved to hear that they did. One woman expressed surprise and relief at the similarities of the experiences described by the women. She had felt alone and doubted her "stability," thinking that she must have been making things up in her head because "doctors couldn't seem to find a reason" for her symptoms.

Physical and Emotional Isolation

The women lived in rural communities or on farms, in areas of few health care resources, and they had little contact with other chronically ill women. The women felt emotionally isolated, afraid to talk about their illnesses with persons who were not ill for fear of alienating them and straining their relationships. They wrote of not being able to tell non-ill persons how they really felt for fear they would tire of hearing from them and "walk away." Although they had the support of family and friends, not being able to share feelings about their illnesses with others who were not ill potentially decreased the support they received and promoted their sense of emotional isolation. As one woman wrote, "This disease accomplishes one thing. It isolates."

Maintaining Balance

This theme referred to the women's roles, responsibilities, and need to balance activities and energies to maintain each role. Eight of the 15 women worked full time outside the home. One commented, "I need to say NO to more things and not get so upset over things that haven't gotten done. I know this but I need to remember it." Limited or no access to health care providers, pharmacies, and other health care services sometimes strained the women's ability to maintain balance. The need to travel to distant cities for specialized health care sometimes required an overnight stay and the driving assistance of a family member or friend. Time away from home and work affected the delicate balance the women were trying to achieve.

Others First

The women in this study put the needs of their communities, employers, and families before their own. They found time to provide community service and participate in civic activities, spend time with friends, and assist neighbors in need. The women worked long hours at home, and for employers, while still finding time to see to the needs of their spouses and children, whether the children were living at home or not. The women wrote about accompanying family members and friends to various activities that often involved long hours in the car. Putting others first affected their ability to maintain balance in their lives by draining their energy and exacerbating their symptoms. Although sometimes uncertain about how their activities would affect them, over time the women learned that they would "pay the price" if they did too much. However, knowing this did not guarantee that they would pull back. Oftentimes they would continue their activities and suffer the consequences.

> I need to share with you ... maybe it is like true confessions ... how I didn't accept responsibility for my recent exacerbation. My employer needed ... my church needed ... my students needed ... and all the time I was getting more tired and nauseated but I kept on going until I was really sick.

Vigilance

We used this theme to describe the alert watchfulness the women displayed toward their physical, emotional, and financial health. Prior to diagnosis, the women actively sought meaning for their symptoms. After diagnosis, the women were alert for any changes that might indicate improvement or deterioration in their conditions, the onset of new problems, or treatment side effects. During the intervention, the women discussed at length their symptoms, queried others to see if they were experiencing similar problems, and shared strategies used to manage them. The most common physical symptoms discussed were pain, sleeplessness, and fatigue. The most common emotions expressed were frustration, depression, and stress.

The cost of care was a frequent topic of discussion among the women. Many shared that they were stressed by the financial burden of health care and uncertain about how they would pay for their care. The women spent a considerable amount of their time dealing with this issue. Online, the women shared strategies to cut costs, finance care, and navigate the bureaucratic red tape of the programs that assist persons with chronic illness. Some expressed their appreciation for health insurance and concern for those who did not have coverage. They welcomed assistance from husbands who would "handle all that."

Ways of Coping

We used this theme to describe several methods used by the women to cope with their illnesses. Common methods included information gathering and self-care. The women took active roles caring for themselves by learning about their illnesses through reading, attending informational sessions presented by experts in the field, and asking questions of their health care providers. As one woman wrote, taking an active role in her health care and not waiting for the doctors to "tell her what to think and do" provided a sense of "control over her illness." The women participated in their prescribed treatments but also tried new things, such as herbs and special diets, with the hope of improving their well-being. They frequently shared self-care strategies with their online peers. Good communication and positive relationships with their health care providers were viewed as essential to their ability to cope with their illnesses. Women who felt that they were "heard" by their health care provider evaluated them as "good" and "caring." A good relationship with their health care providers was important enough to prompt some women to change doctors.

Faith and humor were frequently used as coping mechanisms. The women's conversations frequently included references to scripture, prayer, and faith. Funny stories, anecdotes, and jokes were also common and well received. The women commented on several occasions how good it was for them to laugh and asked their peers to "Keep the jokes coming."

Keeping busy, even though activity could exacerbate their symptoms, was a common strategy used by the women. Participants attempted to maintain normalcy in their lives by maintaining their usual routines and activities. The women tried to balance their activities with rest periods but often did more than they should have done. Maintaining normalcy also involved not talking about their illness with persons who were not ill.

The support network of family and friends was an important coping mechanism. Although persons without illness might not have fully understood what the women were going through, their help was needed and appreciated. Contact with other chronically ill persons was seen as especially helpful. The women expressed a great deal of appreciation for their online peers. One woman wrote, "I have gotten so used to talking to all of you! It's different than talking to anyone else, because we can 'let it all hang out' and everyone understands. Thanks for listening to me and encouraging me." Reaching out and providing support to others was also important. The women shared information, gave advice, and demonstrated concern and compassion for members of the online group and their families.

DISCUSSION AND IMPLICATIONS

The findings from the qualitative data support what is already known about chronic illness and add knowledge specific to living with chronic illness in a rural setting. The data confirmed that chronically ill persons strive to understand their illnesses, recognize and control symptoms, implement prescribed treatments, adjust to changes in the course of the diseases, deal with uncertainty, attempt to normalize daily life, find ways to fund medical care, and confront emotional and physical problems (Strauss et al., 1984). The findings also corroborate that difficulty in achieving a diagnosis can lead to uncertainty and an erosion of faith in the physician (Mishel, 1988, 1993; Mishel & Braden, 1988). The findings support the emotional isolation commonly felt by persons with chronic illnesses (Davies & Sque, 2002) and the importance of support, understanding, and a sense of collaboration between patient and health care provider (FitzGerald, Pearson, & McCutcheon, 2001).

The findings specific to managing chronic illness in a rural setting were experiences related to physical isolation and limited access to others with a similar condition. The emotional isolation the women in this study experienced may have been complicated by their physical isolation. Distance, weather conditions, and geographical constraints affected the women's access to health care providers and health care resources and potentially decreased the support available to them. For example, some of the women in this study traveled hundreds of miles to reach the closest health care specialists, not because they were the "best," but because they were the closest to them. It was also common for those who attended presentations by health experts to have to travel 3 or more hours to a distant city to attend the seminar.

Distance is an accepted part of rural living (Long & Weinert, 1989). However, traveling can be arduous for ill persons, physically and financially, and often involves careful planning. A trip to the specialist sometimes meant an overnight stay, required the driving assistance of a family member or friend, as well as additional trips for diagnostic testing and follow-up care. Effective time management and advanced planning were essential components of the women's illness management strategies. Health care specialists can help decrease the physical and financial burden of chronic illness with thoughtful scheduling, effective communication, and careful collaboration with the women's local health care providers when appropriate. In some circumstances, the use of telemedicine may be an appropriate alternative to a trip to a distant health care specialist.

The women had the support of family members; however, some lived a distance away. They were also physically isolated from other persons living with similar health problems. The women believed that persons who were not ill were less able to understand what they were going through. They also worried that "compassion fatigue" would become a problem for family and friends who were nearby. As a result, the women "put on a happy face" and "didn't let others know how they felt" and experienced emotional isolation. Health care providers can help their patients cope with their illness by encouraging what has worked—in this case, faith, humor, and keeping busy. Facilitating a phone number or e-mail exchange between interested patients or recommending one of the many professional organizations that have online support groups can be empowering (Burrows, Nettleton, Pleace, Loader, & Muncer, 2000) and should be considered. Given the positive experiences of the 15 women in this study, an online chronic illness support group appears to be a viable solution to the problem of isolation. However, additional research is needed to examine the value and health benefits of virtual communities (Eysenbach, Powell, Englesakis, Rizo, & Stern, 2004).

The women were frustrated by delayed or difficult diagnoses, professionals who "didn't listen," and the high costs of care. The women desired to be understood, to understand what was happening to them, and to be able to implement appropriate self-care strategies. Clear, open, and frequent communication with clients may help to decrease frustration and uncertainty while providing the basis for a positive relationship. Health care providers can help their patients to implement self-care strategies by providing both verbal and written information and recommending reputable online information resources. Providing "virtual office hours" where rural patients can contact their health care providers via e-mail might also be helpful. Although information can decrease uncertainty (Mishel, 1993), health care providers should remind their patients that uncertainty is part of chronic illness.

Although the findings add to our understanding of the chronic illness experiences of rural women, questions remain. For example, do isolated rural women with other diagnoses experience chronic illness differently? Do younger or older women and teens manage their illnesses differently than middle-aged women? Furthermore, more research is needed regarding the role nurses play in the experiences of chronically ill rural women. The women were referring to physician providers in their chat room conversations and never mentioned nurses in their postings. More research is needed to understand the role nurses play in the illness experiences of rural women.

CONCLUSION

Using a computer and the Internet was a manageable and accepted method of providing peer support to a group of isolated rural women with chronic illness. With proper instruction and assistance, even the most novice computer user was able to navigate the computer and participate in online conversations with a group of her peers. The women's illness experiences support the findings of others and illustrate commonalities found among persons living in rural areas. Recognizing the common problems and uncertainties experienced by these women is an important step in planning effective care. Further exploration is needed to understand the complex and multifaceted chronic illness experiences of isolated rural women.

ACKNOWLEDGMENTS

This research was funded by the Center for Research on Chronic Health Conditions in Rural Dwellers (Grant NIH/NINR IP20 NR 07790-01). The authors acknowledge Dr. Clarann Weinert for her assistance with this study.

REFERENCES

About MS. (2004). Retrieved July 2, 2004, from http://www.nationalmssociety.org/about%20 ms.asp

Agency for Healthcare Policy and Research. (1996). *Improving health care for rural populations. Research in Action fact sheet*. (AHCPR Publication No. 96–P040). Washington, DC: U.S. Government Printing Office.

Albright, A. (2008). *Diabetes: 2008 at a glance*. Retrieved October 16, 2008, from http://www.cdc.gov/nccdphp/publications/aag/ddt.htm

Benet, A. (1996). A portrait of chronic illness: Inspecting the canvas, reframing the issues. *American Behavioral Scientist, 39,* 767–776.

Burrows, R., Nettleton, S., Pleace, N., Loader, B., & Muncer, S. (2000). Virtual community care? Social policy and the emergence of computer mediated social support. *Information, Communication and Society, 3*(1), 95–121.

Centers for Disease Control (CDC). (2010, July 7). *Chronic disease overview.* Retrieved July 17, 2012, from http://www.cdc.gov/nccdphp/overview.htm

Centers for Disease Control (CDC). (2011). *Fact sheet: Diabetesatwork.org.* Retrieved July 15, 2012, from http://www.cdc.gov/diabetes/pubs/factsheets/atwork.htm

Davies, M., & Sque, M. (2002). Living on the outside looking in: A theory of living with advanced breast cancer. *International Journal of Palliative Nursing, 8,* 583–584, 586–590.

Eberhardt, M. S., Ingram, D. D., Makuc, D. M., Pamuk, E. R., Freid, V. M., Harper, S. B. et al. (2001). *Urban and rural health chartbook. Health, United States, 2001 with rural and urban chartbook* (NCHS Publication No. PHS 01–1232). Hyattsville, MD: National Center for Health Statistics.

Eysenbach, G., Powell, J., Englesakis, M., Rizo, C., & Stern, A. (2004). Health related virtual communities and electronic support groups: Systematic review of the effects of online peer to peer interactions. *British Medical Journal, 328*(7449), 1166–1170.

FitzGerald, M., Pearson, A., & McCutcheon, H. (2001). Impact of rural living on the experience of chronic illness. *Australian Journal of Rural Health, 9,* 235–240.

Gesler, W., Hartwell, S., Ricketts, T., & Rosenberg, M. (1992). Introduction. In W. Gesler, & T. Ricketts (Eds.), *Health in rural North America* (pp. 1–22). New Brunswick, NJ: Rutgers University Press.

Health & Human Services (HHS) Rural Task Force. (2002). *One department serving rural America: Report to the secretary.* Washington, DC: Author.

Hootman, J., Bolen, J., Helmick, C., & Langmaid, G. (2006). Prevalence of doctor-diagnosed arthritis and arthritis-attributable activity limitation— United States, 2003–2005. *Morbidity and Mortality Weekly Report, 55*(40), 1089–1092.

Husaine, B., & Moore, S. (1990). Arthritis disability, depression, and life satisfaction among black elderly people. *Health and Social Work, 15,* 253–259.

Hwu, Y. J. (1995). The impact of chronic illness on patients. *Rehabilitation Nursing, 20,* 221–225.

Ingram, D. D., & Franco, S. J. (2012). NCHS urban-rural classification scheme for counties. National Center for Health Statistics. *Vital Health Statistics, 2*(154), 2012.

Jensen, A. (1991). Psychosocial factors in breast cancer and their possible impact upon prognosis. *Cancer Treatment Reviews, 18,* 191–210.

Kung, H. C., Hoyert, D. L., Xu, J. Q., & Murphy, S. L. (2008, April 24). Deaths: Final data for 2005. *National Vital Statistics Reports, 56*(10). Retrieved July 17, 2012, from http://www.cdc.gov/nchs/data/nvsr/nvsr56/nvsr56_10.pdf

Long, K. A., & Weinert, C. (1989). Rural nursing: Developing the theory base. *Scholarly Inquiry for Nursing Practice, 3*, 113–127.

Marks, J. S. (2003). *The burden of chronic disease and the future of public health.* Retrieved June 28, 2004, from http://www.cdc.gov/nccdphp/burden_pres/

Mast, M. E. (1995). Adult uncertainty in illness: A critical review of research. *Scholarly Inquiry for Nursing Practice, 9*, 3–24; discussion 25–29.

Meit, M. (2004). *Bridging the health divide: The rural public health research agenda.* Pittsburgh, PA: University of Pittsburgh Center for Rural Health Practice.

Miles, M. B., & Huberman, A. M. (1994). *Qualitative data analysis* (2nd ed.). Thousand Oaks, CA: Sage.

Mishel, M. H. (1984). Perceived uncertainty and stress in illness. *Research in Nursing and Health, 7*, 163–171.

Mishel, M. H. (1988). Uncertainty in illness. *Image: Journal of Nursing Scholarship, 20*, 225–232.

Mishel, M. H. (1993). Living with chronic illness: Living with uncertainty. In S. Funk, E. Tornquist, M. Champagne, & R. Wiese (Eds.), *Key aspects of caring for the chronically ill: Hospital and home* (pp. 46–58). New York, NY: Springer Publishing.

Mishel, M. H., & Braden, C. J. (1988). Finding meaning: Antecedents of uncertainty in illness. *Nursing Research, 37*, 98–103, 127.

Muskie School of Public Service and Kaiser Commission on Medicaid and the Uninsured. (2003). *Health insurance coverage in rural America.* Washington, DC: Kaiser Family Foundation.

QSR NUD*IST. (1998). *QSR NUD*IST*, Version 4. Melbourne, Australia: QSR International Pty Ltd.

Ries, L. A. G., Melbert, D., Krapcho, M., Stinchcomb, D. G., Howlader, N., Horner, M. J. et al. (2008). *SEER stat fact sheets.* Retrieved October 16, 2008, from http://seer.cancer.gov/statfacts/html/all.html

Robinson, C. A. (1993). Managing life with a chronic condition: The story of normalization. *Qualitative Health Research, 3*(1), 6–28.

Scott, J. (2000). A nursing leadership challenge: Managing the chronically ill in rural settings. *Nursing Administration Quarterly, 24*(3), 21–32.

Strauss, A., Corbin, J., Fagerhaugh, S., Glaser, B., Maines, D., Suczek, B. et al. (1984). *Chronic illness and the quality of life* (2nd ed.). St. Louis, MO: Mosby.

Stuifbergen, A. (1995). Health-promoting behaviors and quality of life among individuals with multiple sclerosis. *Scholarly Inquiry for Nursing Practice, 9*, 31–50.

Sullivan, T., Weinert, C., & Cudney, S. (2003). Management of chronic illness: Voices of rural women. *Journal of Advanced Nursing, 44*, 566–574.

United States Census Bureau. (2000). *United States—Urban/rural and inside/outside metropolitan area.* Retrieved June 15, 2009, from http://www.census.gov

Weiner, C. (1975). The burden of rheumatoid arthritis: Tolerating the uncertainty. *Social Science and Medicine, 9*, 97–104.

Weinert, C. (2000). Social support in cyberspace for women with chronic illness. *Rehabilitation Nursing, 25*, 129–135.

Winters, C. A. (1997). *Living with chronic heart disease: A pilot study.* Retrieved March 31, 2004, from http://www.nova.edu/ssss/QR/QR3-4/winters.html

Winters, C. A. (1999). Heart failure: Living with uncertainty. *Progress in Cardiovascular Nursing, 14*, 85–91.

Wu, S. Y., & Green, A. (2000). *Projection of chronic illness prevalence and cost inflation.* Santa Monica, CA: RAND Health.

Chapter 12

NEGOTIATION OF CONSTRUCTED GENDER AMONG RURAL MALE CAREGIVERS
Chad O'Lynn

NEARLY 20% OF ALL AMERICANS will be over age 65 by 2030 (United States [U.S.] Census Bureau, 2004). Associated with increased age is the increased incidence of chronic health conditions requiring caregiving services. Many aspects of caregiving have been studied; however, family caregiving in rural communities remains poorly understood. In addition, health care resources and support in rural communities are stretched thinly compared to urbanized communities. Consequently, the growing number of intervention studies based on current descriptions, theoretical models, and urban assumptions of caregiving may not apply to rural caregivers. Additional research is needed to explore the unique needs of rural caregivers. Among rural caregivers, men have been particularly ignored by researchers and policy makers.

SIGNIFICANCE OF THE PROPOSED STUDY

The reported percentage of family caregivers who are male ranges between 34% (National Alliance for Caregiving & American Association of Retired Persons [NAC & AARP], 2009) and 44% (Strength for Caring, 2005). Conservatively, over 12.5 million American men are caring for dependent adults (U.S. Census Bureau, 2002). The number of male caregivers is expected to increase as the number of older Americans increases and the number of female family members who have traditionally filled caregiver roles decreases (Kramer, 2002). Just as with women, caregiving is associated with negative health changes for men (Russell, 2008; Vitaliano,

Zhang, & Scanlan, 2003). Consequently, increasing numbers of men providing caregiving may present a growing men's health concern.

Few rural studies have included male caregivers in their samples; yet knowledge of their needs and perspectives is essential to optimize their health and success as caregivers. It is hypothesized that healthy and successful rural male caregivers will provide better care to their care recipients, and thus reduce morbidity and premature institutionalization of dependent elders. The specific aims of this study were to

1. Explore the meanings and experiences of caregiving from the perspectives of rural male caregivers;
2. Explore the processes used by rural male caregivers as they progress through the caregiving experience;
3. Explore the effects of caregiving on rural male caregiver health and caregiver success; and
4. Develop a theoretical understanding of how male gender and rurality affect caregiving.

LITERATURE REVIEW

Caregiving

The experience of caring for family members has been correlated with numerous negative and positive psychological and physical health consequences, although greater attention has been given to negative consequences. Researchers' tendency to examine negative aspects of caregiving has been criticized (Acton & Winter, 2002; Archbold, Stewart, Greenlick, & Harvath, 1992; Kramer, 1997); however, the evidence for negative consequences of caregiving is strong and unequivocal (National Institute of Nursing Research [NINR], 1994; Pinquart & Sorenson, 2006; Vitaliano et al., 2003; Yee & Schulz, 2000). Commonly, aspects of caregiving that yield negative health consequences include limitations placed upon the caregiver's life, competing roles and time demands for caregivers, and demands placed on caregivers stemming from the care recipient's emotional and physical needs (NAC & AARP, 2009; NINR, 1994). Other documented aspects include lack of social support and deterioration of the relationship between caregiver and recipient. In sum, these aspects lead to increased caregiver burden and caregiver strain, which in turn elevate levels of stress among caregivers to the point of threatening caregiver health. In fact, 17% of caregivers rate their health as fair to poor, compared to 13% in the general U.S. population, and 17% of caregivers reported that caregiving has worsened their health (NAC & AARP, 2009).

Caregiver burden and caregiver strain are constructs that have been poorly defined and variably operationalized among researchers. *Burden* refers to the distress experienced by caregivers and has been operationalized in tools such as the Zarit Burden Inventory (Zarit, Reever, & Bach-Peterson, 1980). Using Lazarus' Stress Theory as a foundation, we can say that caregiver strain is a state that results from enduring problems that are appraised as threats to caregiver well-being and require a coping response (Lawton, Kleban, Moss, Rovine, & Glicksman, 1989; Pearlin & Schooler, 1978; Robinson, 1983). Caregiver strain is categorized as emotional, physical, financial, or familial in nature. Emotional strain is the category best supported in the literature and has been most frequently operationalized as caregiver depression (NINR, 1994). It is estimated that the stress of caregiving can reduce a caregiver's life by as many as 10 years (Arno, 2006).

Positive aspects of caregiving reported in the literature include feeling useful and needed and achieving a sense of personal affirmation (operationalized as caregiver satisfaction) and personal meaning (operationalized as reciprocity, mutuality, affection, or attachment) (NINR, 1994). Theoretically, positive affirmation and meaning may ameliorate negative health consequences of caregiving.

The literature of male caregiving primarily focuses on quantitatively measured differences between male and female caregivers. A number of researchers reported that male caregivers have less depression, fewer role conflicts, less caregiver burden and strain, and greater satisfaction than their female counterparts (Carpenter & Miller, 2002; Gitlin et al., 2003; Pinquart & Sorenson, 2006; Yee & Schulz, 2000). However, several researchers provided opposing findings or reported no significant differences between male and female caregivers on selected measures (Baillie, Norbeck, & Barnes, 1988; Ladner & Cuellar, 2002; Schulz et al., 2001). Explanations for variable findings illuminate methodological limitations of these studies, such as an over-reliance upon cross-sectional designs (Bookwala, Newman, & Schulz, 2002; Carpenter & Miller, 2002) and lack of reporting of effects sizes or clinical significance of findings (Miller & Cafasso, 1992); and sampling procedures that hide unique findings for men or for subcategories of male caregivers (Harris, 2002; Houde, 2002; Thompson, 2002). Theoretical limitations in which findings unique to male subjects are compared to normative female data are also prevalent in the literature (Kramer, 2002; Miller & Cafasso, 1992; Thompson, 2002; Young & Kahana, 1989). These limitations have promoted, at worst, the invisibility of male caregivers, and at best, an unreliable understanding of male caregivers (Stoller, 2002; Thompson, 2002). As such, the knowledge base from these studies is not sufficient to develop support strategies and interventions that are applicable and acceptable to male caregivers (Gwyther, 1992; Thompson, 2002).

Rural Health and Rurality

A lack of agreement on the definition of *rural* among researchers has led to great variation in study samples, thus making comparison among studies difficult. However, the term *frontier* is consistently used to describe the most rural of areas, generally considered to have a population density of less than six persons per square mile (Hewitt, 1992; Wagenfeld, 2000, 2003). Frontier areas may exemplify commonly reported barriers to health services in rural communities and the unique cultural aspects of rural dwellers (Hewitt, 1992; Lee, 1998b; Wagenfeld, 2000). Studies using frontier samples may yield findings most applicable to rural communities as a whole.

Despite great variation among rural communities, health disparities for rural dwellers are well-documented. Published reviews have noted that rural dwellers have higher rates of chronic illness, mental illness, obesity, social and physical limitations, death from motor vehicle accidents, and smoking and alcohol consumption than their urban counterparts (Center on an Aging Society, 2003; Eberhardt, Ingram, & Makuc, 2001). In addition, rural dwellers pay more out-of-pocket expenses for health services, use preventative health services less frequently, and, for elders, report a lower quality of life (Ballantyne & Buehler, 1998; Center on an Aging Society, 2003; Goins & Mitchell, 1999; Kumar, Acanfora, Hennessy, & Kalache, 2001; Lishner, Richardson, Levine, & Patrick, 1996; Morgan, Semchuk, Stewart, & D'Arcy, 2002; National Rural Health Association [NRHA], 2007). Chief explanatory factors for these disparities include a lack of accessible, affordable, available, and diverse health services in rural areas; increased distance to services; inadequate transportation; concerns about privacy; and increased poverty rates for rural dwellers (Ballantyne & Buehler; Center on an Aging Society, 2003; Lishner et al., 1996; Morgan et al., 2002; NRHA, 2007). Unfortunately, many social and governmental programs implemented to address disparities are founded on knowledge derived from urban-based research models, often rendering these programs unacceptable to rural dwellers and inappropriate to the unique needs and realities of rural communities (Bull, Krout, Rathbone-McCuan, & Shreffler, 2001; Ryan-Nicholls, 2004). Rural disparities combined with poorly suited services provide a context in which rural caregivers are likely to experience greater challenges and health risks than their urban counterparts.

Bigbee (1993) identified literature support for the existence of a rural culture. Rural culture is characterized by relatively close and long-term relationships with family and neighbors that result in a lack of anonymity and a blurring of social roles. Rural dwellers tend to be more morally and politically conservative and traditional in their values than urban dwellers. Rural dwellers value individualism, hard work, independence, and self-sufficiency. Bigbee reported that geographical isolation substantially shapes rural culture and enhances the visibility of other rural attributes, such as a keen perception of and distrust of outsiders (Bailey, 1998; Lee, 1998a), ethnocentrism (Dybbro, 1998), and an increased reliance upon nonformal health resources to manage health and illness (Buehler, Malone, & Majerus, 1998; O'Lynn, 2006). However, Wagenfeld (2003) indicated that the cultural divide between urban and rural dwellers is narrowing, especially as communication technology and migration patterns change. This narrowing is not uniform and is likely to be slower in more isolated or frontier rural communities. It is the nexus of rural demographics and rural culture that defines the construct *rurality*, in that rural residence alone does not account for the unique context and experiences of rural dwellers (Wagenfeld, 2003). Wagenfeld questioned whether an urban individual who relocates to a rural area is truly rural, a consideration that is congruent with the perspective of insider/outsider status common among rural dwellers (Lee, 1998a).

Rural Masculinity

Some literature is available on how masculinity is manifested in men living in rural communities, though much of the literature reflects theoretical summaries, observations, and anecdotes or focuses on interpretations discerned from the social messages embedded in portrayals of rural masculinity found in popular literature and film (Anahita & Mix, 2006). Although cognizant of the complexity of gender and multiple masculinities within subgroups of men, including rural men, Levant and Habben (2003) proposed that rural men are likely more traditional in their masculine ideology than are urban men, an ideology characterized by toughness, self-reliance, homophobia, avoidance of feminine behaviors and emotionality, and a high value placed on accomplishment and work. In addition, due to the lack of anonymity typical in rural communities, the actions and reputations of rural men are highly visible and carry much weight. "As a result, rural men are more likely to try to adhere to a higher moral code or else keep their problems very private" (p. 177). Connell (1993) described a frontier masculinity that is based on the myths and stories of characters such as Daniel Boone, Paul Bunyan, and cowboys. This masculinity is based in a context of wilderness, in which men battle and conquer all the challenges and treasures Mother Nature may offer. It is a masculinity characterized by ruggedness, self-sufficiency, control, courage, and physical strength (Anahita & Mix, 2006; Gorman et al., 2007; Hogan & Pursell, 2008). Important to the present study, adherence to a more traditional masculine ideology may encourage rural men to avoid assistance from others, especially health and human service assistance.

METHOD

Sample

In this study, participants were recruited from frontier areas in two northwestern states in the United States with flyers and newspaper advertisements. *Frontier* was defined as a county of less than six persons per square mile. Inclusion criteria required that participants reside within a community with a population of fewer than 15,000 residents and be a male caregiver who provided (or had provided) daily assistance with activities of daily living to a relative. Twelve non-Hispanic Caucasian men participated in this study. The men ranged in age from 45 to 87 years, with a mean of 58.9 years. Caregiving experience ranged from 1 to 28 years, with 8 of the 12 men providing care for 5 years or less. Nine of the men were caregivers for their wives and 3 of the men were caregivers for two family members each, resulting in a total of 15 care recipients for the 12 men. In addition to nine wives, care recipients included one adult daughter, one sister, three mothers, and one grandmother.

Ten of the men were lifelong residents of rural communities. The other two had lived in rural settings for 7 and 15 years, respectively. At the time of the study, two of the men lived on farms or ranches, with the others living in towns with populations ranging from 150 to 12,228. Three of the men were retired; the others were working full- or part-time. All the men had careers in service and extractive industries. Generally, the men reported their health as good, with only two participants reporting chronic illnesses that impaired their ability to work in their chosen careers.

Family members receiving care from the study participants required assistance with activities of daily living and could not live independently without such care. Most of the care recipients suffered from musculoskeletal disorders, including three with spinal cord injuries. Five care recipients had dementia, three care recipients had experienced strokes, two had mental health disorders, one had amyotrophic lateral sclerosis, and one had cerebral palsy. All care recipients had primary care providers located within a few miles of their residences, and most required the care of a specialist on a semiannual basis, requiring travel of 58 to 228 miles (one way).

Data Collection Procedures and Analysis

Data were collected using in-depth interviews and observations consistent with constructivist grounded theory method (Charmaz, 2000, 2006). This method was deemed most appropriate since it is congruent with the study aims and assumptions that gender and culture are socially constructed phenomena. The method integrates the knowledge and experiences of participant and researcher as cocreators of a study's findings.

Phenomena were deconstructed to explore hidden meanings, assumptions, and power relationships followed by construction of findings from data using inductive and generative processes. The method yielded an account of the meanings and actions of a social process rather than a simple explanation of a social process typical with other forms of grounded theory.

Participants contributed 18 interviews, conducted both face-to-face and via telephone. Each interview lasted for 45 to 120 minutes. A semistructured interview approach was used to accommodate conversation and optimal exploration. Latter interviews also included specific questions designed to explore emerging data categories, consistent with grounded theory methodology (Charmaz, 2000, 2006). Interviews were audiotaped and transcribed by the author.

Data analysis began following the first interview with line-by-line open coding. Repetition of many of the codes was evident after four interviews. After eight interviews, 285 codes had been identified. These codes were collapsed into 21 broader focused codes. A situational map was used to help discern relationships among the focused codes. Subsequent interviews clarified emerging relationships and meanings in the data. From this process, four categories were constructed from the data: rurality, rural masculinity, caregiver challenges, and negotiating gender roles. Findings were then compared to the extant literature for further clarification and refinement. Ultimately, a theoretical model was developed in which the core category, gender role negotiation, was constructed as the chief explanatory and action category to account for the differences in experiences and perspectives among the participants.

FINDINGS

Rurality

The division between rurality and rural masculinity is obscure, since both gender and culture are socially constructed phenomena and are intertwined in derivation and manifestation. Nevertheless, participants described attributes of rurality as applicable to most long-term residents of rural communities, whereas, attributes of rural masculinity were described as more prevalent or manifested more intensely in rural men than in rural women.

Geographic isolation was the most commonly discussed rural attribute. Although most participants lived within 50 miles of a health care provider, few lived close to health care specialists and comprehensive durable medical equipment providers. For example, one participant's wife had a subcutaneous pump that delivered pain medication continuously. The pump needed to be filled with medication every month, which required a 450-mile round trip to the medical office. All of the participants noted that driving long distances placed great financial, comfort, and time burdens on them and on their care recipients. Two participants depleted their savings to purchase vans to transport their care recipients to medical appointments. One participant reported that he had become a member of a newly created ambulance service, in which an annual fee is paid to have a helicopter land in his community to transport his wife to an urban hospital when needed. Some participants emphasized that urban dwellers and health providers had little understanding or appreciation of such geographical challenges.

The participants described several social attributes of rurality. One attribute is a value for self-reliance and the hard work needed to maintain self-reliance. In discussing this value, participants did not use a vocal tone of admiration but rather a tone of matter-of-factness. One participant noted that his family and his wife's family were "Oregon Trail people," which fostered not only self-reliance but also ruggedness and independence. Related to self-reliance was a value of caring for one's own. Several participants commented that rural family values dictate that one cares for one's family members when needed. Caregiving was not couched in negative terms of obligation or duty, but rather as a cultural norm that was so engrained that the adoption of the caregiver role did not foster much reflection. In answering a question about caregiver roles for spouses, one participant stated, "She'd be doing exactly what I'm doing because we both believe in the same things, the same kind of principles." Later, this participant commented about how someone had approached him at an urban restaurant and complimented him while he was helping his wife to eat. He was perplexed by the compliment and stated

> [T]he way I take care of her and the attention I give her, I figure that's part of it, that's what I'm supposed to do. I told her [his wife] a long time ago that that's why she hired me on forty years ago.

Other participants noted that this value may be generational and worried that younger rural dwellers may be less likely to assume a caregiving role.

Seemingly contrary to self-reliance is the rural attribute of community support. Participants described rural community support as offers for assistance for tasks that would exceed the capacity of any normally self-reliant individual. They also noted that these offers were expected of others as a normative behavior of rural neighbors. An example was the offers of cutting and baling hay for a participant. Community support was described as "good neighborliness" and was viewed as a pervasive and beneficial characteristic typical of rural, but not urban, communities.

In emphasizing the rural/urban difference in community support, one participant commented,

> I'll give you an idea. I had car troubles at 11:30 at night. I opened my hood, and right away some guy from the Forest Service and a retired mechanic comes over. One sheriff guy comes over. Then one other person. I have no idea who he was, but he comes over... I mean everybody sticks up their finger in the air when they wave to you and drive along; your index finger goes up like a peace sign or whatever. In [urban home town], it's the MIDDLE finger that goes up!

However, community support may be predicated on having an insider status. Two participants who had not lived in their communities for many years commented on having an outsider status and perceived themselves as lacking common histories with local residents and having fewer interdependent relationships. Although an outsider status did not impair their ability to receive desired services, being an outsider led to a perception that increased time was needed to establish community connectedness.

Faith communities were an important source of community support. In noting the difference between general community support and faith community support, one participant noted, "I guess [work colleagues] were more analytical, or 'What can we do to help?' Church people were there not only to help with physical things, but spiritual." The importance of faith community support was acknowledged even by those who did not attend a specific church. One participant commented,

> It kind of elevates you..... You depend upon prayer chains from denominations in this community. That's a really nice thing about being in a small town, is you know you're not known in just your faith community. You're known in many groups. And, so, I'd meet folks in the grocery store who'd say, "I'm praying for you, your wife and you." Which, you know, is humbling, uplifting, and it's sustainable.

Another participant noted that rural communities have two kinds of tight-knit families: the "church family" and the "bar [tavern] family," with both families having regular members who spend time together and look out for each other. Each of these smaller communities may provide caregivers focused and ongoing support as opposed to the general support and encouragement provided by the community at large.

Participants identified faith as another rural attribute. Faith was less about church attendance and more about belief in a higher power and spirituality. Participants believed that God provided rural dwellers hardiness to endure life's challenges. For example, "God plants us the seeds to be strong and get us through tough times." In addition, participants articulated a somewhat fatalistic perspective when those challenges were beyond human intervention. For these challenges, rural dwellers accepted God's will. One participant commented, "We said that we married for better or for worse. We just happened to draw the worse card. You [have to] take life as it comes."

Rural Masculinity

The participants described rural masculinity in very personal and visceral language. Participants discussed attributes that not only described themselves but also the perspectives they had of other rural men. No rural masculinity attribute was discussed as much as self-reliance. Participants indicated that self-reliance was a keystone characteristic of rural masculinity. In addition, the participants described self-reliance in more detail as it related to masculinity than they did for rurality.

Participants described masculine self-reliance as a deep sense of independence with a strong unwillingness to ask others for assistance. This unwillingness did not stop at physical assistance with tasks, but included advice or feedback on their plans and actions as well. An unwillingness to ask for assistance is what separated the self-reliance of rural men from the self-reliance of rural women, whom these men perceived to be more willing to seek advice from peers. Self-reliance influenced how men approached work and challenges in all aspects of their lives and how they viewed themselves as men. Self-reliance was also described as including a "can-do" attitude, which promoted ingenuity and a "hands- on" and pragmatic approach to problems. For example, although having access to durable medical equipment and physical therapy services for his injured wife, one participant felt not only an unwillingness to ask for these services but also felt that such services would not be needed because he could provide the services himself. He noted,

> I started manufacturing different things to get her up and walk, and even had her in the shop ... used an engine hoist to get her up in the walker. Yeah, we had all different kinds of things. And when she goes to the potty, why I got an overhead winch that I run on a rail that I transfer her into the bathroom and the shower.

Participants noted that an unwillingness to ask for assistance was present even if it became apparent to the participant that he needed assistance with caregiving. The participants explained this unwillingness as a general resistance to relinquish control of a situation. According to the participants, relinquishing control by having others come in to provide caregiving was a frank admission that they, as men, were unable to complete the work and somehow had failed as caregivers. This belief was most common in terms of the personal and intimate aspects of caregiving, and less prevalent in asking for help with large and highly visible tasks such as farm work.

Discussion of independence, or possibly aversion to dependence, was common in the participants' descriptions of self-reliance. One participant commented on how important it was for him for his wife to become as independent as possible, not as a way to avoid work for himself, but as a way for her to improve self-esteem. One way he fostered independence in his wife was to intentionally fumble at caregiver tasks. He stated,

> And it gives her more incentive to do more for herself. And I'm a firm believer in that 'cause that's just the way it seems. If you do everything for them ... she gets in the habit of it, but if you drag your feet, well, she'll figure out a way of doing it. I used to dress her up until about four or five months ago, and now she says, "I'll do it myself!" And, thank God, she does a pretty good job of dressing herself.

Self-reliance also meant doing all work necessary, regardless of previous or stereotypical gendered divisions of labor. The participants were explicit that they did not see housework as feminine, but rather as work that had to be done, as is all work on a farm or ranch. If their wives could no longer perform housework, they pitched in and did it themselves. A typical comment was that "You gotta do what you gotta do." One participant stated that this "just do it" perspective was modeled to most rural men by their fathers and other men in their communities. One participant commented,

> My father] was just a doer, you know, washing dishes, making dinner and everything. All my life he was like that. If mom worked at the hospital ... how many Thanksgiving dinners did this man make? You know, I mean changing the kids' diapers, he was just a hands-on kind of guy, and at the same time he'd be underneath the car pulling the transmission .... I could take lessons from this guy.

The attribute of focusing on outcomes was also described. Regardless of the specific task, work was simply a process that yielded results. When asked about the increased amount of work they were doing as caregivers, participants paused and stammered to provide a response. The question was nonsensical to them. Participants commented that they did not think much about the work itself. However, participants described in great detail the sense of pride they felt when they completed tasks or met some other work objective.

Another attribute described by several participants was a reluctance to meet their emotional needs. Although somewhat variable among the participants, if any assistance was sought, for most of the participants it was for caregiving tasks, and not for coping with stress. When asked if he shares his feelings with friends during visits, one participant replied, "I don't bring up anything like that ... I don't give them any hard luck stories, because it wouldn't do any good." Three of the participants described themselves as stoic loners, who responded to stress with solitude. They described actions such as leaving the home to go for a walk or drive, distracting themselves with chores, or going for a drink when feeling stressed or overwhelmed. Although many people employ some solitude strategies when stressed, these three men employed these strategies exclusively. Sometimes these actions were beneficial. These men discussed how they used self-talk when alone to help them reframe their problems and motivate themselves for caregiving. However, they also described situations in which they left their care recipients in questionable safety so that they could be alone to "cool off."

Similar to the reluctance to meet emotional needs was the reluctance participants had in meeting their own physical health needs. Although most of the participants described themselves as healthy, several participants reported chronic illnesses that required ongoing medical attention. These participants reported that they only sought medical attention when illness symptoms got in the way of their ability to work for a day or two. Some participants reported new health changes caused by caregiving (e.g., insomnia, back pain), yet did not self-treat or seek medical attention for these new problems.

Participants also commented that rural men value common sense. Several participants provided numerous accounts of how health and human service providers lack common sense by adhering to bureaucratic procedures that impaired efficient delivery of services. These actions caused great frustration among the participants. For example, one participant's wife needed hospitalization for an acute respiratory illness. The participant knew that the local rural hospital would not admit her and would transfer her to a distant urban hospital. When he tried to convince the rural emergency room staff of this, they insisted on a full medical evaluation prior to transfer. This evaluation was then duplicated at the urban hospital when she arrived, thus creating duplicate billing to Medicare and a delay of treatment. Common sense was also described in terms of their own learning of how to be a caregiver. None of the men reported receiving formal instructions from hospital and clinic nurses or home health personnel on how to complete caregiving tasks, such as transferring, medication administration, and personal hygiene. The men stated that they learned these skills by asking other family members, by observation, and by common sense. One participant stated,

> When I first started taking care of her, I got a little bit of information from my stepdaughter. And myself, I got a lot of common sense. I figure myself pretty smart. I've watched other people, picked up a few things here and there. And I'm the type you show me something today, I'll remember ten years from now. I do what is necessary, and most of it is common sense.

The participants expressed pride in their common sense. Common sense served as a foundation for their ingenuity and enabled them to remain self-reliant.

Another attribute of rural masculinity offered by the participants was that of the importance of fulfilling the provider role for one's family. Being a provider meant more than completing immediate caregiving tasks; it also required advocating for an optimal caregiving environment. Some men had to battle agencies to meet the needs of their care recipients, or battle employers to allow for more flexible scheduling to allow for caregiving. Two participants had to contest local zoning ordinances to build additions to their homes to better accommodate caring for sick family members.

Caregiver Challenges

The participants described a myriad of challenges related to caregiving, including hard physical labor, emotional/behavioral problems of care recipients, fatigue, lack of time, poor sleep, disrupted intimate and emotional relationships with their wives, disruptions at work, financial hardship, and detriments to their personal health. These challenges led to a pervasive stress that most of the men recognized, but that most simply chose to endure. The participants described this stress in very few, but very powerful words. One participant commented, "It [the stress] gets pretty tough. (Long pause) It can be real tough."

Gender Role Negotiation

Negotiation, or a redefining of one's gender role, is the core category constructed from the data and best accounts for how these men responded to caregiver stress. Caregiving required that the men confront situations, adopt behaviors, and complete tasks to which they were unaccustomed. For one participant, these changes produced no reported stress. For the rest of the men, some new behaviors and tasks conflicted with their individually constructed gender roles. These men underwent a process, which varied over time, in which various attributes of rural masculinity had to be rectified with caregiving responsibilities. This process was not always completed in a self-reflective manner; indeed, for most of the men, this process occurred in a reflexive manner to sudden care recipient changes, to periods of markedly increased caregiver stress, or to both. However, for others the rectification process became quite overt and adopted a more negotiation-like process that allowed them to reduce any dissonance between caregiving responsibilities and their individual perspectives on their gender roles. Three general patterns of addressing gender role conflict were noted: gender role compromise, gender role conflict preservation, and gender role reconstruction.

Gender Role Compromise: Accommodation

Some men implemented a compromise between necessary caregiving work and one or more attributes of their rural masculinity. Compromise allowed for tolerance of the conflict, made possible by recognizing that compromise would facilitate completion of caregiver tasks. These men perceived themselves as "getting by" or "making do" with the challenges presented to them, resulting in a stage of accommodation with any perceived gender conflict. Any discomfort with conflict was balanced by the personal satisfaction of meeting a challenge and producing an end product, namely effective caregiving. Sometimes, compromise meant reaching out for help from others, but seeking help only occurred in a transient fashion. Such a pattern is analogous to the farmer, who ordinarily is independent in farm work, but seeks assistance only at harvest time. These men did not seek help for purposes of restoration or self-growth. One participant stated,

> The advice I would give anyone taking care of someone is to evaluate the amount of care, then decide if you are able to do the job. Sometimes the care required can be more than one person can give.

The men expressed very pragmatic perspectives. Managing conflicts between caregiving and gender was not an internal, self-reflexive process but rather a visibly external and outcome-focused process.

Gender Role Conflict Preservation: Edge of Crisis

Another group of men stubbornly clung to attributes of their rural masculinity, particularly the attributes of what might be considered an excessive self-reliance, a need for total control of the caregiver context, and neglect of their own physical and psychosocial health needs. These men resisted all assistance offered by others, even to the detriment of the care recipient, accepting help only when it was forced upon them by others. One participant complained bitterly about being forced to go to a nursing home after his own cardiac surgery, which required him to find someone else to take care of his wife during his absence. Another acquiesced to home health services only after his wife (his care recipient) refused to continue with the poor care she was receiving from him. These men reported anger, bitterness, and high levels of stress. Unlike the other men in the study, these men adopted routine patterns of disengagement from others, including their care recipients, when feeling overwhelmed. These men described themselves as loners. Frequently, they would leave the house for drives, walks, or "alone time" in a workshop during periods of stress. Occasionally, this disengagement involved drinking alcohol in their solitude. These men used disengagement as their primary stress reduction measure. None of these men seemed aware that their behavior had negative consequences to themselves and to their care recipients. The men were unable to quantify the length of time of disengagement periods, stating that they returned to the caregiver environment when they had "cooled off." It is noteworthy that care recipients were left unattended during periods of disengagement. One participant admitted that his care recipient wife complained frequently about being left on the commode for as long as an hour while he left the house to "clear his mind." Frequent disengagement often accelerated the caregiving context toward crisis, a situation in which the quality of caregiving becomes so poor that disruptions in the care recipient's health could require institutionalization or human service intervention.

Gender Role Reconstruction: Resiliency

This transformational process represents the third pattern of gender negotiation among the men. Men in this group had experienced caregiver trajectories in which the intensity of caregiver challenges had eventually overwhelmed them, overloading any gender compromise that may have been in place. Unlike men who employed a gender compromise pattern, men using gender reconstruction sent out more frequent, less task-specific calls for help. These men sought assistance from all sources, including friends, neighbors, faith communities, as well as assistance from professional service organizations. The diversity of support addressed a plethora of needs, not just immediate or transient caregiver tasks. As support was utilized, these men reported that they had time to reflect upon recent changes in the caregiver dynamic, how they felt about caregiving, and how caregiving was affecting them as men.

These men described individual epiphanies of awareness of the benefits of assistance-seeking and assistance-accepting in enhancing the quality of the caregiving work, the improvement in their emotional health, and ultimately their abilities as caregivers. They acknowledged that the value they had placed in being independent, self-reliant and in control was excessive to the point of making them ineffective as caregivers. They realized that letting go of control and asking for help was essential to avoid crisis. Importantly, these men identified these specific rural masculinity attributes as something their peers had in common, not as things that were uniquely characteristic of themselves. One participant commented,

> You know, I'm macho, and I'm a guy, and I figured I could do it all. So, in retrospect, I could have had hospice in here two or three months sooner ... it would have been nice.

Continuing with his advice to other men, this participant shared,

> Don't be afraid to ask for help. Just know that there are resources out there... don't be as fussy as I was.... There is always somebody, and you don't know who that is. It might be somebody you don't expect.

These men reported that they had become much more adept at identifying personal emotional and instrumental needs and at locating appropriate resources to meet their needs. Importantly, these men did not seek help to remove themselves from the primary caregiver role. Instead, these men remained active in the day-to-day hands-on care of the care recipient and described their new roles as caregiver team leaders. These men also described a newly found resiliency to stress stemming from caregiver challenges. This resiliency was not a result of experience, but rather as a result of changed self-perceptions and changed behaviors. The men employing the gender role reconstruction pattern did not describe their individual transformations as an emasculating experience. Instead, these men described a reprioritization of rural masculinity attributes. They described how they learned to de-emphasize the importance of self-reliance and emphasize the importance of being a good provider to loved ones. Being a good provider meant that they had to seek and accept assistance.

Gender-Cultural Model of Caregiving: Rural Male Caregivers

A preliminary model was constructed from the data to illustrate the process of gender negotiation (see Figure 12.1). The model depicts the rural male caregiver imbedded in overlapping cultural and gender contexts. Attributes of caregiving, rural masculinity, and rurality serve as challenges and resources for caregivers. The interplay between challenges and resources moves the caregiver between episodes of high stress and caregiver crisis and episodes of low stress and caregiver success. At individualized points on a caregiver's trajectory, a stress point is reached in which he must respond to noncongruence between constructed gender and caregiver work. This response, gender role negotiation, can take one of three pathways: gender role conflict preservation, resulting in an approach to crisis; gender role compromise, resulting in a state of accommodation; and gender role reconstruction, resulting in the development of resiliency.

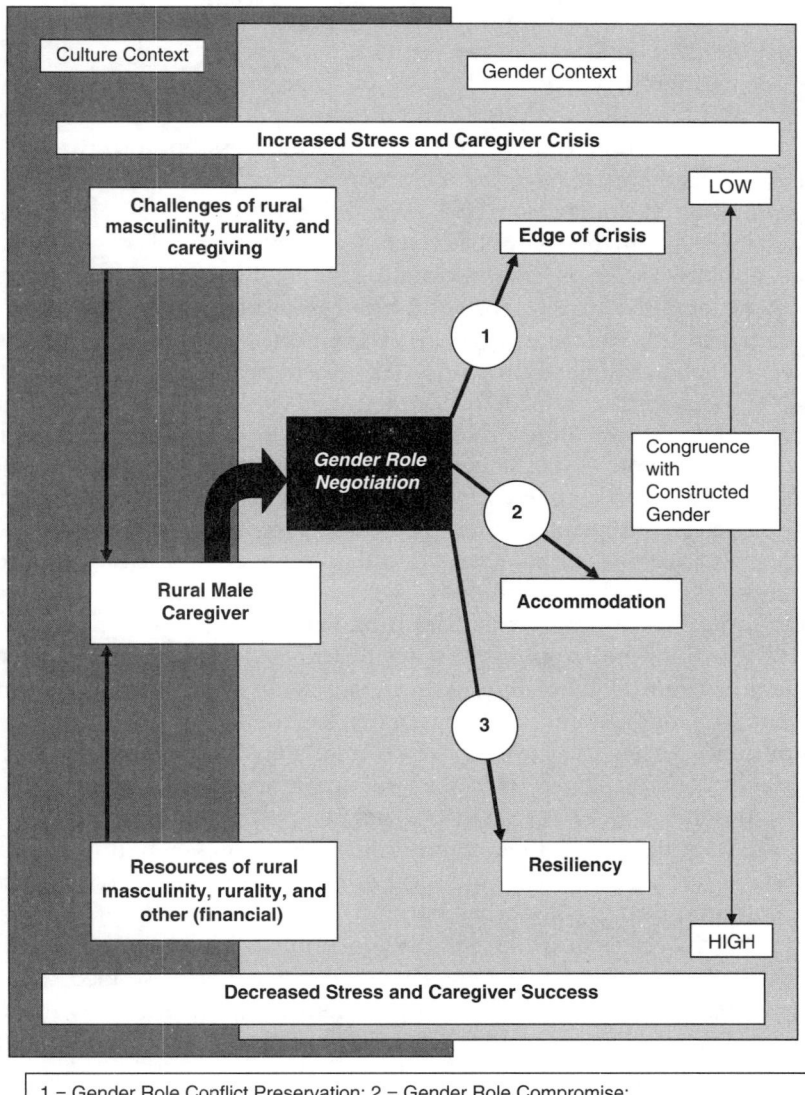

1 = Gender Role Conflict Preservation; 2 = Gender Role Compromise; 3 = Gender Role Reconstruction

FIGURE 12.1 Theoretical model of gender role negotiation in rural male caregivers.

DISCUSSION

Several attributes of rurality were evident in the study data, all of which are consistent with the extant literature. Pervasively, participants described geographic isolation consistent with rural areas (Bigbee, 1991; Wagenfeld,

2003). This isolation permeates the other rural attributes identified, both historically and influentially. In terms of caregiving services, although most of the men lived relatively close to emergency care services, other routine and specialty services were miles away. Travel to these services placed great emotional, financial, and physical stress on both caregivers and care recipients, a hardship common among rural dwellers (Bales, 2006; Findholt, 2006; Henson, Sadler, & Walton, 1998). Geographic isolation has perhaps made self-reliance necessary among rural dwellers. Self-reliance, according to the men, was valued among both men and women, and incorporated a strong sense of hardiness and hard work; this is well supported in the literature (Bigbee, 1991; Gorman et al., 2007; Hammer, Vogel, & Heimerdinger-Edwards, 2012; Koehler, 1998; Lee & Winters, 2004; Leipert & Reutter, 2005; Wathen & Harris, 2007; Weinert, 2005; Wells, 2009). The attribute of community support suggests the interdependence common in rural communities. Community support comes from a variety of sources, from individuals as well as from social groups such as faith communities. Although potential sources of community support are present in all communities, the pervasiveness of community support in rural communities is noteworthy, as described by the men who had moved to rural areas from urban areas. High levels of community support in rural communities are described in the literature (Bales, Winters, & Lee, 2006); however, in some instances, access to this community support may depend upon having an insider status within the rural community. A few of the men who were new to their communities described a "clannish" aspect to their rural neighbors and perceived challenges in obtaining desired support. This perspective was not mentioned by those who resided in their communities for many years. It is possible that long-time residents were unaware of their insider status within their own communities. On the other hand, it is possible that men who perceived themselves as outsiders simply were not socialized in local behaviors and customs for help-seeking, since one newcomer described selfless offers of assistance from friends and strangers alike. The men described a strong faith in God as central to rural communities. This faith was evident in fatalistic perspectives, acknowledging that God sometimes sends challenges that cannot be overturned by hardworking people. As such, people must trust that God will see them through. Faith and prayer were central to these communities and have been described by others (Arcury, Quandt, McDonald, & Bell, 2000; Bennett & Lengacher, 1999; Gaskins & Lyons, 2000; Irvin, Sutherland, & Harris, 2006; Schoenberg et al., 2009).

As a socially constructed phenomenon, it is not surprising that attributes of rural masculinity identified in this study overlap with attributes of rurality. Most pervasive in overlap is the attribute of self-reliance. However, the men provided detailed clarifications of how self-reliance is different for rural men than for rural women. The men described self-reliance solely in positive terms for rural residents in general, namely hardworking, hardy, and independent. In relation to rural men, the men described additional characteristics of self-reliance that were both positive and negative. The participants believe that rural men are more likely to add a strong work orientation to self-reliance, incorporating a strong can-do attitude and doing anything and everything to accomplish desired work outcomes. These characteristics of self-reliance were described in very glowing terms and were a source of great pride among the men. On the other hand, with the exception of those men using a gender role conflict preservation pattern of gender negotiation, the men noted that rural men took the independence aspect of self-reliance to the extreme, describing rural men as characteristically too independent, resistant to relinquishing control of their home caregiving context, and likely to display an excessive unwillingness to seek help. Awareness of this negative side of self-reliance appears to be an essential step to adopting a gender role reconstruction pattern of gender negotiation. Other attributes of rural masculinity (see Table 12.1) were common, and served as either sources of challenges or resources within the caregiving context.

The academic literature is sparse on the topic of rural masculinities (Campbell & Bell, 2000), though some have proposed that traditional and hegemonic types of masculinity are challenged by economic and social changes occurring in rural settings (Anahita & Mix, 2006; Jones & Curtin, 2011; Sorensen & Cooper, 2010). Masculinity ideology among rural men is likely different, namely more traditional and hegemonic, than that of nonrural men (Anahita & Mix, 2006; Beynon, 2002; Courtenay, 2000;

TABLE 12.1 Attributes of Rural Masculinity

Attributes and Sub-attributes	Source of Challenge	Source of Resource
1. Self-reliance: Overly independent		
a. Resists relinquishing control	X	
b. Unwilling to seek help	X	
2. Self-reliance: Work-action orientation		
a. Can-do attitude		X
b. Focus on outcomes		X
c. Will do all work necessary		X
3. Reluctance to address emotional needs		
a. Loner perspective	X	
b. Isolation from male peer caregivers	X	
4. Neglects personal health	X	
5. Values outdoors/engages in hobbies		X
6. Values common sense/ingenuity		X
7. Values provider role		X

Good et al., 1995; Gorman et al., 2007; Hammer et al., 2012; Hogan & Pursell, 2008; Levant & Habben, 2003; Levant et al., 1992; O'Neil, Good, & Holmes, 1995); however, few scholars have provided clear descriptions or empirical evidence of these differences. Among the commonly understood traditional masculinity attributes (O'Neil et al., 1995; Pleck 1995), the men did not provide evidence of support for homophobia and objectification of sexuality, probably due to the topics and directions of the interviews conducted. Support, however, was provided for the characteristics of toughness, self-reliance, restricted emotionality, and an importance on accomplishments and work.

The lack of empirical analyses of rural masculinities from the research literature, the examination of the popular media for support of the study's findings is reasonable, and has been used as a means of discernment by others (e.g., Bell, 2000; Hogan & Pursell, 2008). There is no shortage of presentations of rural western men in print, film, and song. Often these presentations are stereotypes or caricatures of rural men; however, topical themes are evident within these media. The popular media tend to portray rural men in ways consistent with conceptions of traditional masculinity, with possibly the additional characterizations that rural men are unrefined, poorly educated, and cling to common sense as the primary source for personal knowledge. A couple of examples are illustrative.

In music, Michael Martin Murphey sings about rural masculinity in his song, Cowboy Logic (Cooks & Rains, 1990). The song's lyrics describe how cowboys solve problems, namely through common sense, a focus on outcomes, hard work, and simplicity. The chorus of the song provides a list of maxims that highlight the values of hard work, toughness, and simple functionality. These values were expressed by the men in the study as well. Additionally, Murphey sings that these maxims are well-known to the point of universality. Again, the song matches the comments of the men. The men were remarkably similar in naming these values as attributes of rural masculinity.

In literature, many fictional accounts present an overly dramatic and inaccurate characterization of rural men. Notable historical exceptions are the stories of Charles ("Charlie") Russell, who was identified by field placement community members as the best source for understanding both rural men and rural western culture. Although C. M. Russell lived nearly a century ago, his stories of rural men adapting to the changes of the twentieth century mimic the experiences of today's rural men adapting to increased technology and changing economic realities (Cristy, 2004). Challenges of social roles and work adaptation were expressed by a number of men in this study.

In C. M. Russell's stories (1927), the similarities in the thinking and actions of his characters to the cowboy logic noted earlier are seen. The basic plot of many of C. M. Russell's stories centers on a rugged and self-reliant man who is ranching, cowboying, hunting, or doing some other work endeavor. While working, the character comes across a surprising and often dangerous problem, which requires swift and creative thinking. The character relies upon a response seemingly based on common sense, but the response does not quite solve the problem. Some calamity or unexpected series of events results, informing the reader that the character did not really have the common sense he thought he had. C. M. Russell twists this plot with humor to help drive home his point. This story line provides a helpful allegory for the collective experiences for the men in this study. These caregivers experienced new and unforeseen challenges. Approaches to these challenges were generally based on common sense and hard work (and perhaps a bit of luck). A focus on task outcomes made the hard work palatable, at times even enjoyable, and led to a great sense of pride when outcomes were met. However, these approaches were variably successful, often falling short of meeting outcomes if challenges were particularly intense or frequent. Calamity and near calamity were evident in the caregiver trajectories of some of the participants. Like C. M. Russell, who informs the reader how expanded perspective might avert calamity, the men undergoing gender role reconstruction developed insight that transformed their experiences.

In terms of caregiver challenges, the men in the study recounted burdens typical of those described at length in the literature. However, there was great variability in the interpretation of how these burdens affected them as individuals and how these interpretations changed over time. This variation lends support to the criticism made of the numerous quantitative caregiver studies that have examined phenomenon using cross-sectional designs (Coe & Neufeld, 1999; Harris, 1993; Kramer, 2000). In terms of caregiver rewards, rewards were most often described in terms of work accomplishment. These rewards served to strengthen or validate preexisting rurality and rural masculinity. Of notable exception were the men who used the gender role reconstruction pattern of gender role negotiation. These men described additional rewards much more characteristic of personal growth, such as a strengthening of faith, a new and more balanced perspective on life, and a deeper discernment of one's personal strengths and limitations.

Two studies were located in the literature that noted a process of negotiating gender role as a means to rectify conflicts between rural men's constructed genders and subsequent behaviors in the context of caregiving. Sorensen and Cooper (2010) reported that rural Australian grandfathers negotiated previously held gender identities to adopt new and nurturing behaviors toward their grandchildren. Jones and Curtin (2011) explored the experiences of rural Australian men who assumed primary caregiver roles for family members with traumatic brain injury. They noted that men went through a process of reformulation of their masculinities. This process took one of three paths: nonacceptance of the reformulated masculinity, acceptance of the reformulated masculinity but only for the sake of others, and acceptance and personally valuing the reformulated masculinity. Their experiences were remarkably similar to the men interviewed in the present study.

Although informative, other qualitative studies examining male caregivers are generally thematic in nature and do not present well-defined processes men adopt to respond to conflicts with constructed gender (Archer & MacLean, 1993; Coe & Neufeld, 1999; Harris, 1993; Hilton, Crawford, & Tarko, 2001; Mays & Lund, 1999; Neufeld & Harrison, 1998; Parsons, 1997; R. Russell, 2004, 2007). However, most of the themes identified in these previous studies are supported by the focused codes constructed in the present study.

LIMITATIONS

The small sample size and exploratory nature of this study present significant limitations to the generalizability of findings. The constructed findings are representative of a homogeneous subsample of rural male caregivers. The model constructed from the findings provides a very preliminary framework for understanding how men might negotiate conflicts between gender roles and caregiving. In this study, men negotiated gender roles but not rurality. It is likely that in other ethnic and racial groups, negotiation of both gender roles and culture might occur. Also, the study did not provide findings that adequately explain possible shifts in gender role negotiation patterns as one journeys along a caregiver trajectory. Further research is needed to investigate possible pattern shifts and factors that facilitate pattern shifts to more fully develop the model. Further research is also needed in other subgroups of caregivers to more fully understand gender attributes and their effect on caregiver and care recipient health and quality of life.

IMPLICATIONS FOR PRACTICE

R. Russell (2007) noted the importance of constructed gender in our understanding of caregiving. Such understanding is essential in developing strategies that will enhance men's ability to experience and provide caregiving with greater satisfaction and quality. Although individual participants variably adopted identified rural masculinity attributes, findings from this study suggests possible attributes of masculinity that may differ from those of other subgroups of men. In terms of a caregiving context, attributes of overly independent self-reliance (characterized by a strong resistance to seek help and an unwillingness to relinquish perceived control of the caregiving context) and reluctance to meet emotional needs (characterized by lonerism and escapism) promoted negative caregiving experiences and outcomes that may result in poor caregiver and care recipient health. Men who became aware of the potential harm caused by these gender attributes and who reconstructed their perspectives on these attributes were able to adopt new behaviors that provided improved caregiving quality and satisfaction. However, this awareness and behavior change occurred after enduring much stress.

Health and human service providers could potentially identify men who cling strongly to attributes associated with negative caregiver experiences and assist them to develop awareness and behavior change before reaching caregiver crisis. Identification might occur through questioning men on how they (a) feel about asking for and accepting help from others, (b) access sources of support, (c) manage their stress, and (d) take care of their own health and emotional needs. Such questioning can serve as an initial exploration for caregiver and provider alike and determine baseline perspectives and strategies caregivers possess as they progress through their caregiver trajectories. It is important to note that gaining awareness of one's perspectives on gender roles and adopting new behaviors are not easy tasks; for these participants, they occurred only as they approached a perceived crisis. Crisis can be averted, however, if providers work cooperatively with caregivers early in their caregiver trajectories.

Providers must not use an approach that negates a caregiver's baseline constructed gender. Simply pointing out attributes held by the caregiver that are problematic in a caregiving context will only result in an emasculating tone that will possibly be rejected by the caregiver. Therefore, providers should offer information and assistance that emphasize attributes of rural masculinity and rurality associated with positive experiences that might already fall within an individual's constructed gender and culture. Such attributes include a self-reliance that is outcome-focused and celebratory of hard work, the value for caring for one's own family, the value of a common-sense approach to work, recognition and acceptance of available community support, and the value of being a good provider. Helping caregivers elevate these attributes may serve as a deterrent to less helpful attributes held by the caregiver. For example, for the participants in this study who adopted a gender role reconstruction pattern, the value of being a good provider deterred their tendency to resist asking for help. Providers might focus a discussion on how reaching out for help yields better outcomes and is not a sign of personal failure, similar to the need to seek assistance at harvest time. Services that respect the caregiver's desire to provide caregiving, but let him maintain privacy and dominance in the home setting may also be beneficial. These services might include in-home services in which the caregiver is taught necessary caregiving skills and is mentored to adopt a team-leader role. It is troubling that none of the participants in this study received any instruction from health and human service providers on how to provide caregiving. Home health workers who come into a home and only provide assistance to the care recipient foster caregiver escapism, denounce caregiver personhood, and are perceived as highly intrusive. By refocusing the caregiving context on positive attributes, providers will help reduce the stress of caregiving and allow the caregiver the respite needed to facilitate gender reconstruction and personal growth.

Routine family assessment and service intake procedures may need to be examined to accommodate the exploration of the constructed genders of clients. Many providers may need continuing education on established theoretical foundations of gender and may require mentoring on how to conduct gender role assessments in a sensitive and respectful manner. In addition, educators in health and human service academic programs need to instruct students on the importance of gender and the clinical complexities resulting from variable and competing gendered attributes. Most likely, such content is rare in academic programs. However, educators may find using current academic content on culture to be an effective conduit for gender content, since culture also includes variable and competing constructed attributes that affect health and wellness. Use of this type of conduit can provide students an appropriate bridge from relatively familiar to unfamiliar content.

SUMMARY

This study provides initial insight into the processes used by a group of male rural caregivers. It used qualitative methods and a constructivist approach. The findings suggest that the men experienced conflict with personal gender roles as they adopted necessary caregiver work. This conflict produced variable levels of stress. The men managed their stress in one of three patterns: gender role conflict preservation, in which men avoided conflict resolution by employing actions of detachment; gender role compromise, in which men accepted conflict by doing what was necessary to get the caregiving work completed; and gender role reconstruction, in which men reframed their perspectives on gender so that caregiving work no longer provided conflict with personal gender roles. Men using the gender role reconstruction pattern reported greater caregiver success and personal growth. Implications of this study for health and human service providers include the need to explore the constructed genders of male caregivers to optimize caregiver success and health.

ACKNOWLEDGMENTS

The author acknowledges Deborah Messecar, PhD, RN, and Judy Kendall, PhD, RN, from the School of Nursing, Oregon Health & Science University, and Helen Lee, PhD, RN, who served as dissertation committee members for this study, for their guidance, and their support.

REFERENCES

Acton, G. J., & Winter, M. A. (2002). Interventions for family members caring for an elder with dementia. *Annual Review of Nursing Research, 20,* 149–179.

Anahita, S., & Mix, T. L. (2006). Retrofitting frontier masculinity for Alaska's war against wolves. *Gender and Society, 20*(3), 332–353.

Archbold, P. G., Stewart, B. J., Greenlick, M., & Harvath, T. A. (1992). The clinical assessment of mutuality and preparedness in family caregivers to frail older people. In S. Funk, E. Tornquist, M. Champagne, & R. Wiese (Eds.), *Key aspects of elder care: Managing falls, incontinence, and cognitive impairment* (pp. 328–339). New York, NY: Springer Publishing.

Archer, C., & MacLean, M. (1993). Husbands and sons as caregivers of chronically ill elderly women. *Journal of Gerontological Social Work, 21*(11/2), 5–23.

Arcury, T. A., Quandt, S. A., McDonald, J., & Bell, R. A. (2000). Faith and health self-management of rural older adults. *Journal of Cross Cultural Gerontology, 15*(1), 55–74.

Arno, P. S. (2006, January). *Economic value of informal caregiving.* Paper presented at the Care Coordination and the Caregiving Forum, Department of Veterans Affairs, NIH, Bethesda, MD.

Bailey, M. C. (1998). Outsider. In H. J. Lee (Ed.), *Conceptual basis for rural nursing* (pp. 139–148). New York, NY: Springer Publishing.

Baillie, V., Norbeck, J. S., & Barnes, L. E. (1988). Stress, social support, and psychological distress of family caregivers of the elderly. *Nursing Research, 37*(4), 217–222.

Bales, R. L. (2006). Health perceptions, needs, and behaviors of remote rural women of childbearing and childrearing age. In H. J. Lee, & C. A. Winters (Eds.), *Rural nursing: Concepts, theory, and practice* (2nd ed., pp. 66–78). New York, NY: Springer Publishing.

Bales, R. L., Winters, C. A., & Lee, H. J. (2006). Health needs and perceptions of rural persons. In H. J. Lee, & C. A. Winters (Eds.), *Rural nursing: Concepts, theory, and practice* (2nd ed., pp. 53–65). New York, NY: Springer Publishing.

Ballantyne, J., & Buehler, J. (1998). Experiences of HIV-infected men with rural health care. In H. Lee (Ed.), *Conceptual basis for rural nursing* (pp. 366–377). New York, NY: Springer Publishing.

Bell, D. (2000). Farm boys and wild men: Rurality, masculinity, and homosexuality. *Rural Sociology, 65*(4), 547–561.

Bennett, M., & Lengacher, C. (1999). Use of complementary therapies in a rural cancer population. *Oncology Nursing Forum, 26*(8), 1287–1294.

Beynon, J. (2002). What is masculinity? J. Beynon (Ed.), *Masculinities and culture* (pp. 1–25). Philadelphia, PA: Open University Press.

Bigbee, J. L. (1991). The concept of hardiness as applied to rural nursing. In A. Bushy (Ed.), *Rural nursing* (pp. 39–58). Thousand Oaks, CA: Sage.

Bigbee, J. L. (1993). The uniqueness of rural nursing. *Nursing Clinics of North America, 28*(1), 131–144.

Bookwala, J., Newman, J., & Schulz, R. (2002). Methodological issues in research on men caregivers. In B. J. Kramer, & E. Thompson (Eds.), *Men as caregivers: Theory, research, and service implications* (pp. 69–98). New York, NY: Springer Publishing.

Buehler, J., Malone, M., & Majerus, J. (1998). Patterns of responses to symptoms in rural residents: The symptom-action-time-line process. In H. Lee (Ed.), *Conceptual basis for rural nursing* (pp. 318–328). New York, NY: Springer.

Bull, C. N., Krout, J. A., Rathbone-McCuan, E., & Shreffler, M. J. (2001). Access and issues of equity in remote/rural areas. *Journal of Rural Health, 17*(4), 356–359.

Carpenter, E. H., & Miller, B. H. (2002). Psychological challenges and rewards experienced by caregiving men: A review of the literature. In B. J. Kramer, & E. H. Thompson (Eds.), *Men as caregivers: Theory, research, and service implications* (pp. 99–126). New York, NY: Springer Publishing.

Center on an Aging Society. (2003, January). Data profile: Rural and urban health. *Challenges for the 21st century: Chronic and disabling conditions* (pp. 1–6). Washington, DC: Institute for Health Care Research and Policy, Georgetown University.

Charmaz, K. (2000). Grounded theory: Objectivist and constructivist methods. In N. K. Denzin, & Y. S. Lincoln (Eds.), *Handbook of qualitative research* (2nd ed., pp. 509–536). Thousand Oaks, CA: Sage.

Charmaz, K. (2006). *Constructing grounded theory: A practical guide through qualitative analysis.* Thousand Oaks, CA: Sage.

Coe, M., & Neufeld, A. (1999). Male caregivers' use of formal support. *Western Journal of Nursing Research, 21*(4), 568–588.

Connell, R. W. (1993). The big picture: Masculinities in recent world history. *Theory and Society, 22,* 597–623.

Cook, D., & Rains, C. (1990). "Cowboy Logic" [Recorded by M. M. Murphey] [Music]. New York, NY: Warner Bros. Records.

Courtenay, W. H. (2000). Constructions of masculinity and their influence on men's well-being: A theory of gender and health. *Social Science and Medicine*, 50(10), 1385–1401.

Cristy, R. J. (2004). *Charles M. Russell: The storyteller's art*. Albuquerque, NM: University of New Mexico Press.

Dybbro, J. A. (1998). Ethnocentrism. In H. J. Lee (Ed.), *Conceptual basis for rural nursing* (pp. 287–296). New York, NY: Springer Publishing.

Eberhardt, M., Ingram, D., & Makuc, D. (2001). *Urban and rural health chartbook, health, United States*, 2001 (No. 76-641496). Hyattsville, MD: National Center for Health Statistics.

Findholt, N. (2006). The culture of rural communities: An examination of rural nursing concepts at the community level. In H. J. Lee, & C. A. Winters (Eds.), *Rural nursing: Concepts, theory, and practice* (2nd ed., pp. 301–312). New York, NY: Springer Publishing.

Gaskins, S., & Lyons, M. A. (2000). Self-care practices of rural people with HIV disease. *Online Journal of Rural Nursing and Health Care*, 1(1). Retrieved July 29, 2012, from http://www.rno.org/journal/index.php/online-journal/article/view/64/63

Gitlin, L. N., Belle, S. H., Burgio, L. D., Czaja, S. J., Mahoney, D., Gallagher-Thompson, D. et al. (2003). Effect of multicomponent interventions on caregiver burden and depression: The REACH multisite initiative at 6-month follow-up. *Psychology & Aging*, 18(3), 361–374.

Goins, R. T., & Mitchell, J. (1999). Health-related quality of life: Does rurality matter? *Journal of Rural Health*, 15(2), 147–156.

Good, G. E., Robertson, J. M., O'Neil, J. M., Fitzgerald, L. F., Stevens, M., DeBord, K. A. et al. (1995). Male gender role conflict: Psychometric issues and relations to psychological distress. *Journal of Counseling Psychology*, 42(1), 3–10.

Gorman, D., Buikstra, E., Hegney, D., Pearce, S., Rogers-Clark, C., Weir, J. et al. (2007). Rural men and mental health: Their experiences and how they managed. *International Journal of Mental Health Nursing*, 16(5), 298–306.

Gwyther, L. (1992). Research on gender and family caregiving: Implications for clinical practice. In J. Dwyer, & R. Coward (Eds.), *Gender, families and elder care*. Newbury Park, CA: Sage.

Hammer, J. H., Vogel, D. L., & Heimerdinger-Edwards, S. R. (2012, January 23). Men's help seeking: Examination of differences across community size, education, and income. *Psychology of Men and Masculinity*. Advance online publication. Doi: 10.1037/a0026813.

Harris, P. B. (1993). The misunderstood caregiver? A qualitative study of the male care-giver of Alzheimer's disease victims. *Gerontologist*, 33(4), 551–556.

Harris, P. B. (2002). The voices of husbands and sons caring for a family member with dementia. In B. J. Kramer, & E. Thompson (Eds.), *Men as caregivers: Theory, research, and service implications* (pp. 213–233). New York, NY: Springer Publishing.

Henson, D., Sadler, T., & Walton, S. (1998). Distance. In H. J. Lee (Ed.), *Conceptual basis for rural nursing* (pp. 51–60). New York, NY: Springer Publishing.

Hewitt, M. (1992). Defining 'rural' areas: Impact on health care policy and research. In W. Gesler, & T. Ricketts (Eds.), *Health in rural North America: The geography of health care services delivery* (pp. 25–54). New Brunswick, NJ: Rutgers University Press.

Hilton, B., Crawford, J., & Tarko, M. (2001). Men's experiences of coping with their wives' breast cancer involved focusing on the cancer and treatment and focusing on family to keep going. *Evidence-Based Nursing*, 4(1), 31.

Hogan, M. P., & Pursell, T. (2008). The 'real Alaskan': Nostalgia and rural masculinity in the 'last frontier'. *Men and Masculinities*, 11(1), 63–85.

Houde, S. C. (2002). Methodological issues in male caregiver research: An integrative review of the literature. *Journal of Advanced Nursing*, 40(6), 626–640.

Irvin, T., Sutherland, M., & Harris, G. (2006). A faith-based arthritis self-help program for rural African-American. *American Journal of Health Studies*, 21(1/2), 107–114.

Jones, J. A., & Curtin, M. (2011). Reformulating masculinity: Traumatic brain injury and the gendered nature of care and domestic roles. *Disability and Rehabilitation*, 33(17–18), 1568–1578.

Koehler, V. (1998). The substantive theory of protecting independence. In H. J. Lee (Ed.), *Conceptual basis for rural nursing* (pp. 236–256). New York, NY: Springer Publishing.

Kramer, B. J. (1997). Differential predictors of strain and gain among husbands caring for wives with dementia. *Gerontologist*, 37(2), 239–249.

Kramer, B. J. (2000). Husbands caring for wives with dementia: A longitudinal study of continuity and change. *Health and Social Work*, 25(2), 97–107.

Kramer, B. J. (2002). Men caregivers: An overview. In B. J. Kramer, & E. Thompson (Eds.), *Men as caregivers: Theory, research, and service implications* (pp. 3–19). New York, NY: Springer Publishing.

Kumar, V., Acanfora, M., Hennessy, C. H., & Kalache, A. (2001). Health status of the rural elderly. *Journal of Rural Health*, 17(4), 328–331.

Ladner, C., & Cuellar, N. (2002). Depression in rural hospice family caregivers. *Online Journal of Rural Nursing and Health Care*, 31(1). Retrieved July 29, 2012, from http://www.rno.org/journal/index.php/online-journal/article/view/108

Lawton, M. P., Kleban, M. H., Moss, M., Rovine, M., & Glicksman, A. (1989). Measuring caregiver appraisal. *Journal of Gerontology, 44*(3), P61–P71.

Lee, H. J. (1998a). Concept comparison: Old-timer/newcomer/insider/outsider. In H. J. Lee (Ed.), *Conceptual basis for rural nursing* (pp. 149–155). New York, NY: Springer Publishing.

Lee, H. J. (1998b). Lack of anonymity. In H. J. Lee (Ed.), *Conceptual basis for rural nursing* (pp. 76–88). New York, NY: Springer Publishing.

Lee, H. J., & Winters, C. A. (2004). Testing rural nursing theory: Perceptions and needs of service providers. *Online Journal of Rural Nursing and Health Care, 4*(1). Retrieved September 6, 2006, from http://www.rno.org/journal/index.php/online-journal/article/view/128

Leipert, B. D., & Reutter, L. (2005). Developing resilience: How women maintain their health in northern geographic isolated settings. *Qualitative Health Research, 15*(1), 49–65.

Levant, R. F., & Habben, C. (2003). The new psychology of men: Application to rural men. In B. Stamm (Ed.), *Rural behavioral health care: An interdisciplinary guide* (pp. 171–180). Washington, DC: American Psychological Association.

Levant, R. F., Hirsch, L. S., Cozza, T. M., Hill, S., MacEachern, M., Marty, N. et al. (1992). The male role: An investigation of contemporary norms. *Journal of Mental Health Counseling, 14*(3), 325–337.

Lishner, D. M., Richardson, M., Levine, P., & Patrick, D. (1996). Access to primary health care among persons with disabilities in rural areas: A summary of the literature. *Journal of Rural Health, 12*(1), 45–53.

Mays, G. D., & Lund, C. H. (1999). Male caregivers of mentally ill relatives. *Perspectives in Psychiatric Care, 35*(2), 19–28.

Miller, B., & Cafasso, L. (1992). Gender differences in caregiving: Fact or artifact? *Gerontologist, 32*(4), 498–507.

Morgan, D. G., Semchuk, K. M., Stewart, N. J., & D'Arcy, C. (2002). Rural families caring for a relative with dementia: Barriers to use of formal services. *Social Science and Medicine, 55*(7), 1129–1142.

National Alliance for Caregiving and American Association of Retired Persons [NAC & AARP]. (2009). *Caregiving in the U.S. 2009.* (Report). Washington, DC: National Alliance for Caregiving.

National Institute of Nursing Research [NINR]. (1994). *Family caregiving.* Retrieved April 8, 2003, from http://www.nih.gov/ninr/research/vol3/FamCare.htm

National Rural Health Association [NRHA]. (2007). *What's different about rural health care?* Retrieved December 21, 2008, from http://www.ruralhealthweb.org/go/left/about-rural-health/what-s-different-about-rural-health-care

Neufeld, A., & Harrison, M. J. (1998). Men as caregivers: Reciprocal relationships or obligation? *Journal of Advanced Nursing, 28*(5), 959–968.

O'Lynn, C. (2006). The symptom-action time line: A literature review and recommendations for revision. In H. J. Lee, & C. A. Winters (Eds.), *Rural nursing: Concepts, theory, and practice* (2nd ed., pp. 138–152). New York, NY: Springer Publishing.

O'Neil, J. M., Good, G. E., & Holmes, S. (1995). Fifteen years of theory and research on men's gender role conflict: New paradigms for empirical research. In R. F. Levant, & W. S. Pollack (Eds.), *A new psychology of men* (pp. 164–206). New York, NY: Basic Books.

Parsons, K. (1997). Male experience of caregiving for a family member with Alzheimer's disease. *Qualitative Health Research, 7,* 391–407.

Pearlin, L. I., & Schooler, C. (1978). The structure of coping. *Journal of Health and Social Behavior, 19,* 2–21.

Pinquart, M., & Sorensen, S. (2006). Gender differences in caregiver stressors, social resources, and health: An updated meta-analysis. *Journals of Gerontology. Series B: Psychological Sciences and Social Sciences, 61B*(1), P33–P45.

Pleck, J. H. (1995). The gender role strain paradigm: An update. In R. F. Levant, & W. S. Pollack (Eds.), *A new psychology of men* (pp. 11–32). New York, NY: Basic Books.

Robinson, B. C. (1983). Validation of a caregiver strain index. *Journal of Gerontology, 38*(3), 344–348.

Russell, C. M. (1927). *Trails plowed under.* Lincoln: University of Nebraska Press.

Russell, R. (2004). Social networks among elderly men caregivers. *The Journal of Men's Studies, 13*(1), 121–142.

Russell, R. (2007). Men doing "women's work": Elderly men caregivers and the gendered construction of care work. *Journal of Men's Studies, 15*(1), 1–19.

Russell, R. (2008). Their story, my story: Health of older men as caregivers. *Generations, 32*(1), 62–67.

Ryan-Nicholls, K. (2004). Health and sustainability of rural communities. *Rural and Remote Health, 4*(242), 1–11. Retrieved July 30, 2012, from http://www.rrh.org.au/articles/subviewnew.asp?ArticleID=242

Schoenberg, N. E., Hatcher, J., Dignan, M. B., Shelton, B., Wright, S., & Dollarhide, K. T. (2009). Faith moves mountains: An Appalachian cervical cancer prevention program. *American Journal of Health Behavior, 33*(6), 627–638.

Schulz, R., Beach, S. R., Lind, B., Martire, L. M., Zdaniuk, B., & Hirsch, C. (2001). Involvement in caregiving and adjustment to death of a spouse: Findings from the caregiver health effects study. *JAMA, 285*(24), 3123–3129.

Sorensen, P., & Cooper, N. J. (2010). Reshaping the family man: A grounded theory study of the meaning of grandfatherhood. *The Journal of Men's Studies, 18*(2), 117–136.

Stoller, E. (2002). Theoretical perspectives on caregiving men. In B. J. Kramer, & E. Thompson (Eds.), *Men as caregivers: Theory, research, and service implications* (pp. 51–68). New York, NY: Springer Publishing.

Strength for Caring, Johnson & Johnson Consumer Products. (2005). Attitudes and beliefs about caregiving in the U.S.: Findings of a national opinion survey. Survey conducted by Opinion Research Corporation, Princeton, NJ. Retrieved from www.strengthforcaring.com/util/press/research/index.html

Thompson, E. H. (2002). What's unique about men's caregiving? In B. J. Kramer, & E. H. Thompson (Eds.), *Men as caregivers: Theory, research, and service implications* (pp. 20–50). New York, NY: Springer Publishing.

U.S. Census Bureau. (2002). *U.S. summary: 2000* (Census profile No. C2KPROF/00- US). Washington, DC: U.S. Department of Commerce.

U.S. Census Bureau. (2004). *U.S. interim projections by age, sex, race, and Hispanic origin*. Retrieved February 27, 2007, from http://www.census.gov/ipc/www/usinterim- proj/

Vitaliano, P. P., Zhang, J., & Scanlan, J. M. (2003). Is caregiving "hazardous to one's physical health"? A meta-analysis. *Psychological Bulletin, 129*, 946–997.

Wagenfeld, M. O. (2000). Delivering mental health services to the persistently and seriously mentally ill in frontier areas. *Journal of Rural Health, 16*(1), 91–96.

Wagenfeld, M. O. (2003). A snapshot of rural and frontier America. In B. Stamm (Ed.), *Rural behavioral health care: An interdisciplinary guide* (pp. 33–41). Washington, DC: American Psychological Association.

Wathen, C. N., & Harris, R. M. (2007). "I try to take care of it myself." How rural women search for health information. *Qualitative Health Research, 17*(5), 639–651.

Weinert, C. (2005). Chronically ill rural women's views of health care. *Online Journal of Rural Nursing and Health Care, 5*(2), 18p. Retrieved July 29, 2012, from http://www.rno.org/journal/index.php/online-journal/article/view/42

Wells, M. (2009). Resilience in rural community-dwelling older adults. *Journal of Rural Health, 25*(4), 415–419.

Yee, J. L., & Schulz, R. (2000). Gender differences in psychiatric morbidity among family caregivers: A review and analysis. *The Gerontologist, 40*, 147–164.

Young, R. F., & Kahana, E. (1989). Specifying caregiver outcomes: Gender and relationship aspects of caregiving strain. *Gerontologist, 29*(5), 660–666.

Zarit, S., Reever, K. E., & Bach-Peterson, J. (1980). Relatives of the impaired elderly: Correlates of feelings of burden. *The Gerontologist, 20*(6), 649–655.

Chapter 13

COMPLEMENTARY THERAPY AND HEALTH LITERACY IN RURAL DWELLERS

Jean M. Shreffler-Grant,
Elizabeth Nichols, Clarann Weinert,
and Bette Ide

ADEQUATE HEALTH LITERACY IS NECESSARY in today's health care marketplace so that consumers are able to understand and evaluate information regarding conventional or allopathic health care (Institute of Medicine [IOM], 2004). Health literacy is defined in *Healthy People 2010* as "the degree to which individuals have the capacity to obtain, process, and understand basic health information and services needed to make appropriate health decisions" (U.S. Department of Health and Human Services, 2000, Section 11-2).

Health literacy is even more important for evaluating complementary and alternative medicine (CAM). Health care consumers usually have some assistance from providers to interpret information about allopathic care and often receive instructions and advice to guide health care decision making and action taking. This is less likely with CAM. These therapies are often self-prescribed or self-directed in nature and are less regulated or controlled by governmental agencies or allopathic providers. Further, studies have found that often there is limited communication between consumers and allopathic providers about consumers' use or potential use of CAM (Eisenberg et al., 1993, 1998; Vallerand, Fouladbakhsh, & Templin, 2003).

During the past several decades, the use of CAM in the United States has grown significantly (Barnes, Bloom, & Nahin, 2008; Eisenberg et al., 1993, 1998; IOM, 2005). CAM has become an important component of the U.S. health care system as consumers, including those living in rural areas, increasingly use CAM as an adjunct to or substitute for conventional health care (Arcury, Preisser, Gesler, & Sherman, 2004; Astin, 1998;

Eisenberg et al., 1998; Harron & Glasser, 2003; McFarland, Bigelow, Zani, Newson, & Kaplan, 2002). In addition, the recent downturn in the economy has fueled an increase in the use of CAM products in place of allopathic treatments because of the lower cost of CAM (Associated Press, 2009). The National Center for Complementary and Alternative Medicine (NCCAM, 2006) defines CAM as a group of diverse health care systems, practices, and products that are not presently considered a part of allopathic health care. The CAM therapies and products are not considered part of allopathic care in large part because there is insufficient evidence that they are safe and effective (NCCAM, 2008). Types of CAM range from therapies provided by practitioners such as naturopathic physicians and acupuncturists to self-care practices, such as herbs and magnets.

In 2007, approximately 40% of adults in the United States used some form of CAM in the past 12 months (Barnes et al., 2008), which is slightly more than the 36% use rate found in a comparable national study conducted in 2003 (Barnes, Pewell-Griner, McFann, & Nahin, 2004). In addition, the results of the Barnes et al. study demonstrated that approximately one in nine (11.8%) children used CAM in the past 12 months. Not surprisingly, use among children whose parents used CAM was significantly higher (23.9%) than among children whose parents did not use CAM (5.1%). In 2007, when cost concerns caused a delay in seeking allopathic care, CAM was more likely to be used by both adults and children than when cost was not a concern (Barnes et al., 2004). Despite the widespread use and acceptance of CAM in the general population, consumers are reluctant to inform allopathic providers that they used CAM (Eisenberg et al., 1993, 1998).

On the basis of the literature, the demographics of those in the general United States population who use CAM vary; but in general, CAM is used more often for chronic than acute health conditions and use is more common among women than men, younger adults than older, those with higher incomes and more education, and those living in the West than in other parts of the country (Astin, 1998; Astin, Pelletier, Marie, & Haskell, 2000; Cherniack, Senzel, & Pan, 2001; Eisenberg et al., 1998). Studies have found that individuals with chronic illness have a variety of reasons for using CAM, including (a) symptom relief, (b) ineffectiveness of allopathic treatments, (c) side effects of allopathic treatments, (d) dissatisfaction with allopathic care, (e) concerns about adverse effects of allopathic care, (f) desire for control, and (g) the ready availability of CAM (Johnson, 1999; Montbraind & Laing, 1991; Rao et al., 1999; Vincent & Furnham, 1996).

Despite extensive searches, no empirical studies have been located in the literature specifically on health literacy about CAM. There is also very limited evidence in general about how much CAM users know about the products and treatments they use, what sources of information they use, or how they evaluate and use the information they have or acquire (IOM, 2005). Evidence is also lacking about how consumers in the United States decide when and how to use CAM and whether or not they comply with instructions from CAM providers or product labels. One study found that while 80% of older study participants reported using two or more CAM therapies, their self-rated knowledge about most of the therapies was very low (King & Pettigrew, 2004). The IOM cited three primary sources of information that consumers use about CAM: word of mouth, the Internet, and health food stores. The few studies evaluating the quality of information available from these sources suggested that quality may be a concern.

The purpose of this chapter is to present a summary of a series of research studies conducted by a team of investigators at the Colleges of Nursing at Montana State University (MSU) and the University of North Dakota on the use of CAM by older rural dwellers. The results of these projects have raised a number of researchable questions regarding the health literacy levels about CAM among older rural adults, particularly rural adults with chronic illnesses.

HEALTH CARE CHOICES: A STUDY OF COMPLEMENTARY THERAPY USE AMONG OLDER RURAL DWELLERS

At the time this study was conducted, a number of well-known studies had demonstrated that use of CAM was growing among the general population in the United States, but little was known about use of these therapies among rural residents. Most of the national studies did not report where study participants lived and some used only urban participants. To address this gap in the literature, the Health Care Choices study was conducted with older adults living in sparsely populated rural areas in Montana and North Dakota (Shreffler-Grant, Weinert, Nichols, & Ide, 2005). The purpose of the study was to explore the use, cost of, and satisfaction with the quality and effectiveness of CAM from the perspectives of the older rural adult participants. The study was conducted during 2000 to 2003 and funded by NCCAM (1R15AT09501). A descriptive survey design was used to generate data from a random sample of older adults in 19 rural communities in Montana and North Dakota. An interview instrument was developed to elicit data addressing the specific aims; it was piloted prior to use. Telephone interviews were conducted with 325 older adults. Participants ranged in age from 60 to 98 years ($m = 71.7$). Most of the participants (67.7%, $n = 202$) reported having one or more chronic illnesses. Only 17.5% ($n = 57$) reported using CAM providers, while 35.7% ($n = 116$) used self-prescribed CAM practices. When these two categories of use were combined, a total of 45.2% of the participants used some form of CAM, or used CAM providers, self-prescribed CAM practices, or both. This finding demonstrated that these older rural residents were using as much or more CAM than participants in national studies (36%–40%) that included all adult age groups.

Relevant to the issue of health literacy about CAM, the participants in this study most often learned about the CAM therapies by word of mouth from relatives or friends, consumer marketing, or reading, rather than from health care professionals (Shreffler-Grant et al., 2005). Much of the CAM used by participants of this study was self-prescribed, raising questions about whether the participants had sufficient knowledge and information for safe and effective use of the CAM products. In addition, a majority (64.6%, $n = 210$) of the participants reported that they had at least one significant acute or chronic health problem and 32.3% ($n = 105$) had two or more significant health problems. The research team wondered about the potential for adverse drug–herb or drug–vitamin interactions with this population of vulnerable older adults, who likely were taking multiple prescription medications and had aging, impaired physiological responses impaired physiological responses.

Health Care Choices: Older Rural Women

Additional analyses were conducted on a portion of the data set generated in the first Health Care Choices study to answer the following research question: What factors predict use of CAM among older rural women (Shreffler-Grant, Hill, Weinert, Nichols, & Ide, 2007). Men were excluded from this analysis because too few men in the larger data set used CAM, which is consistent with the literature about CAM use. Potential predictors were selected from the literature and observations from practice and included education, age, rurality, marital status, income, spirituality, number of chronic illnesses, and health status. Logistic regression analysis was used to examine factors associated with use of CAM by the rural women participants ($n = 156$). A total of 25.6% of the women had used CAM recently and most of the therapies they used were self-prescribed. Women most likely to use CAM were those who were fairly well educated, not currently married, and in their early older years (60–69 years of age). They had one or more significant chronic illnesses and lower health-related quality of life due to emotional concerns such as depression or stress.

Although this analysis did not yield additional information about health literacy about CAM per se, the results reinforced and expanded the findings of the main study discussed above. The women who reported use of CAM in this analysis used primarily self-prescribed CAM, which again raises concern about their level of knowledge about CAM. Women with one or more chronic illnesses were more likely to use CAM than those without chronic illness. Specifically, for each additional chronic illness reported the odds of CAM use increased by 46%. By identifying characteristics of older rural women who are more or less likely to use

CAM, the results can be used to tailor educational interventions to improve health literacy about CAM.

Health Care Choices: Chronic Illness

The purpose of this study was to provide a better understanding of older rural adults' use of CAM, their perceptions of efficacy of the CAM they used, and the sources of information they used about CAM (Nichols, Sullivan, Ide, Shreffler-Grant, & Weinert, 2005). The study was conducted during 2003 to 2004 and funded by the Center for Research on Chronic Health Conditions in Rural Dwellers (CRCHC) at MSU College of Nursing (NIH/NINR IP20NR07790-01). Ten participants between 60 and 80 years of age who reported using CAM in the original Health Care Choices study and who had two or more chronic illnesses were interviewed by telephone. Qualitative analysis was used to organize content and identify themes. Participants primarily used self-prescribed CAM therapies such as dietary supplements and herbs, taken to compensate for perceived dietary deficiencies. Participants were generally satisfied with the results they attributed to the CAM. With regard to health literacy about CAM, the participants attempted to use reputable sources of information about the CAM products they used, but it was clear that some used the products in an inconsistent manner and did not understand what the products did. Some individuals reported seeking information about CAM from sources other than their allopathic providers due to a perception that the providers were too busy to answer their questions about CAM.

Health Care Choices: CAM Providers in Rural Locations

The CAM Providers in Rural Locations study was motivated by the results of the first Health Care Choices study, in which the older rural adults reported limited use of CAM providers, in contrast to self-prescribed CAM. The study's purpose was to determine the availability of CAM resources in 20 small rural towns in Montana and North Dakota and to explore the contribution of one type of CAM provider, naturopathic physicians, to rural health care (Nichols, Weinert, Shreffler-Grant, & Ide, 2006). The study was conducted during 2004 to 2005 and funded by the Center for Research on Chronic Health Conditions (CRCHC) in Rural Dwellers at MSU College of Nursing (NIH/NINR IP20NR07790-01). CAM resource data were collected by Internet and telephone directory searches and by an online survey of naturopaths in Montana. Seventy-three CAM providers were identified in the 20 towns. Most naturopaths were located in population centers, but some offered outreach clinics to rural communities. Based on the results, the team concluded that local availability is not the critical factor in use of CAM providers by older rural adults. Although there were likely fewer choices of CAM providers in these small rural towns than in larger towns or cities, there were CAM providers available if the rural residents chose to use them. Rural residents are also known to travel outside their local communities to see health care providers who are acceptable to them (Shreffler-Grant, 2006).

Health Care Choices: The MSU CAM Health Literacy Scale

Owing to the questions concerning CAM health literacy revealed in the results of the studies discussed above, the research team identified the need for an intervention to improve health literacy about CAM among older rural adults, particularly those with chronic health conditions. A measure of CAM health literacy is needed to determine whether or not the intervention is effective. The existing health literacy measures were not suitable for this purpose since they essentially evaluate basic reading and math skills in a health care context (IOM, 2004) and not the more complex aspects needed to make reasoned decisions about the use of CAM. Accordingly, the research team designed and sought funding for the next Health Care Choices project, the purpose of which is to develop a psychometrically sound instrument to measure CAM health literacy. In this project, CAM health literacy is operationally defined as the information about CAM needed to make informed self-management decisions regarding health.

The research team initiated work on the project with funding from an Intramural Block Grant (2008–2009) from MSU College of Nursing. The instrument development process being used is based on DeVellis' (2003) well-established guidelines for scale development. A conceptual model was developed and is being used to guide item construction for the new instrument (Shreffler-Grant, Nichols, Weinert, & Ide, in press). The conceptual model was reviewed and critiqued by a panel of CAM and health literacy experts and revised based on their input. A large pool of initial items for the new instrument was developed and critiqued by nationally known experts on scale development. The items consist of a list of statements about herbal products; participants are instructed to indicate whether or not they agree or disagree with the statements, based on their knowledge or understanding.

Support for continuing development and psychometric evaluation of the MSU CAM Health Literacy Scale was obtained in 2011 from NIH/NCCAM (1R15T006609-01 for 2011–2013). After funding began, focus group meetings were convened involving two groups of older adults and two groups of allopathic and CAM health care providers, who critiqued the new instrument. Following revisions based on the focus groups, another review by experts was conducted and the instrument was refined again. The refined MSU CAM Health Literacy Scale was recently administered by telephone interview to 1,200 randomly selected older adults living in rural areas in the northwestern quadrant of the United States. Psychometric evaluation of the new instrument using the data from the telephone interviews is currently being implemented. The instrument will be revised and refined again, based on these procedures.

A validation assessment will be conducted in the near future by administering the latest draft of the MSU CAM Health Literacy Scale and an established health literacy instrument (S-TOFHLA) to a convenience sample of 75 community-dwelling older adults. The results will be compared and will be used to make additional revisions as appropriate. Following the procedures described above, the team will make decisions about the final scale length and items to retain and discard.

The research team anticipates that this study will contribute to a fuller understanding of health literacy as it relates to CAM among older rural dwellers, particularly those with chronic health conditions. The current study will result in a first-generation measure of CAM health literacy that can be used in the research team's planned intervention as well as in other clinical and research applications. Improved CAM health literacy can help individual consumers avoid risks and harm as well as increase their options for care of their health and illness. We also anticipate that the MSU CAM Health Literacy Scale will have scientific and clinical application for assessing health literacy in other self-care decision-making situations.

DISCUSSION

Over the past decade, this research team conducted the series of studies discussed above on the use of CAM among older rural adults. This work has led us to ask compelling questions about the level of health literacy about CAM among this population, particularly those with chronic illnesses. Health care consumers in any location, particularly those with chronic illnesses, make numerous decisions about health care and use a wide variety of self-care health products and therapies, decisions often made independent of allopathic providers. This is particularly true of older rural adults, who are known to be more independent, engage in more self-care, and have less access to allopathic care than those living in urban areas (Shreffler-Grant et al., 2007). Those with chronic illnesses are also more likely to use CAM therapies (Astin, 1998; Astin et al., 2000; Barnes et al., 2004; Eisenberg et al., 1998; Shreffler-Grant et al., 2007).

Making informed decisions about the use of CAM requires a sophisticated level of health literacy on the part of the consumer. Without adequate CAM health literacy, older rural consumers may not know of all the appropriate health care choices that may benefit them, may fall victim to scams or unscrupulous sales practices, or may ingest potentially harmful substances. Informed use of CAM can increase health and illness management options and support well-reasoned decision making in regard to self-care for older rural adults living with chronic illnesses.

ACKNOWLEDGMENTS

These research studies were funded in part by grants from the National Institutes of Health, National Center for Complementary and Alternative Medicine (1R15AT095-01) (1R15T006609-01), the Center for Research on Chronic Health Conditions at MSU College of Nursing (NIH/NINR IP20NR07790-01), and an Intramural Block Grant (2008–2009) from MSU College of Nursing.

REFERENCES

Arcury, T. A., Preisser, J. S., Gesler, W. M., & Sherman, J. E. (2004). Complementary and alternative medicine use among rural residents in western North Carolina. *Complementary Health Practice Review, 9*(2), 93–102.

Associated Press. (January 13, 2009). With economy sour, consumers sweet on herbal medicines. *Washingtonpost.com.*

Astin, J. (1998). Why patients use alternative medicine: Results of a national study. *Journal of the American Medical Association, 279*(19), 1548–1553.

Astin, J., Pelletier, K., Marie, A., & Haskell, W. (2000). Complementary and alternative medicine use among elderly persons: One-year analysis of a blue shield Medicare supplement. *Journal of Gerontology, 55A*, M4–M9.

Barnes, P. M., Bloom, B., & Nahin, R. L. (2008). *Complementary and alternative medicine use among adults and children: United States, 2007. National health statistics reports, No. 12.* Hyattsville, MD: National Center for Health Statistics.

Barnes, P. M., Pewell-Griner, E., McFann, K., & Nahin, R. L. (2004). *Complementary and alternative medicine use among adults: United States, 2002. National health statistics reports, No. 343.* Hyattsville, MD: National Center for Health Statistics.

Cherniack, E. P., Senzel, R. S., & Pan, C. X. (2001). Correlates of use of alternative medicine by the elderly in an urban population. *Journal of Alternative and Complementary Medicine, 7*, 277–280.

DeVellis, R. (2003). *Scale development: Theory and applications* (2nd ed.). Thousand Oaks, CA: Sage.

Eisenberg, D., Davis, R., Ettner, S., Appel, S., Wilkey, S., Van Rompay, M. et al. (1998). Trends in alternative medicine use in the United States, 1990–1997: Results of a follow-up national survey. *Journal of the American Medical Association, 280*(18), 1569–1575.

Eisenberg, D., Kessler, R., Foster, C., Norlock, F., Calkins, D., & Delbanco, T. (1993). Unconventional medicine in the United States. *The New England Journal of Medicine, 328*, 246–252.

Harron, M., & Glasser, M. (2003). Use of and attitudes toward complementary and alternative medicine among family practice patients in small rural Illinois communities. *The Journal of Rural Health, 19*(3), 279–284.

Institute of Medicine (IOM). (2004). *Health literacy: A prescription to end confusion.* Washington, DC: The National Academies Press.

Institute of Medicine (IOM). (2005). *Complementary and alternative medicine in the United States.* Washington, DC: The National Academies Press.

Johnson, J. (1999). Older rural women and the use of complementary therapies. *Journal of Community Health Nursing, 16*(4), 223–232.

King, M. O., & Pettigrew, A. C. (2004). Complementary and alternative therapy use by older adults in three ethnically diverse populations: A pilot study. *Geriatric Nursing, 25*(1), 30–37.

McFarland, B., Bigelow, D., Zani, B., Newsom, J., & Kaplan, M. (2002). Complementary and alternative medicine use in Canada and the United States. *American Journal of Public Health, 92,* 1616–1618.

Montbraind, M., & Laing, G. (1991). Alternative health care as a control strategy. *Journal of Advanced Nursing, 16,* 325–332.

National Center for Complementary and Alternative Medicine (NCCAM). (2006). *What is complementary and alternative medicine (CAM)?* Retrieved June 10, 2006, from http://nccam.nih.gov/health/whatiscam/

National Center for Complementary and Alternative Medicine (NCCAM). (2008). *Expanding horizons of health care: Strategic plan* 2005–2009. Retrieved July 20, 2012, from http://nccam.nih.gov/sites/nccam.nih.gov/files/about/plans/2005/strategicplan.pdf

Nichols, E., Sullivan, T., Ide, B., Shreffler-Grant, J., & Weinert, C. (2005). Health care choices: Complementary therapy, chronic illness, and older rural dwellers. *Journal of Holistic Nursing, 23*(4), 381–394.

Nichols, E., Weinert, C., Shreffler-Grant, J., & Ide, B. (2006). Complementary and alternative providers in rural locations. *Online Journal of Rural Nursing and Health Care, 6*(2). Retrieved July 20, 2012, from http://www.rno.org/journal/index.php/online-journal/article/viewFile/4/171

Rao, J., Mihaliak, K., Kroenke, K., Bradley, J., Tierney, W., & Weinberger, M. (1999). Use of complementary therapies for arthritis among patients of rheumatologists. *Annals of Internal Medicine, 131,* 409–416.

Shreffler-Grant, J. (2006). Acceptability: One component in choice of health care provider. In H. J. Lee, & C. A. Winters (Eds.), *Rural nursing: Concepts, theory, and practice* (2nd ed., pp. 166–176). New York, NY: Springer Publishing.

Shreffler-Grant, J., Hill, W., Weinert, C., Nichols, E., & Ide, B. (2007). Complementary therapy and older rural women: Who uses and who does not? *Nursing Research, 56*(1), 28–33.

Shreffler-Grant, J., Nichols, E., Weinert, C., & Ide, B. (in press). Montana State University conceptual model of complementary and alternative medicine (CAM) health literacy. *Journal of Health Communication: International Perspectives.*

Shreffler-Grant, J., Weinert, C., Nichols, E., & Ide, B. (2005). Complementary therapy use among older rural adults. *Public Health Nursing,* 22(4), 323–331.

U.S. Department of Health and Human Services. (2000). *Healthy people 2010, section 11-2: Health communication objective.* Retrieved July 14, 2005, from www.healthypeople.gov

Vallerand, A. H., Fouladbakhsh, J. M., & Templin, T. (2003). The use of complementary/alternative medicine for self-treatment of pain among residents or urban, suburban, and rural communities. *American Journal of Public Health,* 93, 923–925.

Vincent, C., & Furnham, A. (1996). Why do patients turn to complementary medicine? An empirical study. *British Journal of Clinical Psychology,* 35, 37–48.

Chapter 14

ACCEPTABILITY: ONE COMPONENT IN CHOICE OF HEALTH CARE PROVIDER
Jean M. Shreffler-Grant

SINCE THE EARLY 1980s, ACCESS to health care has deteriorated in many rural areas in the United States as a result of the closure of rural hospitals and the associated loss of local providers and services that often accompany hospital closure. Historically, much of the blame for closures has been attributed to factors external to rural communities, such as limited Medicare reimbursement, the declining rural economy, and provider shortages. In contrast, a substantial volume of evidence now indicates that the closures may, in part, be due to influences closer to home. Some rural hospitals are underutilized by local residents, who bypass them to seek care in larger towns and cities (Amundson, 1993; DeFriese, Wilson, Ricketts, & Whitener, 1992; Escarse & Kapur, 2009; Liu, Bellamy, Barnet, & Weng, 2008; Liu, Bellamy, & McCormick, 2007; Radcliff, Brasure, Moscovice, & Stensland, 2003).

Since the early 1990s, variations of critical access hospitals (CAHs) have been implemented as alternatives to hospitals that are at risk for closure. CAHs must be located in remote rural areas, are limited to short-stay lower-acuity services, and are allowed more flexibility in staffing and other licensure requirements. They are also reimbursed by Medicare on the basis of reasonable cost instead of prospective payment, as compared with traditional rural hospitals. Cost-based Medicare reimbursement is considered advantageous for small hospitals that often serve a high proportion of older patients and are less likely to be able to average risk across large numbers of admissions, as may be necessary under prospective payment (Christianson, Moscovice, Wellever, & Wingert, 1990). Following implementation of the Rural Hospital Flexibility Program, passed into law in 1997, CAHs became a national model and have gained broad support in rural areas across the nation (Shreffler, Capalbo, Flaherty, & Heggam, 1999). By 2006, less than a decade after the CAH model was passed into law, a large majority (80%) of small rural hospitals and more than 60% of all rural hospitals had converted to CAHs (Pink, Holmes, Thompson, & Slifkin, 2007). As of March 31, 2011, there were 1,327 certified CAHs nationwide (Rural Assistance Center [RAC], 2012). Whether these new CAH models will be any more viable than traditional rural hospitals will likely be tied to how they are viewed and used by the rural residents they are intended to serve.

Improving equity in access to care has been an ongoing concern throughout most of the past half-century (Aday, Bagley, Lairson, & Slater, 1993; Patrick & Erickson, 1993), and rural access to care has been a particularly persistent problem (Gamm & Hutchison, 2003). Although equitable access to health care in and of itself may be intuitively desirable, it is through presumed links between access to quality health services, appropriate use, and resulting positive health outcomes that access becomes important (Millman, 1993). I conducted a study (1996) to examine rural residents' perspectives on access to health care in six communities in Montana with CAHs. The concept of "acceptability" is one dimension of access to care that can be used to explain why people do or do not use local rural health care services. As part of the larger study, a scale to measure acceptability was developed and validated. In this chapter, I will focus on the Acceptability Scale (see Table 14.1).

CONCEPTUAL FRAMEWORK

Access to care was the conceptual framework guiding this study. I conceptualized access to care as having two dimensions. Potential access to care includes properties of the population and health care system that affect opportunities to enter into the health care system. Actual or realized access to care includes utilization and willingness to use the health care system and satisfaction with the care received (Aday & Andersen, 1975; Andersen, McCutcheon, Aday, Chiu, & Bell, 1993).

In several studies published in the 1980s on the relationship between access to care and utilization of care, Penchansky and Thomas (1981; Thomas & Penchansky, 1984) defined access as the fit between clients and the health care system. An adequate degree of fit was measured by objective utilization and subjective satisfaction. They identified five components of potential access that are referred to as "the 5 A's":

1. Availability—the supply of providers and services relative to clients' needs;
2. Accessibility—where services are located relative to where clients are;
3. Accommodation—how services are organized to accept clients;

TABLE 14.1 Individual Items Included in the "Acceptability Scale"

	Circle One Answer for Each Category					
	Excellent	Good	Average	Fair	Poor	
1. How would you rate [facility name] in each of the following categories?						
a. Overall quality of care	5	4	3	2	1	Don't know
b. Medical care	5	4	3	2	1	Don't know
c. Nursing care	5	4	3	2	1	Don't know
d. Staff concern/compassion	5	4	3	2	1	Don't know
e. "Personal" aspects of care	5	4	3	2	1	Don't know
f. Building cleanliness and condition	5	4	3	2	1	Don't know
g. Acceptability as source of care	5	4	3	2	1	Don't know
2. How would you rate each of the following aspects of overall medical care provided in your community? (Care provided by physicians, nurse practitioners, physician assistants, or other primary care providers at their office or local hospital).						
a. Competence of primary care providers	5	4	3	2	1	Don't know
b. Concern/compassion for patient	5	4	3	2	1	Don't know
c. "Personal" aspects of care	5	4	3	2	1	Don't know
d. Competence of support staff	5	4	3	2	1	Don't know
e. Acceptability of provider as source of care	5	4	3	2	1	Don't know

4. Affordability—costs of services relative to resources of clients; and finally,

5. Acceptability—the clients' attitudes and opinions about the characteristics of providers and services.

Discriminant validity of Penchansky and Thomas' (1981; Thomas & Penchansky, 1984) components of access to care was supported in their studies, and subsets of clients were found to differ significantly in utilization of health care, based on how satisfied they were with the components that were salient for them. Although these investigators measured acceptability chiefly by consumers' attitudes and opinions about the physical environment in which care was delivered, they proposed that attitudes about personal and technical practice characteristics of providers and services were also relevant.

METHODS

In the larger study to examine rural residents' perspectives on access to health care (Shreffler, 1996), I employed a descriptive survey design. I sent surveys to a random sample of 100 households in each of the six communities with CAHs, and I interviewed a subset of respondents by telephone. I obtained a 63.5% response rate on the mail survey ($n = 381$).

My principal aims in this study were to identify the predictors of use and willingness to use local health care, and respondents' satisfaction with care. In interpreting the term *predictors*, it should be noted that I sought significant statistical relationships rather than cause and effect relationships. It was not possible to determine from the data whether people used local health care because they thought it was acceptable or whether they thought it was acceptable because they had used it.

There were four dependent variables in the analyses to address actual access to care. They were (a) use of the local CAH, (b) use of the local primary care provider, (c) willingness to use the local CAH, and (d) willingness to use the local provider. These use variables were dichotomous yes or no indicators of whether or not the respondents reported actual use of the CAH and the local provider in the recent past. The willingness to use variables were dichotomous yes or no indicators constructed from responses to a question about where respondents would first seek care for a variety of future health concerns. The future health concerns counted as "yes, willing to use" were concerns for which the local CAH and provider(s) offered health care services, rather than other services included in the question that were not available locally and for which patients would need to be referred elsewhere.

The major independent variables, or potential predictors, included potential access to care factors. All were measured by respondents' self-report and from their perspectives (versus from the perspectives of the hospitals or providers). These included characteristics of the population (e.g., age, income, health insurance, and health status) and characteristics of the health care system that I operationalized according to "the 5 A's" from Penchansky and Thomas' work (1981; Thomas & Penchansky, 1984) (i.e., availability, accessibility, accommodation, affordability, and acceptability).

The Acceptability Scale comprised the summed values of responses to twelve 5-point Likert-type rating questions related to the concept of acceptability, included on the mail survey. I based my selection of the questions for inclusion in the scale on Penchansky and Thomas' work (1981;

Thomas & Penchansky, 1984). I then validated the questions in telephone interviews from responses to the question: "When you and your household members choose a medical care provider and a hospital to use, can you tell me what factors are important to you?" Responses were related to the technical quality of care, the "art" of care, and the appearance of the facility or office.

The Acceptability Scale items were components of two questions that asked respondents to rate a wide variety of aspects of health care in their local communities (see Table 14.1). Response options included excellent, good, average, fair, poor, and don't know. The scale had a possible point range of 12 to 60. The reliability coefficients for the Acceptability Scale were Cronbach's alpha = 0.97 and the Standardized item alpha = 0.97; the inter-item correlations analysis ranged from 0.54 to 0.88.

To identify the predictors of use and willingness to use local health care, I built four separate multivariate logistic regression models (one for each dependent variable) in which I first regressed the dependent variable on a set of six community (dummy) variables to control for confounding by community. Then I added independent variables to the model together as a group (not stepwise). Next, I calculated odds ratios and 95% confidence intervals for the independent variables with $p \leq .05$.

I analyzed qualitative comments on several short-answer questions on the mail survey and open-ended questions from the telephone interview regarding access to care by using content analysis methods. I read all qualitative data multiple times and sorted them into similar categories based on the words used in the comments (manifest content) and the apparent meaning of the words (latent content; Catanzaro, 1988). I sought patterns and categories that might add to the understanding of rural residents' views on access to health care in their local communities. I then summarized these themes and categories and identified relevant themes using the actual phrases of the respondents.

RESULTS

Table 14.2 shows the descriptive results of the "use of" and "willingness to use" the dependent variables I examined. As can be seen on the table, relatively few respondents ($n = 37, 9.7\%$) reported that anyone in their household had used the local CAH for inpatient care in the prior 2 years, whereas roughly two-thirds of the respondents ($n = 260, 68\%$) reported use of the local provider in the past year. Less than half of the respondents indicated willingness to use the CAH ($n = 162, 43\%$) or local providers ($n = 182, 48\%$) for future health concerns.

I computed Acceptability Scale scores for 261 of the total 381 households; I excluded the remaining because of missing values or "don't

TABLE 14.2 Frequencies of Dependent Variables "Use of" and "Willingness to Use" Local Health Care (n = 381)

Variable	n	%
"Used the CAHs" for inpatient care in prior 2 years	37	9.7
"Used local provider(s)" in the past year	260	68.0
"Willing to use the CAH" in the future	162	43.0
"Willing to use the local provider(s)" in the future	182	48.0

Note: CAHs = critical access hospitals.

know" answers. The mean Acceptability Scale score was 46.48 (SD = 9.87; range = 18–60 points [possible range = 12–60 points]).

On the basis of the logistic regression analysis (summarized in Table 14.3), respondents for households most likely to use the CAH for inpatient care were those who rated their knowledge of local health care highly, were older in age, and reported lower incomes. The odds ratio indicates the factor by which the odds of "use" or "willing to use" change when the corresponding variable is changed by one unit. Because in this chapter I focus on the Acceptability Scale, I do not discuss the other results at length, but just as illustration, for every unit increase in the knowledge rating

TABLE 14.3 Results of Multivariate Logistic Regression Models to Identify Predictors of "Use of" and "Willingness to Use" Local Health Care

	β	SE	OR	95% CI
Use of CAHs and				
• Knowledge of local health care	.836*	.400	2.308	(5.05, 1.06)
• Respondent age	.035*	.017	1.036	(1.07, 1.01)
• Household income	−.533*	.221	.587	(0.61, 0.56)
Use of local provider and				
• Acceptability scale score	.096**	.024	1.100	(1.15, 1.05)
Willing to use CAHs and				
• Acceptability scale score	.065**	.021	1.067	(1.11, 1.02)
• Use local provider	.936*	.452	2.549	(6.18, 1.05)
Willing to use local provider and				
• Acceptability scale score	.088**	.023	1.092	(1.14, 1.04)
• Used provider in the past	1.879**	.504	6.546	(17.58, 2.44)
• Community affiliation	1.540**	.549	4.664	(13.69, 1.59)

Note: SE = standard error; OR = odds ratio; 95% CI = 95% confidence interval of the odds ratio. Data include significant independent variables only.
*$p \leq .05$.
**$p \leq .01$.

category with an odds ratio of 2.308, the odds of use of the CAH increased by 130%. An odds ratio of 1 is equal odds, so anything significantly over or less than 1 is considered. The Acceptability Scale as well as other variables in this model (distance from CAH, use of local provider, ease of transportation, and community affiliation) were not significant predictors of use of the CAH. I anticipated that few if any covariates would be significant in this model, with only 37 households who had reported use of the CAH.

Households most likely to use the local provider(s) were those that had higher Acceptability Scale scores. For each additional point on the scale, the odds of use of the provider increased by 10%. Other variables in this model (knowledge of local health care, distance from CAH, respondent age, income, transportation, and community affiliation) were not significant predictors of use of the local provider.

Households most likely to be willing to use the CAH for future health problems were those with higher Acceptability Scale scores and those that had used the local provider(s) in the past year. Based on the odds ratios for each additional point on the Acceptability Scale, the odds of indicating willingness to use the CAH increased by 7%. Other variables in this model (knowledge, distance from CAH, age, income, transportation, and community affiliation) were not significant predictors of willingness to use the CAH.

Residents most likely to be willing to use the local provider(s) in the future were also those with higher acceptability scores, who used the local provider(s) in the past year, and reported that they were affiliated with the local community. Each point on the Acceptability Scale increased the odds of willingness to use the provider by 9%. Other variables in this model (knowledge, distance from CAH, age, income, and transportation) were not significant predictors of willingness to use the local provider.

Among those who used local health care, the Acceptability Scale score was also a significant predictor of satisfaction with care. Because I included only those households that had used both the CAH and local provider(s) in the recent past ($n = 36$) in this analysis, I used Mantel–Haenszel chi-square tests to examine relationships between satisfaction and selected covariates. There was insufficient power to analyze this relationship using multivariate logistic regression models. The Acceptability Scale score was significantly associated with satisfaction with the local CAH, emergency care, local primary care provider(s), and the availability of night or weekend care ($p \leq .01$). Other variables examined were not significantly associated with satisfaction with care.

In the qualitative comments, the rural respondents offered many perspectives related to the relationship between acceptability and use of local health care. "He knows what he's doing. He knows my son and my son knows him and that's comforting." "He's a country type doctor. I like that." "The way a hospital is equipped. I want a doctor who is top of the line." "For the doctor—that you have rapport with him, that he gives you accurate information, that you're comfortable that he knows what he's doing." "For the hospital—the nursing care, cleanliness. The doctor—personality. I go to see him the first time—did the medicines help, did the care help the problem?" "They don't have the services, the doctor's not as good, and it's not as good a hospital."

DISCUSSION AND CONCLUSIONS

In this study, the Acceptability Scale was the most consistent predictor of "use of" and "willingness to use" local rural health care, as well as of satisfaction with care. Acceptability is that component of access to care that reflects potential client's attitudes and opinions about the characteristics of providers and services. Unlike other aspects of access, acceptability reflects opinion, judgment, and personal preferences on the part of consumers. The current rural reality for obtaining most goods and services including health care is that with access to vehicles, modern highways, and health insurance, rural residents are not as affected by distance in choosing health care as they once were. This study suggests that those who do not find local health care acceptable go elsewhere.

It is interesting to note that a large majority (95%) of the respondents in this study indicated that having local health care was very or somewhat important to their household members; "keeping" or maintaining the health services and providers they had was the predominant theme in the qualitative comments—yet only 9.7% of the households had a family member hospitalized in the CAH in the prior 2 years, and only 68.2% had used the local provider(s) in the prior year. A clarification of this discrepancy may be found by considering a second theme that emerged from the data—"just in case," as the following quotes show:

> "You always have certain people who are doubters ... but they still want emergency care available in case they need it, even though they don't support it for everyday things." "I know that it's not paying its way in taxes but we need it. It's like having an insurance policy. Insurance policies don't pay for themselves either but you need it just in case."

Clearly there was support in these six communities for keeping their local health care, but acceptability was associated with use of local health care—support or indicating its importance were not associated.

By improving researchers' understanding of what rural consumers deem acceptable in terms of services and providers, the Acceptability Scale can be used to improve health care access for rural residents. In the practice arena, attending to community residents' perceptions of competence, quality, the art of care, and appearance of facilities as well as developing strategies to strengthen and improve these perceptions may reduce out-migration from health care that is available locally. In the policy arena, as new models of care are developed or refined, paying substantial attention to features or characteristics that influence acceptability to consumers can make the difference between services that will be used and valued and services that will be bypassed by the residents they are intended to serve. When it comes to rural health care, Kinsella's (1982) old baseball adage, and "If you build it, [they] will come" does not necessarily hold, unless what is built is acceptable to rural residents.

ACKNOWLEDGMENTS

This research was funded by Health Care Financing Administration Dissertation Grant 30-P-90510/0-01, Hester McLaws Award, Sigma Theta Tau Zeta Upsilon Research Award, and Montana State University College of Nursing.

REFERENCES

Aday, L. A., & Andersen, R. (1975). A framework for the study of access to medical care. In L. A. Aday, & R. Andersen (Eds.), *Development of indices of access to medical care* (pp. 1–14). Ann Arbor, MI: Health Administration Press.

Aday, L. A., Bagley, C. E., Lairson, D. R., & Slater, C. H. (1993). *Evaluating the medical care system: Effectiveness, efficiency, and equity*. Ann Arbor, MI: Health Administration Press.

Amundson, B. (1993). Myth and reality in the rural health service crisis: Facing up to community responsibilities. *The Journal of Rural Health, 9*, 176–187.

Andersen, R. M., McCutcheon, A., Aday, L. A., Chiu, G. Y., & Bell, R. (1993). Exploring dimensions of access to medical care. *Health Services Research, 18*(1), 49–74.

Catanzaro, M. (1988). Using qualitative analytical techniques. In N. F. Woods & M. Catanzaro, *Nursing research: Theory and practice* (pp. 437–456). St. Louis, MO: C.V. Mosby.

Christianson, J. B., Moscovice, I. S., Wellever, A. L., & Wingert, T. D. (1990). Institutional alternatives to the rural hospital. *Health Care Financing Review, 11*(3), 87–97.

DeFriese, G. H., Wilson, G., Ricketts, T. C., & Whitener, L. (1992). Consumer choice and the national rural hospital crisis. In W. M. Gesler, & T. C. Ricketts (Eds.), *Health in rural North America* (pp. 206–225). New Brunswick, NJ: Rutgers University Press.

Escarse, J. J., & Kapur, K. (2009). Do patients bypass rural hospitals? Determinants of inpatient hospital choice in rural California. *Journal of Health Care for the Poor and Underserved. 20*(3), 625–644.

Gamm, L., & Hutchison, L. (2003). Rural health priorities in America: Where you stand depends on where you sit. *The Journal of Rural Health, 19*(3), 209–213.

Kinsella, W. P. (1982). *Shoeless Joe Jackson comes to Iowa.* New York, NY: Ballantine Books.

Liu, J. J., Bellamy, G., Barnet, B., & Weng, S. (2008). Bypass of local primary care in rural counties: Effect of patient and community characteristics. *Annals of Family Medicine, 6*(2), 124–130.

Liu, J., Bellamy, G. R., & McCormick, M. (2007). Patient bypass behavior and critical access hospitals: Implications for patient retention. *The Journal of Rural Health, 23*(1), 17–24.

Millman, M. (Ed.). (1993). *Access to care in America.* Washington, DC: National Academy Press.

Patrick, D. L., & Erickson, P. (1993). *Health status and health policy: Quality of life in health evaluation and resource allocation.* New York, NY: Oxford University Press.

Penchansky, R., & Thomas, J. W. (1981). The concept of access: Definition and relationship to consumer satisfaction. *Medical Care, 19*, 127–140.

Pink, G. H., Holmes, G. M., Thompson, R. E., & Slifkin, R. T. (2007). Variations in financial performance among peer groups of Critical Access Hospitals. *The Journal of Rural Health, 23*(4), 299–305.

Radcliff, T. A., Brasure, M., Moscovice, I. S., & Stensland, J. T. (2003), Understanding rural hospital bypass behavior. *The Journal of Rural Health, 19*(3), 252–259.

Rural Assistance Center (RAC). (2012). *CAH frequently asked questions.* Retrieved July 2 2012, from http://www.raconline.org/topics/hospitals/cahfaq.php

Shreffler, M. J. (1996). Rural residents views on access to care in frontier communities with medical assistance facilities. *Dissertation Abstracts International, 57*, 3131. (No. 9630109).

Shreffler, M. J., Capalbo, S. M., Flaherty, R. J., & Heggam, C. (1999). Community decision-making about critical access hospitals: Lessons learned from Montana's Medical Assistance Facility program. *The Journal of Rural Health, 15*, 180–188.

Thomas, J. W., & Penchansky, R. (1984). Relating satisfaction with access and utilization of services. *Medical Care, 22*, 553–568.

Chapter 15

HEALTH DISPARITIES IN RURAL POPULATIONS ACROSS THE LIFE SPAN

Angeline Bushy

The Terms Risk, Vulnerability, and Social Determinants often are used synonymously in the literature. This chapter examines each of the concepts relative to health disparities; rural perspectives are included in the discussion. Four rural populations that are particularly vulnerable are highlighted.

DEFINITIONS

Risk

The term "risk" emerges from writings on the natural history of diseases. In epidemiological models, risk refers to health conditions that result from the interaction of many factors, including a person's genetic makeup, lifestyle, as well as the physical and social environments in which the individual lives and works (Webster's Online Dictionary, 2012). Risk exposure subsequently makes it more or less likely that a person will develop a particular outcome. Rarely does one risk factor act in isolation. Rather, the interaction of multiple risks exacerbates the possibility of an individual, family, or even a community to be more susceptible (vulnerable) to less than optimal consequences (Bushy, 2009; Leight, 2003).

Vulnerability

The term "vulnerability" has its origins in the Latin word *vulnerare*, which means "to wound." Broad definitions of the term include the notion of susceptibility to injury; a potential for attack and being insufficiently defended; being liable to censure and criticism; or, more liable to succumb to persuasion and temptation (Webster's Online Dictionary, 2012). Vulnerability can be used in reference to an individual as well as a family or even a community that experiences multiple interfacing risk(s); which, in turn, can impact the health of one or all of its members. Vulnerability implies that some individuals or groups may be more sensitive to risk factors that can impact health status, usually for the worse. The vulnerable are not a homogeneous group, but rather represent all segments of society. Essentially, at various times in life, every person is vulnerable for one or more untoward conditions or outcomes (Bushy, 2009; Leight, 2003).

Families who experience intense clustering of risks (stressors) also can become vulnerable. As a unit, family stressors include unanticipated situational life events as well as normal maturational transitions in individual members. Examples of families at high risk and who are particularly vulnerable include those having a member who has a chronic physical or mental illness, one who abuses alcohol or drugs, or a pregnant teenager. Examples of an unexpected event could include a family member receiving a diagnosis of a fatal disease, a death in the family, or the head of household becoming unemployed, and the spiraling consequences associated with lack of financial resources. Trauma-related events could include a farm-related accident or motor vehicle accident, domestic violence, sexual abuse, and violent crimes, and these could predispose a family to manifest a variety of physical, emotional, and social conditions. The combination of intense and multiple stressors (risks) coupled with the depletion of resources can push the family beyond its ability to cope, impacting each family member in a unique manner. Rural families, because they interface with the community, are particularly sensitive to risks that originate from economic, physical, social, biological, and genetic factors, and these in turn can impact lifestyle behaviors (Bushy, 2009; Rural Assistance Center [RAC], 2012).

Ultimately, multiple risks, coupled with poor lifestyle choices by an individual or a family, can evolve into a spiraling "snowball" of negative events. Repeated bombardment from stressful situations perpetuates feelings of powerlessness, hopelessness, and helplessness, evidenced by low self-esteem, anxiety, chronic depression, and physical manifestations in individuals or all members of a family. Given spiraling out-of-control life events, it is not unusual for a family, neighborhood, or community to become immobilized. In other words, the individual, family, or community does not have the wherewithal to respond effectively. Sometimes they do not have adequate energy to deal with day-to-day activities, associated with depression, to confront even the routine activities of daily living. Rather, the affected go from crisis to crisis, and try to cope as best they can. As coping abilities are strained by unpredictable and unrelenting events, vulnerable individuals' ability to master multiple stress-producing situations is significantly compromised, which can be a detriment to their health, and even lead to illnesses (Bushy, 2009; RAC, 2012).

Vulnerable communities or neighborhoods characteristically have high rates of poverty, unemployment, and crime. In these contexts, residents tend to have low educational achievement and are less likely to engage in health-promoting behaviors. Along with persistent environmental risks, natural or ma-made disasters—for instance, a major fire, massive oil spill, severe drought, a destructive hurricane, tornado, earthquake, or a flood—can have devastating consequences for already vulnerable individuals and families in these communities (Leight, 2003; United States Department of Agriculture [USDA], 1997).

Social Determinants

Social determinants are conditions of the environment into which people are born, live, learn, work, play, worship, and age that can affect health status, functioning, and quality of life. Social determinants include environmental (contextual) attributes of place (i.e., social, economic, physical, resources) in various settings (e.g., school, church, workplace, and neighborhood). Place further alludes to a community's preferred patterns of social engagement, which can impact individuals' and families' sense of security and well-being. Resources that enhance quality of life could have a positive influence on individuals' health (Centers for Disease Control [CDC], 2011; Institute of Medicine [IOM], 2002; Secretary's Advisory Committee on Health Promotion and Disease Prevention Objectives for 2020 [SACHPDP], 2010; World Health Organization, Commission on Social Determinants of Health [WHO], 2008).

Examples of place-based resources that could impact health include safe and affordable housing, access to education, public safety, and availability of healthy food options, local emergency and health care services, and an environment that is free of threatening toxins (CDC, 2011; IOM, 2002). The manner in which an individual, family, and community experience place, as it influences health, is inherent in the notion of social determinants. Examples of place-related social determinants include, among others:

1. Availability of resources to meet daily needs (e.g., safe housing and local food markets).
2. Access to educational, economic, and job opportunities.
3. Access to health care services.
4. Quality of education and job training.
5. Availability of community-based resources that support opportunities for employment, social support, lifelong learning, and leisure-time activities.
6. Transportation options.
7. Public safety.
8. Social norms and attitudes (e.g., discrimination, racism, and distrust of government).

9. Exposure to crime, violence, and social disorder (e.g., presence of trash and lack of cooperation in a community).
10. Socioeconomic conditions (e.g., concentrated poverty and the stressful conditions that accompany it).
11. Residential segregation.
12. Language/literacy skills/culture.
13. Access to mass media and emerging technologies (e.g., cell phones, the Internet, and social media).

Policies that positively influence social and economic conditions can support changes in individual behavior and, ultimately, can improve and sustain the health of a family or a community over time. Improving conditions in which individuals live, learn, work, and play in turn can enhance the quality of relationships, thereby promoting a healthier community.

Healthy People 2020 focuses on social determinants of health as one of its four overarching goals (SACHPDP, 2010). Topic areas related to this goal focus on creating social and physical environments that promote good health for all. Advances are needed not only in health care but also in education, childcare, housing, business, law, media, community planning, transportation, and agriculture. When a community (or subpopulation) experiences deficits in one or more of these dimensions, it becomes more susceptible (vulnerable to an outcome that could result in a health disparity). Risks that contribute to a health-related disparity include, among others, disadvantaged socioeconomic status, risky lifestyle behaviors, low self-esteem, and a sense of powerlessness. Age, race, ethnicity, and gender are demographic variables that might diffuse or enhance the potential for a particular outcome and hence contribute to a health disparity within a particular aggregate. Conversely, intervening to diffuse one or more of these variables could reduce or eliminate a particular disparity (Agency for Healthcare Research and Quality [AHRQ], 2009, 2010; National Partnership for Action [NPA], 2011; National Prevention and Promotion Strategy [NPHPS], 2011).

Resilience

Resilience is the effect of an interaction among individual, social, and demographic assets that can contribute to a higher likelihood better health. Resilience plays a noteworthy role within an individual, family, or community to alleviate vulnerability. For example, the trait of hardiness has been used to describe a dimension of human resilience (Bartone, 2008; Kobasa, 1979). Conceptual dimensions of hardiness theory include control, commitment, and challenge (Low, 1996). For instance, faced with stressful life events, a person possessing the hardiness attribute could change or modify an event (control) into something that is consistent with his or her life purpose (commitment), which subsequently could result in learning and personal growth (challenge). Hardiness refers to a combination of characteristics that deters a person or group from developing a particular health outcome, even after experiencing multiple risks. Hardiness serves as a potential intervening variable that helps individuals, families and, perhaps, even communities to overcome adverse conditions and still lead meaningful lives (Kulig, 2000; Leight, 2003). For example, hardiness might be an attribute that explains why some individuals with a diagnosis of human immunodeficiency virus (HIV) infection remain in relatively good health for decades while other people succumb shortly after exposure to the virus. There may be additional aspects of hardiness that are relevant to rural populations, and this needs further examination by scholars of rural nursing.

Support networks and services also can counterbalance, buffer, or mediate risks that contribute to vulnerability (Lauder, Reel, Farmer, & Griggs, 2006). Preference and use of support varies by individuals, families, communities, and may be culturally defined. For instance, some groups promote and rely heavily on extensive social support networks, as is the case for many Native Americans, African American, and Latino families. The extent of these networks often becomes evident when an individual seeks health care at a community health clinic or is hospitalized, accompanied by a contingent of extended family representing several generations. Such an extensive network does not exist for everyone, however. Some individuals are not able to identify even one person in their support network, which intensifies their vulnerability and may contribute to a health disparity within and among a select group (Bushy, 2009; Kulig, 2000; Leight, 2003).

Health Disparities

Health disparity refers to the disproportionate incidence (frequency of new cases), prevalence (frequency of all existing cases), mortality rate, or morbidity rate for a condition within a population (CDC, 2011; IOM, 2002). Disparities often are characterized by gender, age, ethnicity, race, education, income, social class, disability, geographic location, or sexual orientation (Cole & Fielding, 2007). For more than a half century, the CDC (2011) has monitored the health of U.S. residents, noting, over time, gaps between the least and the most vulnerable. The CDC routinely publishes rates of illness, injury, risk behaviors, use of preventive health services, exposure to environmental hazards, and premature death. It is important to stress that race/ethnicity in and of itself does not lead to health disparities. Rather social determinants have a significant role in the health behaviors of vulnerable individuals, families, and communities (AHRQ, 2009, 2010; McDavid-Harrison & Dean, 2011). For instance, disparities in life expectancy between Blacks and Whites are related to socioeconomic factors rather than to race or ethnicity. The perspective that health is an outcome of the combination of personal attributes (e.g., heredity, lifestyle, and social dynamics) and place-bound features (i.e., access to health care, health-promoting living, and working environment) is not new, but is receiving greater attention in policy and research arenas.

The CDC's (2011) report, *Health Disparities and Inequalities in the United States—2011* highlights disparities in select social and health indicators. Since the early 1980s, there has been progress in improving the nation's health status and reducing a number of disparities (AHRQ, 2009, 2010). Without differentiating rural from urban populations, some disparities persist within the total population as a whole. For example,

1. Individuals with lower incomes report having fewer healthy days. The correlation between health inequalities persists at all levels of income.

2. Air-pollution-related disparities associated with fine particulates and ozone are determined by geographical location. Air pollution can impact the health of people who live or work near the polluting source(s). Regardless of socioeconomic status, individuals in select geographical regions can experience negative health effects of air pollution.

However, racial and ethnic minority groups experience disparate health consequences associated with social determinants (AHRQ, 2009) (i.e., place).

1. Significant disparities in infant mortality rates persist in the U.S. Of note, infants born to Black women are up to 3 times more likely to die than infants born to women of other races/ethnicities.

2. Male individuals of all races/ethnicities are up to 3 times more likely to die in motor vehicle accidents, compared to women. Vehicular mortality rates are twice as high among American Indians/Alaska Natives (AI/AN).

3. Male individuals of all ages and race/ethnicities are up to 4 times more likely to die by suicide, compared to female individuals. Of note, AI/AN male adolescents and young male adults have a particularly high rate of suicide. Of all suicides by male individuals in the United States, AI/AN account for only 1% of such deaths. However, suicide rates among AI/ANs and non-Hispanic Whites are more than twice that of Blacks, Asian Pacific Islanders, and Hispanics.

4. Between 2003 and 2007, the rate of drug-induced deaths increased among men and women of all races/ethnicities, with the exception of Hispanics, but rates were highest among

non-Hispanic Whites. In 2010, more people succumbed from prescription drug abuse than from illicit drugs, a notable trend reversal from the early 1990s.

5. Coronary heart disease and stroke are leading causes of death in the U.S. population, accounting for the highest proportion of inequality in life expectancy between Whites and Blacks, despite the availability of low-cost, highly effective preventive treatment. Overall, male individuals are more likely than women to die from coronary heart disease. Black men and women, however, are more likely to die of heart disease and stroke than their White counterparts.

6. Preventable hospitalizations increase as income decreases. The preventable hospitalization rate for Blacks is more than double that of Whites.

7. With the exception of Asians/Pacific Islanders, racial/ethnic minorities experience disproportionately higher rates of new HIV diagnoses compared to Whites and compared to men who have sex with men (MSM). Disparities are noted among Black male individuals, AI/AN male individuals, and MSM compared to rates holding steady or decreasing in other groups.

8. Hypertension disparities persist among non-Hispanic Blacks (42%) compared to Whites (29%); levels of hypertension control are lowest for Mexican Americans. Male and female individuals have a similar prevalence of hypertension, but women are significantly more likely to control the condition. Individuals who are uninsured are less likely to have their hypertension under control, compared to those with health insurance.

9. Rates of adolescent pregnancy and childbirth have been decreasing for all racial/ethnic minorities in all age groups. However, birth rates for Hispanics and Blacks are up to 3 times higher, compared to Whites.

10. More than half of alcohol consumption by adults is in the form of binge drinking (defined for women as consuming four or more alcoholic drinks per episode and, for men, five or more drinks per episode). Male individuals are more likely to binge drink and consume more alcohol than older people and women. Binge drinking is higher in groups with higher incomes and higher educational levels. Individuals with lower incomes and less educational attainment who binge drink do so more frequently and, when binging, drink more heavily. Notably, AI/AN report more binge drinking episodes per month and higher alcohol consumption per episode than other groups.

11. Tobacco use is a leading cause of preventable illness and death. Over the decades, smoking rates have significantly declined with increasing income and educational attainment. Cigarette smoking rate disparities persist among AI/AN, as well as among some rural groups.

Disparities that are particular to rural rural populations in general are noted are noted as well; for instance, compared to urban counterparts (RAC, 2012):

1. Rural communities represent about 20% of America's population; however, less than 10% of physicians practice in those communities.
2. Rural residents are less likely to have employer-provided health care coverage or prescription drug coverage.
3. Rural poor are less likely to be covered by Medicaid benefits.
4. One-third of all motor vehicle accidents occur in rural areas; however, two-thirds of deaths attributed such accidents occur on rural roads.
5. Fewer dentists and behavioral health professionals practice in rural areas.
6. The majority of Emergency Medical Services (EMS) first responders in rural communities are volunteers.
7. Rural residents are poorer than their rural counterparts.
8. Alcohol abuse is a significant problem among rural youth.
9. Methamphetamine use and admission treatment rates are higher in rural, nonmetro areas.
10. Rural residents are nearly twice as likely to die from unintentional injuries other than motor vehicle accidents.
11. Suicide rates among rural male individuals are significantly higher than rates in urban areas; and, rates among rural women are rapidly becoming equal to male counterparts.

Poverty

Socioeconomic status (i.e., level of education and subsequent employment opportunities) is a critical risk for vulnerability; and, ultimately affects health behaviors and health status of individuals as well as families and communities (CDC, 2011; IOM, 2002; WHO, 2010). Albeit often hidden, poverty even exists within communities that are seemingly quite affluent. Low socioeconomic status (poverty within the context of social determinants), rather than race and ethnicity per se, is a precursor to health disparities. In other words, poverty in and of itself potentiates other risks and vulnerability. Financial resources, or the lack thereof, can counterbalance or intensify situational and maturational risks and, ultimately, health status. Correlates of poverty include increased rates of communicable disease, especially tuberculosis and HIV, premature death, occupational hazards, unsafe and sometimes deplorable housing, and homelessness. Be it urban or rural, children in single-parent households are poorer in income and other resources compared to counterparts in communities with higher average family incomes. Particularly unfortunate correlates for impoverished children include delayed development, depression, anxiety, increased incidences of separation from families, and placement in foster care.

A multitude of definitions are offered for poverty and for determining who truly is "poor" (Bushy, 2009). Various disciplines describe poverty in terms related to the culture of a particular profession. For instance, social scientist use the term "impoverished" to describe a number of less-than-optimal conditions, such as lack of adequate housing, and lack of relationships, education, and financial resources. Health care professionals understand poverty in terms of not having sufficient financial resources for basic living expenses such as food, clothing, shelter, transportation, and medical care.

The U.S. federal government has put into place an absolute economic standard to define poverty using a standard poverty index based on an adequate living wage for a family with a specified number of household members (U.S. Department of Human Services, 2012). The poverty index is determined by calculating the cost of housing, goods, services, and food for a minimum–adequate diet for an individual. Poverty guidelines are derived from the consumer price index and are revised annually. Subsequently, the poverty index is used to determine whether or not a person or family qualifies for an entitlement program such as Medicaid, Women, Infants, and Children (WIC), Head Start, Children's Health Insurance Program (CHIP), and the school lunch program. Families who fall below the poverty index usually qualify for public assistance programs. Families who have a higher income than delineated by the poverty index do not qualify for benefits; they are often referred to as "near poor" or "working poor" (RAC, 2012).

A high proportion of the uninsured in rural areas are among the working poor. The working poor usually are employed, sometimes holding one or more part-time jobs to make ends meet, but do not have the resources to purchase health insurance (Bushy, 2009). Furthermore, their annual income exceeds the poverty index, thus they do not qualify for public assistance (i.e., Medicaid benefits). For those who have health insurance, premiums are escalating as are the copayments, but benefits are reduced. Consequently, it is not unusual for a family to believe they have adequate coverage until there is a catastrophic illness or chronic disability; then they are confronted with astronomical medical expenses.

The poverty index also is used to compare and contrast national, state, and county socioeconomic status. For instance, the classification of persistent poverty for families, neighborhoods, and counties is used to describe place(s) where average annual salaries are below the poverty index level for a number of years. For rural areas, "persistent poverty" has been a classification for rural county type used since 1977 by the USDA (2004) to characterize counties in which the average salary has been below the poverty index for decades. Some persistent poverty counties have been classified as such for more than half century, and poverty there is intergenerational in nature. Common demographic features of persistent poverty groups include a high proportion of minorities and single mothers, a high rate of unemployment, substandard housing, and low wages for those who are employed. Persistent poverty communities often have higher rates of crime and substance abuse with a lower quality and level of education. In persistent poverty rural counties, it is not unusual to find families living in condemned buildings, in a vehicle, in a storage facility, or as "squatters" in vacated houses or a farmstead building. Such living conditions expose residents to any number of environmental hazards (risks), including inadequate heat in cooler seasons, heat exposure in warm seasons, poor sanitation, lack of hygiene facilities, vermin, pests, unsafe drinking water, landfills, toxic waste sites, and drug-related activity. Poverty is a persistent comorbid risk for chronic health conditions with corresponding high(er) rates of morbidity and mortality, sometimes evidenced by a disparity within particular groups (CDC, 2011; USDA, 2004).

To reiterate, those who are poor are faced with multiple risks associated with chronic stressors, such as frustration over employment options, inadequate and unsafe housing conditions, repeated exposure to violence and crime, inadequate child care assistance, and the insensitive attitudes of health and social service agencies. Clinicians must be aware that the working poor and near poor in rural areas are likely to under-use preventive services. For many, symptoms often go untreated until there is an acute manifestation of illness or an emergency. For example, medical conditions often are exacerbated because the person or family has limited access to health professionals, especially primary health care services. Access to care entails more than simply having a service available in a small community. Rather, it implies that existing health care or social services must fit with the needs and preferences of a particular population for these to be deemed as acceptable and appropriate. Other barriers to access to care include:

1. Inability to pay for services
2. Lack of inadequate health care insurance
3. Language and cultural barriers
4. Inequitable distribution of health care providers (more often in inner cities and remote rural counties)

5. Geographic, social, and sometimes cultural isolation
6. Challenges associated with transportation and communication infrastructures (great distances to providers, poor travel conditions, and lack of telephone services)
7. No public transportation
8. Inconvenient hours at a clinic or community health center
9. Insensitive attitudes by health care providers toward clients who are poor or of another racial/ethnic/cultural background

VULNERABLE GROUPS IN RURAL COMMUNITIES

Demographically, rural communities have a number of at-risk vulnerable groups in their midst. In most of the cases, one finds disproportionate numbers of children and adolescents, elderly, women, and individuals who are disenfranchised. Obviously, extensive discussion about each is limited within space constraints of a single chapter. The next section presents a brief overview of concerns for each of these four groups that are more likely to be vulnerable (Bushy, 2009). Those who are vulnerable often experience comorbidity and may be in more than one of these demographic groups.

Children and Adolescents

Children of all ages are among the most vulnerable people, especially those born and living with less favorable social determinants (CDC, 2011; IOM, 2002). In both rural and urban settings, the number of children living in poverty has dramatically increased since 2001. A growing number of children live in single-parent households; they are twice as likely to be poor compared to those living in two-parent homes. Of all children who are poor, about one-third are African American; poverty among Latino children also is significant. However, AI/NA children probably are the poorest of the poor in the United States. Most AI/NA children are likely to reside in substandard living conditions, especially those on Indian reservations, which are located predominately in more remote rural regions. Unemployment on many reservations is extremely high, as are the rates of alcoholism and violence; thus, healthy role models for AI/NA children are absent (Bushy, 2009; RAC, 2012).

With respect to disparities among rural children, low-income, low educational level, and low-wage occupations correlate with infant mortality, low birth weight, birth defects, and infant deaths. Poverty also increases the risk in young children for developing chronic diseases, trauma-induced injuries and death, developmental delays, poor nutrition, inadequate immunizations, iron-deficiency anemia, and elevated serum lead levels. Compared to nonpoor children, their counterparts who are poor are more likely to go hungry, suffer from fatigue, dizziness, irritability, headache, and ear infections. Impoverished children have a higher prevalence of upper respiratory infections, weight loss, inability to concentrate, and absenteeism from school. The youngest are vulnerable to development delays and physical conditions stemming from inadequate nutrition and routine preventive health care.

Disadvantaged adolescents often do not have the opportunity to acquire the skills and to master knowledge associated with success in adulthood. Correspondingly, they lack sense of personal mastery and self-esteem. Compared to adolescents in families of higher socioeconomic status, counterparts who are poor possess below-average academic skills and are more likely to drop out of school. Regardless of race or setting, adolescents living in socioeconomically deprived situations are about 6 times more likely to have children than counterparts in better financial circumstances. A number of reasons cited for this disparity include lack of knowledge about sexual development and practicing safe sex, limited access to family planning services, and the lack of responsible adult role models (CDC, 2011; IOM, 2002).

Elderly

Like children, the elderly make up a significant segment of many rural communities, and a high proportion of the elderly are poor (CDC, 2011; IOM, 2002). Associated with rural economics, many of the elderly owned or worked in small businesses that did not have a retirement plan (RAC, 2012). Consequently, it is not unusual for older persons in small rural towns to rely on social security benefits. On fixed incomes that are very low, options are limited, especially when it comes to obtaining health care. A disproportionate number of rural elderly have chronic health problems and disabilities and are unable to live alone or manage personal affairs. It is not unusual for an elderly individual to lack transportation, either because he or she no longer is able to drive, does not have a personal vehicle or someone who can transport him or her, or has no public transportation (Bushy, 2009). Elderly people who reside in extended care facilities are particularly vulnerable if they are displaced from their home and family. Some elderly individuals who are eligible for Medicare and Social Security benefits may not know how to access these services. This phenomenon occurs most often when an individual is socially or geographically isolated, cannot speak or read English, or has English as a second language. Rural elderly individuals who are members of a minority group experience higher rates of chronic illness, in particular, African Americans, Latinos, and AI/AN, and significant disparities are noted within these vulnerable populations.

Women

Another highly vulnerable group is women (CDC, 2011; IOM, 2002). The term triple jeopardy is sometimes used in reference to women who are of color and also are poor. Two additional risk factors for women are rural residency and being old (RAC, 2012). Poverty has particularly serious negative consequences for women of childbearing age. Rural women are more likely than urban and nonpoor women to receive late or no prenatal care and have poor pregnancy outcomes. The health status of women has a direct effect on perinatal outcomes and an indirect effect on the health and well-being of the family. In rural areas, women who are mothers tend to be the primary caregivers and health-related decision makers in a family. Women have an important role in transmitting health information from professional sources to their family as well. Older women experience many of the same things described in the previous section on the elderly. This is further complicated by the reality that women are likely to outlive their spouses, oftentimes by more than a decade. This demographic feature further exacerbates impoverishment among rural elderly women (Bushy, 2009; USDA, 2004).

The Disenfranchised

Disenfranchisement alludes to feeling separated from mainstream society and not experiencing an emotional connection with society in general or to any group in particular (Webster's Online Dictionary, 2012). The disenfranchised usually do not have support systems to effectively cope with stress or to engage in a health-promoting lifestyle. Among the disenfranchised in both rural and urban areas, for instance, are individuals who have a chronic mental illness, are homeless, have a prison record, or have a stigma-related diagnosis such as HIV/AIDS (acquired immune deficiency syndrome), along with refugees who have recently immigrated to the United States. As with other vulnerable groups, the disenfranchised often have comorbid conditions. For example, a person with a mental illness may also be homeless, addicted to drugs and alcohol, and without any support system. Veterans, particularly those who served in the Vietnam War and suffer from posttraumatic disorder, are among the disenfranchised that are sometimes seen in more remote rural areas. The disenfranchised, be it by choice or due to an inability to relate to others, often have no connections with informal support such as friends or family or to formal support services such as social service agencies and primary care providers (Bushy, 2009). Although many are highly vulnerable, that is not to say that all rural people without homes are disenfranchised. Rather, many individuals and families report that they recently became "down on their luck" but also have reliable support from a faith community, extended family, neighbors, and the community. Nonetheless, the day-to-day stress of trying to survive makes these families, along with disenfranchised individuals, vulnerable to any number of negative health outcomes—physical, mental, and emotional.

SUMMARY

In summary, while general information exists on disparities among rural populations related to access to care, there is a paucity of evidence focusing on risk, vulnerability, and social determinants in select rural aggregates (AHRQ, 2009, 2010; CDC, 2011; IOM, 2002; RAC, 2012). For rural nursing scholars, this information deficit offers an extensive venue for research, which ultimately is needed to expand and refine a theory for rural nursing practice (Kulig, 2000; Lauder et al., 2006; Lee & Winters, 2004; Leight, 2003).

REFERENCES

Agency for Healthcare Research and Quality (AHRQ). (2009). *National healthcare disparities report—2008*. Washington, DC: National Academies Press. Retrieved January 7, 2013 from http://www.ahrq.gov/qual/nhdr08/nhdr08.pdf

Agency for Healthcare Research and Quality (AHRQ). (2010). *2009—National healthcare quality and disparities report*. Washington, DC: National Academies Press. Retrieved January 7, 2013 from: http://www.ahrq.gov/qual/qrdr09.htm

Bartone, P. (2008). *Hardiness-resilience.com*. Retrieved January 7, 2013 from http://www.hardiness-resilience.com/

Bushy, A. (2009). Vulnerability: An overview (chapter 25). In K. Saucier-Lundy, & S. Jaynes (Eds.), *Community health nursing: Caring for the public's health* (2nd Ed.). Boston, MA: Jones & Bartlett.

Centers for Disease Control (CDC). (2011). *CDC health disparities and inequalities report—United States, 2011*. Retrieved April 6, 2012, from http://www.cdc.gov/mmwr/pdf/other/su6001.pdf

Cole, B., & Fielding, J. (2007). Health impact assessment: A tool to help policy makers understand health beyond health care. *Annual Review of Public Health, 28*, 393–412. Retrieved April 6, 2012, from http://www.annualreviews.org/doi/abs/10.1146/annurev.publhealth.28.083006.131942

Institute of Medicine (IOM). (2002). *Disparities in health care: Methods for studying the effects of race, ethnicity, and SES on access, use, and quality of health care*. Retrieved April 6, 2012, from http://www.iom.edu/~/media/Files/Activity%20Files/Quality/NHDRGuidance/DisparitiesGornick.pdf

Kobasa, S. C. (1979). Stressful life events, personality, and health: Inquiry into hardiness. *Journal of Personality and Social Psychology, 37*(1), 1–11.

Kulig, J. C. (2000). Community resiliency: The potential for community health nursing theory development. *Public Health Nursing, 17*(5), 374–385.

Lauder, W., Reel, S., Farmer, J., & Griggs, H. (2006). Social capital, rural nursing and rural nursing theory. *Nursing Inquiry, 13*(1), 73–79.

Lee, H. J., & Winters, C. A. (2004). Testing rural nursing theory: Perceptions and needs of service providers. *Online Journal of Rural Nursing and Health Care, 4*(1), 51–63.

Leight, S. B. (2003). The application of a vulnerable populations conceptual model to rural health. *Public Health Nursing, 20*(6), 440–448.

Low, J. (1996). The concept of hardiness: A brief but critical commentary. *Journal of Advances in Nursing, 24*(3), 588–590.

McDavid-Harrison, K., & Dean, H. (2011). Guest editorial: Use of data systems to address social determinants of health: A need to do more. *Public Health Reports, 126*(3), 1–6. Retrieved April 6, 2012, from http://www.publichealthreports.org/issueopen.cfm?articleID=2718

National Partnership for Action. (2011). *HHS Action plan to reduce racial and ethnic health disparities.* Retrieved April 6, 2012, from http://www.minorityhealth.hhs.gov/npa/files/Plans/HHS/HHS_Plan_complete.pdf

The National Prevention and Health Promotion Strategy (NPHPS). (2011). *The National prevention strategy: America's plan for better health and wellness.* Retrieved April 6, 2012, from http://www.healthcare.gov/prevention/nphpphc/strategy/report.html

Rural Assistance Center (RAC). (2012). *Rural health disparities resource.* Retrieved April 6, 2012, from http://www.raconline.org/topics/disparities/

Secretary's Advisory Committee on Health Promotion and Disease Prevention Objectives for 2020 (SACHPDP). (2010). *Healthy People 2020: An opportunity to address the societal determinants of health in the United States.* Retrieved April 6, 2012, from http://www.healthypeople.gov/2010/hp2020/advisory/SocietalDeterminantsHealth.htm

U.S. Department of Agriculture (USDA). (2004). *Understanding rural America: County types.* Retrieved April 6, 2012, from http://www.ers.usda.gov/publications/rdrr89/rdrr89.pdf

U.S. Department of Health and Human Services (DHHS). (2012). *2012 HHS Poverty guidelines.* Retrieved April 6, 2012, from http://aspe.hhs.gov/poverty/12poverty.shtml

Webster's Online Dictionary. (2012). Retrieved April 6, 2012, from http://www.webster-dictionary.net/

World Health Organization, Commission on Social Determinants of Health (WHO). (2008). *Closing the gap in a generation: Health equity through action on the social determinants of health.* Retrieved April 6, 2012, from http://whqlibdoc.who.int/publications/2008/9789241563703_eng.pdf

Chapter 16

THE DISTINCTIVE NATURE AND SCOPE OF RURAL NURSING PRACTICE: PHILOSOPHICAL BASES

Jane Ellis Scharff

LOOKING BACK

Plenty and little have changed in 10 years. Rural nursing practice seemed a dichotomous set of the routine and the extraordinary to me back then, as it does now. I was an insider, if not an old-timer, and my findings, although remarkable to some, seemed simply confirmatory to me. Already a budding pragmatist and not yet fully a scientist, I thought, at the time, it was enough to have empiric validation for the practice that I had known and in which my former workplace colleagues continued. For that reason and so many others, I did not publish the findings of my master's thesis in 1987. Subsequently, I have been cited frequently, misrepresented occasionally, and poached a time or two when it comes to references about the world of rural nursing. It is time to uphold my responsibility to nursing science and to set the record straight. The nature and scope of rural nursing *is* distinctive. I am now willing to be quoted on that. Furthermore, rural nursing can now be given a definition based on that distinctiveness.

Rural nursing practice, be it hospital practice, private practice, or community health practice, is distinctive in its nature and scope from the practice of nursing in urban settings. It is distinctive in its boundaries, intersections, dimensions, and even in its core. Ten years ago, I was loath to claim distinctiveness within rural nursing's core. It seemed too bold to proclaim that at the very level of essence, and not attributable to setting alone, rural nursing could be so different. Today, I am determined to claim it: The core of all nursing is care, and care is the substance of the

---

J. Scharff (1998). The distinctive nature and scope of rural nursing practice: Philosophical bases. In H. J. Lee (Ed.), *Conceptual basis for rural nursing* (pp. 19–38). Copyright 1998 by Springer Publishing Company. Reprinted with permission.

relationship between nurse and patient; consequently, what happens at the core of rural nursing is something apart from what happens at the core of nursing anywhere else.

I am still a pragmatist; my job is to get readers as close to the experience as I can. Thankfully, my growth as a scientist makes the job easier than it was some years back. Although no longer in the practice, I understand rural nursing better today than I did then. The importance of rural nursing has not decreased as my worldview has expanded. On the contrary, the more I dissect and reconstruct my thoughts about life and truth and nursing science, the more clearly I see the beauty emanating from the nature and scope of rural nursing, and the more clearly I appreciate its relevance to all of nursing science.

From an ontological viewpoint, I will share some information about what it means to "be" a rural nurse, and from an epistemological viewpoint, I will express a little of what it means to "know" rural nursing practice. What came as primary expression to me, because I lived it, breathed it, and studied it, is secondary expression as I write it; I will do my best to translate the experience through common language. However, the story I tell will require imagination to transcend time and space and to gain a sense of the reality of rural nursing practice. The information for this chapter comes from my ethnographic study of rural hospital nurses in the Inland Northwest, completed in 1987, from dialogue with key informants before then and up until today, and from my personal experiences within rural health care systems over the past 20 years.

In the last 10 or 15 years, I have made some presentations about portions of this work to nurse clinicians, nurse researchers, and non-nurse health care audiences. Inevitably, following such presentations, I was approached by one or two individuals who had been rural nurses who wanted to tell me that the presentation struck a chord. I understood their need, which stemmed from the human desire to be recognized and understood. It stems from the frequent, albeit unintended, distortion of truth about rural nursing communicated by those who do not fully understand what it means to walk a mile in a rural nurse's duty shoes. I may not be able to change that, but I offer my perspective nonetheless.

CONCEPTUALIZING RURAL NURSING PRACTICE

Being Rural

There was a wonderful line in the 1984 science fiction film *The Adventures of Buckaroo Banzai: Across the Eighth Dimension* (Rausch). The line was delivered by the main character, Buckaroo, a multi-skilled neurosurgeon, particle physicist, rock musician, and Zen warrior who, in the midst of chaos matter-of-factly declared, "No matter where you go, there you are." If this sounds simple, I would caution that it is hardly simple. Buckaroo was talking about being in the moment, so imagine for a moment what it means to have *gone* rural. What of rural nursing identity? While the imagery may seem silly or surreal, the truth is real, authentic, important, credible, respectable, and as serious as any nursing practice anywhere. However, as indicated earlier, rural nursing practice is also distinctive from nursing anywhere else. Although I use the analogy of Buckaroo Banzai, hoping it will bring a smile, rural nurses will recognize the script of playing a cool and noble professional, simultaneously enacting multiple roles, and managing the continual transition from one part to another with the frankness of Buckaroo.

Being rural means being a long way from anywhere and pretty close to nowhere. Being rural means being independent or perhaps just being alone. Being a rural nurse means that when a nurse saves a life, everyone in town recognizes that she or he was there; and when a nurse loses a life, everyone in town recognizes that she or he was there. Being rural means turning inward for answers, because there may be nobody to turn to outward. Being rural means that when a nurse walks into the emergency room, it may be her or his spouse or child who needs a nurse, and at that moment, being a nurse takes priority over being anyone else. Being a rural nurse means being able to deal with what she or he has got, where she or he is, and being able to live with the consequences.

Knowing Rural

Certainly every reader has heard that a little knowledge can be a dangerous thing. The adage was probably modified from what Alexander Pope (1711) said in the 17th century: "A little learning is a dangerous thing." I dispute it now and say that a little knowledge can be a lifesaving thing. The demarcation between danger and safety is the difference between having knowledge and *using* knowledge. From time to time, I have had conversations with academic colleagues about dangerous nurses. In these conversations, we have agreed that dangerous nurses are not those who know they do not know what they are doing—although there is certainly an element of danger in that scenario, which ultimately must be addressed. The greater danger, however, emerges with those nurses who think they do know, but actually do not know, what they are doing. Although I have no statistics on the prevalence of such nurses, it is my belief that they hide more easily in urban settings than they do in rural settings.

Knowing rural means knowing that what one knows may be all one has. Knowing rural means personally knowing everyone with whom one works and having knowledge about nearly everyone for whom one cares. As a rural nurse, knowing means sharing knowledge in an informal yet crucially important exchange with other professionals, where the addition of one mind can mean expanding the knowledge base by 100%.

Although *whom* one knows can be important in any setting, the distinction between rural and urban dynamics of whom one knows is that in the urban setting whom one knows is more likely to be related to competitive advantage, whereas in the rural setting whom one knows is more likely to be related to cooperative advantage. Knowing rural means that knowledge can mean the difference between perishing, surviving, and thriving, and therefore knowing is inextricably connected to *being* when one is rural.

THE NATURE AND SCOPE OF NURSING

For practicality, a framework for the study of the nature and scope of rural nursing practice was sought to identify and describe the distinctive characteristics of practice in rural settings. The American Nurses' Association (ANA) Social Policy Statement (1980) provided the framework for a logical sequence of investigation into details of rural nursing practice. The policy statement includes an organized and systematic approach to studying nursing nature and scope.

1. *Nursing's Nature.* Within the policy statement, the nature of nursing is characterized as a relationship between the nursing profession and society that is mutually beneficial, and nursing itself is deemed an essential outgrowth of the society that it serves.

    Nursing is described as existing in response to society's needs. From that standpoint, my study of rural nursing was based on assumptions that rural nursing emerges from and is essential to rural society, and distinctions of rural nursing are due, in part, to distinctive interests and needs of rural society.

2. *Nursing's Scope.* The scope of nursing includes four definitive characteristics that are intersections, dimensions, core, and boundary (ANA, 1980). These four characteristics became conceptual foundation blocks for my study of rural nursing.
    (a) *Intersections.* Nursing intersects with other professions involved in health care. These intersections are points at which nursing meets and interfaces with other professions and expands its practice into the domain of other professions as necessary.
    (b) *Dimensions.* Characteristics such as philosophy, ethics, roles, responsibilities, skills, and authority are examples of nursing dimensions. These are qualities that add depth to nursing practice. They are characteristics underscored and influenced by interpersonal relationships and intimacy as well as the intrapersonal quality of nursing.
    (c) *Core.* The concept of the core of nursing is complex and somewhat more difficult to discuss than are the other concepts. It is

oversimplification to say that the needs of people are the core of nursing, although such is true. Nursing exists to deal with human response to health issues, and human response can be equated to human need with respect to health. The patients' *needs* and their responses are outgrowths of who they are as human *beings*. The nursing care we provide is an outgrowth of who we are as human *beings*. The core of nursing is the dynamic of nursing care juxtaposed with human response.

(d) *Boundaries*. Nursing's boundaries change and expand in direct reflection of the intersections, dimensions, and core of practice. Boundaries are nebulous, unseen, intangible lines of demarcation between what is clearly within the nature and scope of nursing and what is questionably within nursing's scope. Unlike physical boundaries, nursing's boundaries are metaphysical, are relationally and contextually based, and sometimes have origins outside the control of nursing.

METHODS

In an effort to describe the nature and scope of rural nursing, it was determined that an ethnographic method, using participant observation and interviewing techniques, would yield the most pertinent data for analysis. Data were gathered throughout several stages of conceptualization concerning rural nursing phenomena. Field notations, printed news media, and taped interviews were employed. The study of rural hospital nurses included an exploratory phase in which eight rural nurses from northwest Montana were interviewed. These interviews were audiotaped, and from initial open-ended questions, a more refined interview guide was developed that contained both closed and open-ended questions. Twenty-six rural hospital nurses in one of four rural towns in eastern Washington, northern Idaho, or western Montana were interviewed. All interviews were audiotaped and then transcribed verbatim. The findings reported in this chapter are related to many aspects of rural nursing practice and are based on the responses of all 34 rural nurses, as well as several other key rural informants and my own observations. All samples were convenience, and all informants elected to be included in the studies.

FINDINGS

Informant Demographics

All of the informants were women ranging in age from 25 to 61 years, with an average age of 40 years. The number of years actively employed as a registered nurse (RN) was 3 to 35 years. The mean number of years spent working in rural hospitals was 8 years and, for most informants, was roughly half the total of their active nursing years. Most informants were originally diploma-prepared, seven were baccalaureate graduates, and four were associate graduates. Two informants had achieved a master's degree in nursing. Although informants were not asked about marital or parental status, nearly all said during the interview that they were married and were parents.

Most of the informants worked full time, and those who worked part time averaged 23 hours per week. In addition, many were placed "on call" if they were not working. On-call status could be attributed to low census, high census, operating room call, cardiac care call, or emergency department call. Most informants reported 1 or 2 days of overtime per month. In almost every case, informants indicated a need to be flexible about their working schedules with regard to the events of the rural practice setting. Turnover rates were low at all facilities, and the most senior nurses had been on staff from 16 to 25 years.

Hospital Demographics

Information about the hospitals was obtained through interviews with nursing, fiscal, administrative, or other personnel, as well as from public records and the participant observation process. The hospital organizations were between 20 and 60 years in existence, the present structures were between 3 and 35 years old, and all had undergone some renovation over time. Ownership of the hospitals was stated as nonproprietary, public district, or community. Each hospital was governed by a board of directors of 3 to 10 individuals who held fiduciary and decision-making authorities and to whom the administration was accountable. Board membership was either self-perpetuating or community elected. One facility was accredited by what was then the Joint Commission on Accreditation of Healthcare Organizations (JCAHO). Administrative personnel said that there was little to be gained by small rural hospitals having JCAHO accreditation, especially in light of what the JCAHO charged for the process.

The hospitals had licensure ranging from 20 to 44 acute care beds, 0 to 3 intensive or cardiac beds, 5 to 7 newborn bassinets, and 3 to 5 swing beds for extended care. In every case, occupancy was at a fraction of licensure, and occupancy figures averaged to be about 20% to 40% for acute care beds. There was some variability in the use of the other services at each facility. Two had fairly active use of the cardiac or intensive care beds. Two had fairly active obstetrical departments. Three had active surgical departments. Emergency cases at these hospitals ranged from 3 to 13 per 24-hour day during the previous fiscal year. One relied on the constant occupancy of swing beds to maintain financial solvency. The number of physicians on medical staff ranged from 3 to 17. Typically, physicians who held admitting privilege at a given facility did not necessarily live within the community. Undoubtedly, the variety of medical practitioners on staff impacted the occupancy of each facility. Usually, nurses were expected to be able to float from medical–surgical areas to emergency, obstetrical, and intensive care areas, but not to the operating room, which seemed to be the one sacrosanct specialty area.

The Rural Communities

At the time of the study, I spent several weeks traveling to and about four separate communities in western Montana, northern Idaho, and eastern Washington to gather information regarding the nature and scope of rural nursing. Each of these towns fits the operational definition of being geographically isolated and of having less than 5,000 residents. Upon arrival in each community, time was taken to drive about, observe the local terrain, look for indicators of economy, walk around town to observe the pace and lifestyle, note the casual conversations taking place in public areas, and read each community's local weekly newspaper.

There were many similarities and few differences between the communities in terms of how they appeared to the outsider. Each town was located near railroad tracks, all of which were currently used. Three of the towns were on a river in forested mountain terrain and were logging or lumber mill towns. The fourth town was on an expansive plain and was an agricultural community. Each town was inhabited mostly by Caucasian people, and each was laid out in typical western fashion with one main street and several auxiliary streets at which the center of the business district was found. Each town boasted the typical hardware stores, grocery stores, restaurants, farm or logging machinery shops, tool shops, post office, drug store, employment office, beauty shops, ice cream stands, feed stores, junk shops, small motels, bars, and churches. Each town had a well-kept appearance, although each had a few empty buildings or storefronts in the business district.

Residents in these communities were friendly and helpful. They recognized me as an outsider, and, although willing to answer my questions, were curious and wanted to know the purpose of my presence in their town. When I explained myself, the residents registered sincere interest and pleasure that their community had been targeted for this study. They acted like they felt privileged and eagerly conveyed their high regard for nurses in general and *their* nurses specifically. Never did these residents express animosity toward the community of nurses. Most of them had a story to tell about how a friend or relative's life was saved at the local hospital.

Rural Hospital Nurses

The rural nurses I observed and interviewed were a dynamic group of women who could certainly be called *expert generalists*. They moved quickly, and for the most part easily, from one role to another as circumstances required. They explained that most rural nurses have a great deal of knowledge regarding a variety of nursing practice areas. When beginning work in a rural hospital, many nurses suffer reality shock due to the variety of demands placed on them. One seasoned nurse told me, "Although you might start out and you don't have that wide knowledge, you better get it quickly." A relative newcomer nurse expressed admiration about the knowledge level of her rural colleagues, calling them "impressive." The nurses I interviewed routinely worked in three or four different specialty areas of nursing practice every week, and sometimes every day. When talking with one respondent about this phenomenon and how easy certain nurses made it look, she said, "The ones who are experienced in rural nursing seem to be very comfortable in switching back and forth between specialties."

Nursing Staff Tenure and Group Acceptance

At all facilities nurses were heard to use the terms *new* or *newcomer* and *old* or *old-timer* in reference to a given nurse's tenure on the staff. There was no particular time limit identified when a nurse makes the transition from new to old, nor how one arrives at a level of acceptance. However, tenure of less than 2 years was apparently definitely considered new, and tenure of 3 to 5 years in combination with competence generally constituted acceptance. Tenure beyond 10 years was considered seasoned, and in special cases of achieving high proficiency or social acceptance, one of these nurses might be called an old-timer, but usually this term was reserved for someone who had been around for 20 or more years. What I discerned was some gray area depending on a nurse's tenure, level of proficiency, and sociability related to group fit. It seemed that a nurse who was very skillful, flexible, and likeable might reach old-timer status sooner than a nurse who was lacking one of those characteristics.

Although I cannot pinpoint a "typical" rural nurse, certain characteristics were confirmed as traits of distinctive advantage for a rural nurse's success. For example, good common sense, good judgment ability, the ability to set priorities, good physical assessment skills, and physical and emotional strengths were considered of survival significance to these nurses, due, in part, to the aloneness of their practices. They made comments such as, "You have to make all your own decisions. There's no one to do that for you." "You have to be able to be autonomous." "You can't go to somebody for concurrence with decision making." "At any time during your shift, your assignment may change drastically." "You can make the difference between life or death—the judgment calls are yours." All informants were adamant that the prevalent feeling of aloneness and serious responsibility were distinctive to the rural setting. None would concede that the feeling was anything like that experienced in an urban setting. These nurses expressed a very real and pervasive sense of responsibility that rural nurses bear for their patients. The nurses who do not have the ability consistently to carry the burden of such decisional responsibility are the ones who do not survive as rural nurses. Old-timers claimed they could often tell right away, or within a few weeks, if a newcomer was going to catch on or not. Old-timers based such predictions on their assessments of a newcomer's characteristics as mentioned above, combined with evidence of adaptation to the new environment.

Education and Professional Development

The burden for self-responsibility of education is greater in the rural setting than in the urban setting, and most rural nurses accept this burden. There are a wide variety of sources from which rural nurses receive their continuing education, such as out-of-town workshops or conferences, in-service education, journals, textbooks, practice sessions, physicians, and other nurses. The greatest educational needs voiced were in cardiac, trauma, maternal/child, and complex medical nursing.

Informants indicated a thirst for knowledge in accredited professional continuing education. Several respondents reported attending more than 10 continuing education events in a year. Most attended between three and ten events annually. These events were developed and held locally, developed elsewhere but held locally, or developed and held in urban settings. Although expenses were a factor, they were not the central factor in respondents' attending continuing education events.

Nearly all informants also relied on journals for new information, read journals regularly, and reported the most popular journals to be *Nursing, American Journal of Nursing, RN, Journal of Nursing Administration,* and *Nursing Management,* in that order. Current journals were visible in each facility, and notations were seen hanging on bulletin boards in nursing report rooms or locker rooms with a suggestion from one nurse to others that everyone review a given recent journal article germane to a given current case.

Rural nurses, in fact, identify one another as their most important single source of information and education. This was often explained as information being imparted from a peer when it was needed most, so that learning occurred while doing, which tended to heighten the memory. Comments that supported these phenomena included, "We try to share everything we can with each other." "New nurses sometimes come in with great new information or real current ideas. It helps a lot." "Sometimes the new girls expect you to know things, and I don't, and it can be embarrassing. So we look it up together." "When you've been around for a while, you develop camaraderie. We know what we can expect from each other."

Out-of-town workshops were identified as the next most important source of continuing education to rural nurses. Informants qualified this by stressing that the topic or presentation needed to be relevant to the rural environment. One informant said, "It's got to be meaningful. You know, you go up to the city and they tell you how to do something, and they don't realize how different the setup is."

Interpersonal Relationships and Nursing Practice

Rural nurses know everyone who works at the hospital, all of the physicians, and most of their patients. Rural nurses say that the interpersonal closeness of knowing everyone with whom they work and for whom they care generally has a positive influence on their practice. The intensity of this interpersonal dynamic is unique to the rural setting. Although it is likely that nurses in any setting develop close relationships, rural nurses are in the distinctive situation of being personally acquainted with all of those around them, so that the depth of interaction is potentially greater, and the accountability for interpersonal exchange is a constant that is simply not present in other settings. An informant explained the bond she felt with coworkers by saying, "It's nice to know the people you're working with. You work more together, you try harder, and you work closer." Another nurse shared that among many rewarding qualities of rural nursing, "The cooperation of the other nurses and the cohesiveness of the group is probably the biggest."

An old-timer at one hospital said, "I don't have to explain when I say something. They believe me, and they do it without wasting time." It was easy to verify this through observation. Certain old-timers could communicate a virtual reassignment of responsibilities through the tone of their voices as they disappeared momentarily to deal with arisen crises, such as the admission of trauma victims in the emergency room. On occasions it was like watching a dance, the motions of which were so well understood, each dancer so valued and respected, that without missing a step, workers would change places based on available expertise and would back each other up without visible cues. Even physicians were seen deferring to old-timer nurses at such times. Yet, the choreography depended heavily on the direction of the one in charge; and on other occasions, with an inexperienced newcomer directing, the dance was frantic and the flow chaotic.

Practicing Medicine

Rural nurses are understandably reluctant to admit that they practice medicine, but they know their boundaries are sometimes stretched by circumstance. "You take it upon yourself and do what has to be done to make sure the patient's stable before you can call the doctor," said one nurse to me. When patient crises occur, calling the physician is considered important, but it simply does not rank at the top of the list. The nurses I interviewed and watched used a standard A-B-C (airway, breathing, circulation) order of setting priorities to respond to patient needs. Thus, they often began written or unwritten medical protocols while the aide would be sent to summon the physician. Physician response times varied from 5 to 30 minutes at the rural hospitals, resulting in nurses being responsible for considerable decision making during the time lapse. At each site, I heard or saw variations on the themes of nurses stabilizing cardiac or trauma victims and nurses managing precipitous births without the benefit of physicians present. In interviews, nurses were adamant that they had a responsibility to the patients to do whatever was required during an emergency, and although it sometimes felt uncomfortable, inaction would have constituted neglect. The words of one nurse summarize the collective opinion, "We do it because we have to, because it would be wrong if we didn't."

There were also circumstances of newcomer physicians relying on seasoned nurses for insight into or even direction regarding a given patient case. Per physician request, the nurse would literally advise what medications and treatments to order in cases where the doctor did not have the familiarity with a patient's history that the nurse did. This was especially true in after-hours situations of physicians covering for another's patients. My assessment of these circumstances is that each party acted within unseen lines of mutual trust and understanding with the dynamic of trust specific to a given relationship.

Another observation I made at these facilities, which struck me then and which I have informally reconfirmed on multiple occasions since, is that rural physicians seem more likely to read and respond to nurses' notes about patients than do urban physicians. Doubtless there is great individual variability, yet it is tempting to hypothesize that rural professionals have a better grasp than do their urban counterparts of pertinent information that is necessary to communicate to the health care team. Certainly, further study would be required to confirm the probability.

Rural Expertise: Aces and Pinch Hitters

Rural nurses generally believe that no one can be an expert in every area of rural nursing practice. However, a few nurses are extremely proficient in all clinical areas, and these nurses become role models and mentors to the other nurses with whom they work. At two study sites, many informants identified a colleague or two who fit this category. Interestingly, those who were identified by others as *aces* did not identify themselves as such. Each nurse was very modest about her own capability, but the pride toward aces among the staff was obvious. I was aware that talking to or watching these aces in action was as much an honor for the locals as it was for me as an investigating outsider.

All rural nurses interviewed agreed that they must be competent in more than one clinical area to be considered an acceptable staff member.

The top four clinical areas deemed to be most important for competency were emergency nursing, obstetrical nursing, intensive or coronary nursing, and medical–surgical nursing. A supervisory nurse told me, "There's a difference between competent and expert. I think everybody who works in this hospital should be able to walk into any specialty area and function." But there was an expectation held by all informants that they be clinically strong, if not expert, in at least two of the above-named areas and be able to float to any other department and still function well in a pinch.

With regard to functioning in a pinch, in the early 1980s two rural Montana nurse executives who are admitted baseball fans coined the Pinch Hitter Theory of Rural Nursing. One of those persons, Jean Shreffler, now an academic, is author of other chapters in this book. The second person, Maura Fields, was then and remains today the nurse executive at a rural hospital in Montana and is arguably one of the most innovative and masterful nurse leaders I have ever had the good fortune to know. Her rendition of the theory went like this:

> In rural nursing, you have to be like a pinch hitter. You may not perform a task or procedure or work on a very specialized case but once a year. But when you go to do it, you have to do it like you do it every day. In baseball, a batting average of 300 is good. But the pinch hitter, well, you want them to be better than that, really, you want them to bat a thousand. That's what it's like for a rural nurse, when they go to work, you want them to bat a thousand (Maura Fields, 1983, personal conversation).

For those readers who are doubting that there can be that many instances in which the above theory becomes important, rest assured that it happens all the time. Industrial and recreational traumas are frequent in these communities. Rural citizens experience their share of severe burns, drug overdoses, cardiac arrests, head injuries, freak accidents, and critical illness. Although transfer to larger medical centers is sometimes preferred, stabilization is first necessary, and transfer is sometimes not possible. One hospital in this study is 90 road miles from the nearest medical center of any size and 150 road miles from a trauma center. Rotary blade or fixed wing aircraft are often used to transport cases that require more care than can be delivered locally, but northwest mountain weather conditions can be a significant factor in keeping aircraft grounded.

Although rural nurses do not expect an easy routine, frustration is common surrounding the conflict of trying to achieve expertise in such a complex practice. Boredom is rare as they face the constant variety of demands. One informant related the example of the prior day's evening shift. The informant was one of two RNs on duty at the time, assisted by one aide. The scenario she described began after change of shift report and went like this:

> Just yesterday evening there were seven patients in the house with nothing going on. Within an hour, there was one admitted with a depression state, an OB came in, and there were four or five cases in the ER, one being a child with rectal bleeding, which makes you wonder about child abuse.

Although two nurses and an aide would have no difficulty caring for seven stable medical–surgical patients, the admission of the depressed patient was a wrench in the works. Mental health diagnoses are among those which rural nurses feel least appropriately prepared for, and they lack confidence in rural physicians' ability to treat mental health patients appropriately, as well. The depressed patient required suicide precautions for a period of time, which meant that the aide was assigned to remain with the patient at all times. The pediatric patient in the emergency room required careful documentation, delicate interaction, and a social services consultation. The obstetrical patient admission required nurse assessment and individual care until it was determined that the patient was in early labor. One nurse moved back and forth between the emergency room and the general care unit; the other moved back and forth between the labor room, the depressed patient, and the general care unit.

Here is an account from another informant about another evening shift where three RNs were on duty but without assistance from an aide:

> Not long ago we had an OB with a bad baby, small for gestational age; and at the same time we got two ambulances 5 minutes apart, and they were both cardiacs with chest pain. While that was happening, there was surgery going on, and there was somebody in the unit. I don't know if God is watching you or what, but, for the most part, things seem to come out okay in the end.

In this case, one nurse was already assigned to the intensive care unit, and one was required to remain with the obstetrical patient to do monitoring and other procedures. When the first ambulance arrived, the third nurse was dispatched to the emergency room. Fortunately, some ambulance crew members were emergency medical technicians and could help with continued patient monitoring and calling in the physician, laboratory, and respiratory personnel. Also fortunately, the physician arrived within 10 minutes and was designated to care for both patients. The final good fortune is that nothing went wrong on the general care unit while hell was breaking loose elsewhere.

Knowing Patients Personally

Most rural nurses subscribe to the belief that when they know patients personally, they can give better care. The possibility of experiencing fear when caring for family members or best friends notwithstanding, the rewards are considered rich. A gradual loss of anonymity occurs to rural nurses as they become immersed in and assimilated into rural society, making anonymity nonexistent for old-timers. "I can be more supportive emotionally when I know them," one said, and another elaborated, "Let's say in the ER, with chronic lungers, you know them, and they feel secure because they know we remember them." I saw instances of rural nurses informally calling to check on patients after discharge. As far as I know, patients were always glad to have these calls. The loss of anonymity is generally considered reassuring for those professionals who are comfortable with rural life, but it can be constricting as well. It should not be assumed, however, that negative aspects of anonymity loss are necessarily related to poor patient outcomes. On the contrary, one informant told me,

> I know of several situations where knowing my OB patients who had poor outcomes made a difference to them, where I was really able to help them get through the experience. It's a real emotional drain, but you're ahead of the game because the trust is there.

The argument could be made that patients perceive their care to be better based on the close personal contact that is often made in the rural setting. A nurse who believes that her relationship to a patient made a difference in the patient's outcome said,

> I recovered my little neighbor girl after her surgery. Most little kids are scared when they wake up, but when she woke up she knew me and wasn't afraid and recovered really fast. Because fear generates pain, but she wasn't afraid, she recovered faster than usual.

It is a cultural expectation of many rural people to be taken care of by someone they know. This differs from the expectation in urban settings. For the most part, informants agreed that rural people do expect to have their medical needs met, even though they live far from a major medical center. However, one informant said that rural patients often wait until they are "half dead" before they seek intervention and are "grateful for what they get." Another nurse said, "People have told me they were glad I was on when they were here, that if I said it was going to be okay, then it was going to be okay."

Nearly all rural nurses could confirm that sometimes they had patients from out of town who had previously experienced urban hospital admissions. These patients, whether vacationing in the rural setting or passing through the rural area, ended up in rural hospitals for reasons not important to this story. Their comments about the care they received in rural hospitals are important. The nurses were told by these patients that the care was of better quality, that they felt more cared for, that the rural nurses took more time to listen, that care was accomplished more quickly and smoothly, and that they felt more like people and less like numbers in the rural hospital than they did in any urban hospital. The outsider patients often expressed surprise at the high level of competence they encountered in the rural setting.

DISCUSSION

Rural Nursing's Distinctive Nature and Scope

Analyses of the reports of rural nurses show that the nature and scope of rural nursing are clearly distinctive. Using a framework to focus the discussion, the distinctions can apparently be categorized as those pertaining to rural nursing's nature, as well as the four components of rural nursing's scope, those being intersections, dimensions, core, and boundary.

The Nature of Rural Nursing

Most rural nurses have difficulty defining their practice, although they can describe it. Their descriptions are a variety of rich, thoughtful, colorful, and articulate responses. Rural nursing is generalist nursing, not to be mistaken for mundane, and includes an intensity of purpose that makes it distinctive. Rural nurses may feel misunderstood and poorly recognized by the larger nursing community, but they are nonetheless a proud lot.

The Scope of Rural Nursing

The intersections of rural nursing are distinctively marked and fluid. Rural nurses consistently and necessarily practice well within the realm of other health care disciplines, the most notable being respiratory therapy, pharmacy, and medicine. The intersection between nursing and medicine has the most extensive implications. It is a gray area that hinges on circumstances and relationships, and the most complex intersections occur during emergent situations, "until the doctor gets there." Some rural nurses embrace this intersection more willingly than others, but none do it casually. Reflective concern is apparent in comments related to this intersection. One informant said, "It means putting your neck out there on the line, but you have to make the judgment and go on." Another told me, "It sometimes feels uncomfortable, but it's part of my responsibility to the patient."

It is evident that the practice of rural nursing is dimensionally distinctive. Rural nurses embrace an ethic of openness and honesty that is pervasive. The dimension of interpersonal knowing is viewed as a positive feature of rural practice, and it exists between nurses and patients as well as among coworkers. A nurse administrator shared with me that, "in terms of practice outcomes, your accountability is right in front of your face." Rural nurses talked about being able to accomplish goals more quickly with their patients and said that guidance, teaching, and counseling behaviors are automatic to their practice in the rural environment. Communication patterns in the rural setting are more direct and suffer less obfuscation than do those in urban settings. There are fewer barriers to go through when imparting messages from one to another. As a result, there are probably fewer errors of omission and commission related to practice in the rural setting than there are in the urban setting. Confronting and managing conflict is more common in the rural setting, avoidance being an unacceptable dynamic for group cohesiveness that stems from mutual concern and regard for one another. Independent decision making is a given in rural practice, but rural nurses are aware of their limitations. One said, "You have to know when you don't know, and you have to know where to go to find out." Rural nurses are mindful, if not fully informed, about the legal dimensions of their practice. However, with respect to questions of patient safety and survival, rural nurses sometimes decide that their ethical obligation to do what is right for their patients carries more weight than their legal responsibility to uphold the law. These cases generally become lessons of learning, are scrutinized and discussed by the group, and are entered into memory for future reference.

Human responses, which nurses diagnose and treat, are the core of nursing. Some sources have suggested, and informants in this study agreed, that rural dwellers are known to delay health seeking and tend to define health as the ability to get out of bed and go to work. Thinking in terms of nursing diagnosis, one might call this behavior "dysfunctional perceptual orientation to health," which requires distinctive intervention at nursing's core. Rural nurses are faced with determining an appropriate line of demarcation between a rural dweller's rugged individualism and stubborn disregard for health. Inextricable from rural nursing's core are the relational issues of what it means to be rural. As noted earlier in this chapter, from an ontological standpoint, rural nursing is distinctive at its very core.

Boundary being dependent on the intersections, dimensions, and core of nursing, there can be no question as to rural nursing's distinctive boundary. Rural nursing is constantly changing in response to complex intersections and dimensional intricacies distinctive to rural society. The boundary is therefore neither smooth nor even static. When nurses come to a rural setting from an urban setting, they are very aware that the boundary of their practice changes. The transitional period for these nurses is not always easy, and boundary expansion can be accompanied by ambivalence, anxiety, and frustration. Newcomers must become adjusted to the rural culture to function effectively, and not all survive. Rural experts can play a key role in the success of newcomer transition, and those aces who invest themselves in the orientation and mentoring of newcomers know the importance of the payoff.

Defining Rural Nursing

Rural nursing is a special variety of nursing in which the nurse must have a wide range of advanced knowledge and ability, in combination with commitment, to practice proficiently in multiple clinical areas simultaneously along the career trajectory. The practice requires constant and continual personal and professional adaptation in developing identity. A rural nurse has both an ontological sense of being and an epistemological sense of knowing that connect the nurse with the surrounding community, and through which the rural nurse creates a reality of rural professional nursing practice. In no other setting is a nurse's practice so thoroughly and integrally a constant factor in a nurse's life. In a society where separating one's private life from one's professional life is considered obligatory, rural nurses are singularly challenged, stripped of their own anonymity while simultaneously charged with protecting their patients' privacy.

CLOSING THOUGHT

The newcomer practices nursing in a rural setting, unlike the old-timer, who practices *rural nursing*. Somewhere between these spectral extremes lies the transitional period of events and conditions through which each nurse passes at her or his own pace. It is within this temporal zone that nurses experience rural reality and move toward becoming professionals who understand that having gone rural they are not less than they were, but rather they are more than they expected to be. Some may be conscious of the transition and others may not, but in the end a few will say, "I am a rural nurse."

REFERENCES

American Nurses' Association (ANA). (1980). *Nursing: A social policy statement.* Publication No. NP-63 20M 9/82R. Kansas City, MO: Author.

Pope, A. (1711). Essay on criticism. Cited in B. Evans (Ed.), *Dictionary of quotations* (1978). New York, NY: Avenel Books, Delecorte Press.

Rausch, E. M. (screenplay author). (1984). *The adventures of Buckaroo Banzai: Across the eighth dimension*. [Film]. (Available through Vestron Video.)

Chapter 17

MEN WORKING AS RURAL NURSES: LAND OF OPPORTUNITY
Chad O'Lynn

A GROWING BODY OF LITERATURE suggests that rural residency is associated with poorer health outcomes than urban residency (Center on an Aging Society, 2003; Goins & Mitchell, 1999; Kumar, Acanfora, Hennessy, & Kalache, 2001; National Institute of Nursing Research [NINR], 1995). The suggested reasons for this disparity generally relate to barriers of access to health services because of distance and lack of available providers in rural areas. One strategy to address the health disparities in rural settings is to recruit and to retain and then to support health care providers, including nurses. However, amidst the rural health literature, relatively little has been published describing the experiences of nurses who care for rural dwellers.

This gap in the literature is significant in that recruitment and retention of nurses in rural practice is challenging and more difficult than in urban practice because of rural wages, paucity of jobs for spouses, and the negative perceptions of rural nursing (Bushy, 2002; Hopkins & Domrose, 2001; Long, 2000; Trossman, 2001; Vukic & Keddy, 2002). This challenge serves as an overlay for an already well-documented nationwide nursing shortage. To meet projected vacancies, the profession has begun to implement general recruitment strategies targeting groups such as ethnic minorities and men (Buerhaus, Staiger, & Auerbach, 2000; Gordon, 2002). Increasing the number of men in the nursing profession will assist in meeting the demands for future nurses and in improving the diversity of the nursing workforce (American Association of Colleges of Nursing [AACN], 1997, 2001; Anders, 1993; Davis & Bartfay, 2001; Sullivan, 2000; Villeneuve, 1994). However, virtually nothing is known about the experiences of men in rural nursing and the recruitment strategies that might be appropriate to attract men to practice in rural settings.

Because men only comprised 5.4% of the U.S. registered nurse (RN) workforce in 2000, one may assume that there is opportunity for increased recruitment (Spratley, Johnson, Sochalski, Fritz, & Spencer, 2001). However, there is some suspicion that men leave nursing shortly after entering the profession at higher rates than women do (Davis & Bartfay, 2001). The reason for this is unclear. O'Lynn (2004) noted that men in nursing felt that their basic nursing education program did not prepare them well for working primarily with women coworkers.

To recruit and retain men in rural nursing practice, a better understanding of rural nursing from the masculine perspective is needed. This understanding will assist in the development of gender-appropriate strategies to recruit men to critical shortage areas and will assist in the development of gender-appropriate supports to retain men in rural nursing. My purpose in this study was to examine the experiences and perspectives of men working as rural nurses. I asked two research questions: What are the experiences of men working as rural nurses? What would be the appropriate strategies to recruit and retain men in rural nursing practice?

BACKGROUND AND SIGNIFICANCE

Limitations of the Literature on Rural Male Nurses

Houde (2002) and Thompson (2002) reported that invisibility of men occurs when researchers do not include men in study samples or when data generated from men are folded into the data generated mostly by women. Most studies noted in this book do not include men. As such, the findings from these studies have questionable generalizability to men working or considering working in rural nursing. No study located for review described rural nursing practice from a male perspective. In the current study, I addressed this gap by providing an initial understanding of the experiences of men in rural nursing practice and how men may be recruited and retained to work in rural communities.

Significance

The implications of the invisibility of men in the nursing literature are profound. A review of literature by O'Lynn (2004) showed that men experience nursing education and nursing practice differently than women do. These differences stem from a variety of reasons, including historical discrimination of men in nursing, differing gender roles, and different approaches to caregiving. If men are to be recruited and retained in rural practice settings, strategies developed from the current understanding of rural nursing practice may not be gender appropriate.

METHODS

I used the hermeneutic phenomenology in the Heideggerian tradition for this study. According to Koch (1995) and Benner (1999), hermeneutic phenomenology assumes a constructivist reality, in which people encounter phenomena with uniquely individualized preunderstanding and historical knowledge that cannot be stripped away. Phenomena are experienced and understood in a highly contextualized and interpreted world. Consequently, reality is not absolute and cannot be reduced to essential truths, although individuals may have many similar experiences (Koch, 1995; Lincoln & Guba, 2000). From an epistemological perspective, hermeneutic phenomenology assumes that knowledge is co-created among individuals. The researcher cannot be an objective observer, but rather serves as a vehicle through which understanding occurs from transactions with others and the existing world contexts can only be corrected and modified (Benner, 1999). Hermeneutic phenomenology is a research approach appropriate for exploration of poorly understood phenomena and the meaning they hold for persons.

Procedure

I used open-ended interviews with six men working as RNs in frontier communities in Montana. Inclusion criteria for participation were (a) RN licensure in Montana, (b) employment in a frontier county and a community of less than 5,000 residents, and (c) the ability to speak English. I obtained an informed consent from all participants. The Human Subjects Committee of Montana State University-Bozeman and the Institutional Review Board of Oregon Health & Science University approved this study. I completed the study as a partial requirement for research practicum credit at Oregon Health & Science University.

I recruited a purposive sample of participants from a list of all RNs licensed in Montana supplied by the State Board of Nursing. This list provided only the names and residential addresses of the nurses. It provided no indication of the nurse's sex, ethnicity, or race. I examined the list for names of nurses believed to be men residing in frontier counties. If more than one nurse resided in a community, one name was highlighted for enrollment. The rationale for this procedure was to ensure maximum representation of rural communities in the sample. From the screening of the list, I identified 30 potential participants and sent letters in the spring of 2004 inviting them to participate. Seven letters were returned stamped "No longer at this address/No forwarding address." Of the 21 remaining potential participants, seven agreed to participate. However, one withdrew from the study prior to his interview.

The six men in the sample were Caucasian. The men's age range from 34 to 58 years ($m = 40.7$ years). Their years of experience as nurses ranged from less than 1 year to 30 years ($m = 11.4$ years). All had some nursing experience in an urban setting at some point during their careers. The range of time spent working as rural nurses was from less than 1 year to 20 years ($m = 7.7$ years). Five worked in rural hospitals as staff nurses. The sixth worked as a nurse practitioner in a primary care clinic. Nursing was a second career for all of the participants.

The size range of communities in which the men worked was 940 to 2,874 residents ($m = 1,668$; U.S. Bureau of Census, 2002). Two of the six communities were located on or near Indian reservations. The major economic activities of five of the communities was ranching and farming. One community relied on tourism, as it was located near a national park.

Two participants lived in the communities in which they worked. The other four participants commuted 340, 129, 53, and 35 miles one way to the agencies where they worked. The participants working in hospitals and not in their communities grouped their shifts, staying in town either at the hospital or in a motel, and returning home during their off days. One participant had been doing this for 20 years.

The hospitals in which five participants worked were designated as critical access hospitals (CAHs) with a range in beds of 4 to 15. All had long-term care facilities either attached to the hospital or located next door. None of the participants worked as staff nurses in these long-term care facilities at the time of the interviews. All hospitals were served by volunteer ambulance services. As such, local ambulance availability was not guaranteed on a 24-hour basis. Participants noted that it was not uncommon for patients to present to the emergency department (ED) who had transported themselves or were transported by family or friends or by the local sheriff. The nearest emergency services from these hospitals were located from 23 to 65 miles away ($m = 37$ miles). However, the hospital located 23 miles from another emergency facility was accessible only by secondary roads, with a usual driving time of 45 minutes in the best of weather. All hospitals had access to helicopter transport to a regional medical center. Although some had improved heliport pads nearby, one helicopter service was 7 miles away. However, if needed, there was a grassy area next to the hospital upon which a helicopter could land in good weather. For the helicopter to land safely, the participant needed to ensure that the area was clear of debris and turn on the outdoor lights if it was dark.

Data Collection and Data Analysis

I conducted interviews over the telephone at a time and date selected by the participants; the interviews lasted 45 to 100 minutes. Consistent with phenomenological methods, I used loosely structured interview questions, which allowed for free discussion of topics that the participant or I deemed relevant. I asked some general (grand-tour) questions of all the participants to obtain information on rural nursing, gender, and recruitment. These questions included: (a) What is rural nursing? (b) What is your typical work day like? (c) What is it like being a man working in rural nursing? (d) Why do you work in a rural area? and (e) What would attract men to work as rural nurses?

I audiotaped all interviews and then transcribed them. I analyzed transcripts sequentially as each interview occurred. I read transcripts in total to gain a general perspective. I then analyzed each transcript section-by-section for codes. I used direct quotes when possible for codes to represent the participants' responses. I then organized codes into categories that represented emerging themes. I compared categories and themes from each transcript to determine similarities and differences among the transcripts.

After I completed and analyzed interviews with four participants, I noted a redundancy in themes. However, the transcript of one participant, the nurse practitioner, included details of his duties and work day that were very different from the other transcripts. These differences were most likely reflective of the fundamental differences between the nurse practitioner and the staff nurse roles. On the other hand, his discussion of other aspects of rural living and his rural clientele generated findings similar to the transcripts of the rural staff nurse participants. Because of this, I decided to include the transcript but did not pursue further exploration of the practice characteristics of rural advanced practice nurses.

After I conducted the first four interviews, I gave copies of the uncoded transcripts to two experienced rural nurse researchers and a graduate student who resided in a rural community. These peer auditors, working independently, examined these interviews for categories. They contrasted categories with the categories from the original data analysis. Although there were slight differences in the wording of the categories, the meaning of the categories was similar.

With redundancy in the transcripts and similarity in the categories derived from the peer auditors, I enrolled two additional rural hospital staff nurses and interviewed them to ensure that no new themes emerged. The findings were consistent with the previous findings, and I did not conduct any more interviews.

RESULTS

Generally, the participants painted a very positive view of rural nursing and the rural environments in which they worked. For the men who were seasoned nurses, all were happy with rural nursing and had no plans for relocation. The men who were relatively new to rural nursing demonstrated a general excitement and enthusiasm with the characteristics and challenges of rural nursing practice. Although the term "opportunities" was not used by the men, the term captured the overarching sentiment in their discussions. The term reflected the positive accounts provided by the participants and may reflect the desired perspective of a potential nurse recruiter looking to fill vacant nursing positions in rural communities. The specific themes of opportunities include (a) expanded practice, (b) autonomy, (c) meaningful relationships, (d) challenge, (e) rural rewards, and (f) recruitment.

Opportunities for Expanded Practice

All men described rural nursing as a generalist practice that extended beyond the typical generalist practice employed by float or resource pool nurses in larger facilities. Typically, in larger hospitals, nurses who work on multiple units develop generalist skills for select patient populations. Rarely do nurses working in a larger hospital care for all the types of patients seen in that hospital. In rural nursing, the men stated that they work pediatrics to geriatrics, emergency care to long-term care, all within the same shift, and every shift. The term jack-of-all-trades was used by several of the participants. One participant described his typical shift this way:

> Well, I guess a good example would be not too long ago, we had a serious motor vehicle accident involving a motorcyclist that we were stabilizing and trying to transport elsewhere. At the same time, we had a mom and a new-born baby ... postpartum patient, and then with all that, we had an ambulance call with an 89-year old patient who had respiratory distress who died on us that night .... In the meantime, we had two or three patients down the hall, one was on a cardiac monitor, while another was just ... I don't remember what the other one was, but you know, it's every night, and you can see everything all in one night.

Four participants stated that they were the only RN on duty, accompanied by a nurse's aide. As such, they completed all skilled procedures and care coordination for all of the patients present during their shifts.

In addition to the expanded patient population of the rural nurse, all participants described the expanded role of the rural nurse. The specific duties of each of the participants varied depending upon his workplace, but all discussed the completion of roles typically done by ancillary staff in larger hospitals. These roles included emergency department (ED) assistant, respiratory therapist, ward clerk, billing clerk, phlebotomist, electrocardiograph technician, security officer, central supply clerk, pharmacy technician, community educator, social worker, and ambulance personnel. The men noted that as the nurse on duty, they were the "only game in town." One participant described the time-consuming task of taking inventory of all medications and treatments provided to a patient during the previous 24-hour period for billing purposes. Another participant indicated that the RN also served as the hospital's security officer. Another participant provided the following description:

> Of course, in that facility, we do all the paperwork. We do the patient charts, we write out the lab slips. Sometimes if lab's not there, we go ahead and do the blood draw [.] ... We basically do all the ward clerk duties. We do all the transfer paperwork. We dispense medications from what we call the pharmacy. We don't have a pharmacy .... Well, actually, we have the hospital pharmacy, but we're it as far as dispensing and keeping track of what we have and what needs ordering and that kind of stuff. Of course, there's a lot of paperwork there involved in tracking, you know, what medication is going to what patient and that kind of thing .... We copy paperwork. We make sure we have insurance information. We do all the HIPAA (Healty Insurance Portability and Accountability Act of 1996) privacy paperwork, you know, I mean we'll cook the meals if need be. We pretty much are there to do whatever needs doing.

The men discussed a blending of the roles, noted earlier, but in particular, the blending of roles between medicine and nursing. This blending occurred most frequently in the ED and involved tasks such as initiating treatments and diagnostic work while waiting for the physician to arrive. However, all participants noted that they were practicing within their scope of practice as defined by the State of Montana.

Despite the seemingly overwhelming burden patient diversity and expanded roles might create, participants noted the benefits (and hence, opportunities) of these characteristics of rural nursing. One participant stated that working in a rural hospital was "less frustrating" than working in a larger hospital because he did not have to wait on other health care personnel to come and do their task for a patient before he could move forward with nursing care. "Instead," stated another participant, "you just do it yourself." Several participants described the expanded roles as a way to become more involved with their patients, and thus, become more knowledgeable about their individual care needs. They indicated that nurses might treat a patient in the ED, admit that patient to a hospital bed, take comprehensive and holistic care of that patient for several days, and then work with that patient as he transitions to a swing bed or is discharged to the community. The participants criticized the care received by patients in larger hospitals as being disjointed and poorly coordinated, because patients receive care by numerous providers and disciplines as they progress through a hospital stay. The participants felt that the patients in rural hospitals receive more personalized care.

Opportunities for Autonomy

All participants described the increased level of autonomy enjoyed by rural nurses compared with their nonrural colleagues. Several of the men specifically used the term *autonomy*, whereas others used the terms *independence, having more leeway, or freer to make decisions*. One participant noted that rural nursing is a "self-driven practice." All described increased autonomy as a benefit of rural nursing practice.

Autonomy was categorized in two ways: (a) greater freedom to make decisions affecting patient care and (b) greater freedom to use one's own work routines. The participants described using nursing judgment in revising an individual patient's plan of care more freely than they had experienced while working in larger hospitals. Several noted that rural nurses are able to request needed supplies, initiate protocols and deliver necessary treatments that were once a commonplace in nursing practice, but are now becoming increasingly dependent upon the decisions of other professionals (e.g., respiratory therapist required to initiate incentive spirometry). The greater autonomy described by the participants suggests greater integrity of the domains of collaborative and independent nursing practice, whereas the trend in larger hospitals may be increasing the domain of dependent nursing practice.

Some participants described the freedom to set one's own schedule and routines on any given shift as a positive experience. Because they usually worked with only one other individual, how and when specific tasks were to be accomplished during a shift was negotiated. The freedom to set work routines was not only desirable, but also necessary to provide the flexibility for unpredicted ED visits and patient admissions. On hospital units with more staff, an individual nurse has much less freedom for establishing routines, as these types of decisions will impact a larger group of workers and may conflict with preestablished unit routines and cultures. It is interesting that with a perceived increased level of autonomy, none of the participants noted autonomy-based conflicts with coworkers. Instead, the participants described how the staff worked together better than in larger hospitals, hence they described relationships that are more meaningful with coworkers.

Opportunities for Meaningful Relationships

All participants described at length the improved ability to develop and maintain positive and meaningful relationships in rural practice settings with coworkers, clients, and the community. With coworkers, the men described a higher level of teamwork than they had experienced in urban settings. One participant noted,

> Basically, the biggest thing I found with rural nursing is the teamwork. When I worked in [urban setting] for so many

doctors, you never really got to know any of them. I mean, there were some that were easier to work with than others, but you didn't get to know them very well. And in a rural community, your doctors and nurses really work together as a team. They have to because there are only so many of you.

This teamwork not only included nurses and physicians, but all health care workers. Several participants praised the nurse's aides with whom they worked. Because they were sometimes busy in the ED, participants relied upon their aides to "keep an eye on the other patients" for them. They noted the skill and dedication of their aides. The reliance upon and admiration for their aides led to a higher level of trust than they had experienced with the aides with whom they had worked in larger hospitals.

Since there were fewer employees and more frequent contact with other employees, participants stated that they really "got to know" the people with whom they worked. Teamwork was demonstrated by everyone "pitching in and helping out" and doing whatever it takes to "get the job done." As one participant explained,

> If we have something major going on, generally the ambulance crew is there to help. They can do CPR, help start IVs. Usually if it's something major, when the ambulance crew brings them in, they will stay and help.

All participants had access to an on-call nurse or nurse at the nursing home that they could call for assistance. Also, physicians and physician assistants were able to get to the hospital in a very short period of time when needed. This readiness to help each other was such that none of the participants felt isolated when working at the hospital.

Participants commented on how patient the staff and physicians were when asked questions and how willing they were to teach. This milieu facilitated teamwork and collaboration, maintained trust among the staff, created a climate of mutual respect, and enhanced camaraderie. Moreover, although two participants noted that there were occasional conflicts ("everyone is human"), none reported troubled relationships with coworkers that eroded teamwork.

Another benefit of working in a rural practice is direct access to management. Small numbers of staff in the hospitals meant few, if any, layers of middle management that separated frontline workers from hospital administration. One participant sat on the hospital's foundation board; he stated he was able to bring representation directly from the patient care staff to hospital decision makers. Such access can translate into beneficial power that directly affects the nurses' work environments.

All participants talked about meaningful relationships with their patients and with the communities in which they worked. Relationships with patients and communities have been described as inherently different from those in urban settings because of the lack of anonymity many rural health care providers experience (Lee, 1998). Lack of anonymity makes it difficult for rural health care providers to maintain professional role boundaries (Lee, Scharff, 1998). However, all participants in this study described familiarity with their patients as a benefit that improved their ability to provide quality care. One participant stated,

> Generally, patients coming in ... if they recognize somebody, if they know somebody, then they are more confident. They feel more comfortable, you know, and more confident in the care. I don't know how many times that I've had people say that. They come into the ER or they're patients in the hospital and they go, "Oh, it's so nice to see someone I recognize." You know, but it's actually a real benefit for the patients.

Rural nurses "treat generations of families." For example, a woman may be admitted to the hospital. One month later, her son may come to the ED with an injury. Several months later, a grandmother is admitted, and so on. Because of the small population, each rural nurse can affect a relatively large percentage of the community and, unlike urban settings where nurses may never see their patients again, in rural areas, a nurse may encounter former patients several times a week at the store, at a high school sporting event, and so on. Participants did not seem burdened by off-duty contacts from the community.

Several participants remarked how supportive the community was of the hospital. Examples of the support included voluntarily raising taxes to support the local hospital, holding fundraisers to purchase an up-to-date ambulance, stopping by to visit patients and cheering them up, and volunteering a few hours to "do anything that we might need help getting done."

Opportunities for Challenge

All participants remarked that rural nursing was challenging. One stated, "The first eight months were tough .... REALLY tough." Most challenges stemmed from the realities of working with an expanded patient population and in an expanded practice role. In addition, the increased accountability required by working in multiple roles created challenges that the men felt were not as pronounced in nonrural practice settings. Such challenges require that rural nurses be flexible, have excellent triage and prioritization skills, and have broad-based nursing knowledge supplemented by emergency, critical care, and trauma certifications. Preparation for the unexpected was seen as crucial by the participants. One noted, "You don't see a lot of everything, but you see a little bit of everything a lot."

However, despite the challenges of rural nursing, all participants expressed a sense of pride in their accomplishments and their skills. One noted that when urban nurses come to a rural setting, they are amazed at the talent and versatility of rural nurses. Another, who was new to nursing, commented on how much better trained and skilled he was than his former classmates who were working in highly specialized urban practices. Another noted that because of his skill set and experience, he could go "just about anywhere" and be an asset to a potential employer.

Another challenge mentioned by the participants was maintaining confidentiality. As stated previously, some community members are actively involved in hospital activities. In addition, one participant commented that the stereotypes of small towns, like "everyone knowin' everyone's business" and "there are no secrets in a small town," are true. However, maintaining patient confidentiality was not particularly difficult, as long as the nurses stayed vigilant. One participant stated, "You just know that you don't talk about certain things. If someone is persistent in finding out information, you just say 'I'm sorry, I can't share that information.'"

Opportunities for Rural Rewards

I asked each participant why he chose to work in a rural practice. Some commented on the ability to gain diverse nursing experiences, and two reported financial incentives. The nurse practitioner reported receiving a higher salary from the Public Health Service for working in an underserved rural area. The participant just out of nursing school discussed a federally funded loan repayment program available to him for agreeing to work in a critical (rural) shortage area. In addition, all commented on the beneficial aspects of a rural lifestyle. These aspects included picturesque surroundings, less stressful lifestyle, lower crime rate, and friendly people in the rural communities. However, most important were the close proximity to outdoor activities, such as hunting and fishing, and the family-friendly environments of the rural communities. One participant commented,

> Basically, the lifestyle in the small community is more conducive to family. Schools are closer. You have more involvement with the children in school. You can take the kids to the park, or they can go out on their own to the park and play.... So you don't have as much concern in a small town. The kids have much more freedom ... a better way to grow up.

Gender and the Opportunities for Recruitment

Participants did not feel that nursing practice differed between male and female rural nurses. In addition, all felt well received and respected by their employers and their local communities. One participant said, "They told me they were excited to have a male nurse." Men provide physical strength and were able to provide balance to an all-female nursing staff. One participant felt he was able to confront belligerent male patients in the ED better than his female coworkers. He stated,

> I think that in the emergency room ... sometimes just seeing a male quiets them down a little bit. They don't act quite as offensive.... [Although] some of the [female] nurses are pretty tough, some of them will get a little intimidated and walk out and ask me to take care of the patient or ask me to help settle them down.

Other participants stated that their experience with team sports provided a sound foundation for the teamwork necessary for effective rural practice.

All participants felt that rural nursing would be attractive for men. When I asked them about recruitment strategies, the participants stated that autonomy and diversity of experiences are particularly attractive for men. Two noted that in their experience, men tend to like emergency and trauma nursing and believed that rural nursing would routinely provide these experiences. However, a number of participants pointed out that salaries are lower in rural areas than in urban areas and believed that rural hospitals need to be competitive with larger hospitals to attract men to rural practice.

DISCUSSIONS AND IMPLICATIONS

The findings from the current study support those of other studies describing rural nursing practice that primarily used the perspectives of female nurse samples. In particular, the current study found similar descriptions of increased autonomy, collaboration, role expansion, patient diversity, challenges, and lack of anonymity as characteristics of rural nursing practice. Consistent with other studies, the men in this study also reported the need for flexibility, extensive generalist knowledge, emergency and trauma certifications, and a "can-do" attitude to be effective in rural nursing. Not found in the current study was the theme of insider or outsider to the local community. Generally, the men were well received as they came to work in their rural communities.

The study provides new insight on the positive aspects of rural nursing practice (Hegney, McCarthey, Rogers-Clark, & Gorman, 2002; Rosenthal,

1996; Scharff, 1998). The men described potentially negative aspects of rural nursing, such as lack of anonymity and the diversity of patients, as benefits and attractions to rural nursing. The positive depiction of rural nursing provided by the men supports the term "opportunity" as an overarching theme. The participants in the current study took pride in their accomplishments at meeting the challenges of rural nursing and felt that their experiences in rural nursing made them better nurses overall.

In terms of recruitment, the findings are somewhat different from those noted by Australian researchers (Hegney et al., 2002). In terms of recruitment, the findings are somewhat different from those noted by Australian researchers (Hegney et al., 2002). These researchers did not report easy access to outdoor recreation or positive relationships with coworkers and members of the community as positive attributes of rural nursing. In addition, the Australian study reported the physical and emotional demands of rural nursing as factors for leaving rural nursing practice. The men in the current study did not mention emotional or physical demands as part of their practice. In fact, several indicated that their physical strength was of benefit in the practice setting. The only negative aspect of rural nursing mentioned by the current study participants that might dissuade someone from rural nursing practice are the lower wages offered by most employers.

According to participants in the current study, nurse recruiters hoping to fill vacancies in rural settings by accessing the undertapped male nurse labor pool should highlight the following in their marketing strategies: (a) increased autonomy; (b) increased opportunity for diverse patient experiences, including emergency and trauma nursing; (c) more meaningful relationships with coworkers, patients, and the community; and (d) the outdoor recreation and family-friendly environments available in rural settings.

LIMITATIONS AND RECOMMENDATIONS FOR FURTHER RESEARCH

The sample size of the study was small. However, consistent with phenomenology, sample sizes are generally small, but data are rich from lengthy interviews (Creswell, 1998; Patton, 2002). Because I obtained similar findings among the participants, expanding the sample size might not have contributed additional themes. Consistent with qualitative studies, findings from this study cannot be generalized to rural nursing populations (Creswell, 1998; Patton, 2002). Yet, because the findings of this study are consistent with the findings of other qualitative studies of rural nursing practice, the findings may have high transferability to other nurses working in rural hospitals.

Another limitation is self-selection of the participants. It is possible that men working as rural nurses who had very different perspectives chose not to participate in the study. In addition, all of the participants are Caucasian. It is unclear how many male nurses of ethnic minority background are working in rural Montana communities, because the State Board of Nursing did not provide this information with its list of RNs. However, there was some diversity within the sample in terms of years of nursing and rural nursing experience and in terms of the types of communities in which they worked. Further research is needed to understand the experiences of men in other rural locations and practice settings, particularly in long-term care and in advanced practice.

CONCLUSION

My purpose in the current study was to examine the experiences and perspectives of men working as rural nurses. The findings indicate that men find rural nursing practice a very positive experience that can be described as a land of opportunity. These include opportunities for expanded practice, autonomy, meaningful relationships, challenges, and rural rewards. Nurse recruiters trying to attract men to rural nursing should emphasize the positive aspects of rural nursing, the opportunities for outdoor recreation, and the family-friendly environments offered by rural communities.

ACKNOWLEDGMENTS

This research was funded by Montana State University-Bozeman College of Nursing Block Grant Program. The author acknowledges Helen J. Lee and Charlene A. Winters for their assistance with this study.

REFERENCES

American Association of Colleges of Nursing (AACN). (1997). *Diversity and equality of opportunity*. Retrieved March 12, 2002, from http://www.aacn.nche.edu/Publications/positions/diverse.htm

American Association of Colleges of Nursing (AACN). (2001, December Issue Bulletin). *Effective strategies for increasing diversity in nursing programs*. Washington, DC: American Association of Colleges of Nursing.

Anders, R. L. (1993). Targeting male students. *Nurse Educator, 18*(2), 4.

Benner, P. (1999). Quality of life: A phenomenological perspective on explanation, prediction, and understanding in nursing science. In E. C. Polifroni, & M. Welch (Eds.), *Perspectives on philosophy of science in* nursing: An historical and contemporary anthology (pp. 303–314). Philadelphia, PA: Lippincott.

Buerhaus, P. I., Staiger, D. O., & Auerbach, D. I. (2000). Implications of an aging registered nurse workforce. *Journal of the American Mathematical Society, 283*, 2948–2954.

Bushy, A. (2002). International perspectives on rural nursing: Australia, Canada, USA. *Australian Journal of Rural Health, 10*, 104–111.

Center on an Aging Society. (2003, January). *Data profile: Rural and urban health. Challenges for the 21st century: Chronic and disabling conditions* (pp. 1–6). Washington, DC: Institute for Health Care Research and Policy, Georgetown University.

Creswell, J. (1998). *Qualitative inquiry and research design: Choosing among five traditions*. Thousand Oaks, CA: Sage.

Davis, M. T., & Bartfay, W. J. (2001). Men in nursing: An untapped resource. *Canadian Nurse, 97*(5), 14–18.

Goins, R. T., & Mitchell, J. (1999). Health-related quality of life: Does rurality matter? *Journal of Rural Health, 15*, 147–146.

Gordon, S. (2002). *A hemorrhage in the hospitals*. Retrieved June 4, 2002, from http://www.latimes.com/la-000038996jun03.story

Hegney, D., McCarthy, A., Rogers-Clark, C., & Gorman, D. (2002). Why nurses are attracted to rural and remote practice? *Australian Journal of Rural Health, 10*, 178–186.

Hopkins, M., & Domrose, C. (2001). *Remote control*. Retrieved January 11, 2004, from http://www.nurseweek.com/news/features/01–04/rural.asp

Houde, S. C. (2002). Methodological issues in male caregiver research: An integrative review of the literature. *Journal of Advanced Nursing, 40*, 626–640.

Koch, T. (1995). Interpretive approaches in nursing research: The influence of Husserl and Heidegger. *Journal of Advanced Nursing, 21*, 827–836.

Kumar, V., Acanfora, M., Hennessy, C. H., & Kalache, A. (2001). Health status of the rural elderly. *Journal of Rural Health, 17*, 328–331.

Lee, H. (1998). Lack of anonymity. In H. J. Lee (Ed.), *Conceptual basis for rural nursing* (pp. 76–88). New York, NY: Springer Publishing.

Lincoln, Y. S., & Guba, E. (2000). Paradigmatic controversies, contradictions, and emerging confluences. In N. K. Denzin, & Y. S. Lincoln (Eds.), *Handbook of qualitative research* (2nd ed., pp. 163–188). Thousand Oaks, CA: Sage.

Long, C. (2000, October 9). *Rural communities feel sting of nursing shortage*. Retrieved November 28, 2004, from http://community.bouldernews.com/news/statewest/091nurs.html

National Institute of Nursing Research. (1995). *Chapter 2: Rural America: Challenges and opportunities*. Retrieved April 9, 2003, from http://ninr.nih.gov/ninr/research/volq/chapter2.htm

O'Lynn, C. E. (2004). Gender-based barriers for male students in nursing education programs: Prevalence and perceived importance. *Journal of Nursing Education, 43*, 229–236.

Patton, M. Q. (2002). *Qualitative research & evaluation methods* (3rd ed.). Thousand Oaks, CA: Sage.

Rosenthal, K. (1996). *Rural nursing: An exploratory narrative description.* Unpublished dissertation, University of Colorado, Denver.

Scharff, J. (1998). The distinctive nature and scope of rural nursing practice: Philosophical bases. In H. J. Lee (Ed.), *Conceptual basis for rural nursing* (pp. 19–38). New York, NY: Springer Publishing.

Spratley, E., Johnson, A., Sochalski, J., Fritz, M., & Spencer, W. (2001). *The registered nurse population March 2000: Findings from the National Sample Survey of Registered Nurses*. Washington, DC: U.S. Department of Health and Human Services, Bureau of Health Professions, Division of Nursing.

Sullivan, E. J. (2000). Men in nursing: The importance of gender diversity. *Journal of Professional Nursing, 16*, 253–254.

Thompson, E. (2002). What's unique about men's caregiving? In B. J. Kramer, & E. Thompson (Eds.), *Men as caregivers: Theory, research, and service implications* (pp. 20–50). New York, NY: Springer Publishing.

Trossman, S. (2001, July/August). Rural nursing anyone? Recruiting nurses is always a challenge. *The American Nurse, 1*, 18–19.

U.S. Bureau of the Census. (2002). *U.S. summary: 2000* (Census profile no. C2K- PROF/00–US). Washington, DC: U.S. Department of Commerce.

Villeneuve, M. J. (1994). Recruiting and retaining men in nursing: A review of the literature. *Journal of Professional Nursing, 10*, 217–228.

Vukic, A., & Keddy, B. (2002). Northern nursing practice in a primary health care setting. *Journal of Advanced Nursing, 40*, 542–548.

Chapter 18

RURAL NURSES' ATTITUDES AND BELIEFS TOWARD EVIDENCE-BASED PRACTICE

Brenda D. Koessl, Charlene A. Winters, Helen J. Lee, and Lori Hendrickx

EVIDENCE-BASED PRACTICE (EBP) IS A hallmark of professional nursing practice and high-quality patient care (Case, 2004). Melnyk, Fineout-Overholt, Feinstein, Sadler, and Green-Hernandez (2008) defined EBP as a "problem-solving approach to the delivery of care that incorporates the best evidence from well-designed studies in combination with a clinician's expertise and patient preferences and values" (p. 8). EBP is further characterized by the American Nurses Association (ANA, 2004) as practice that occurs within the context of available resources. Evidence-based nursing deemphasizes ritual, isolated, and unsystematic clinical experiences, ungrounded opinions, and tradition as a basis for practice. It stresses the use of research findings and other operational and evaluation data, the consensus of recognized experts, and affirmed experience to substantiate clinical practice (American Nurses Credentialing Center [ANCC], 2005). Most nursing leaders would agree that EBP should be usual and customary in their organizations (Munroe, Duffy, & Fisher, 2006). As a case in point, the Joint Commission (JC, 2008) requires the use of evidence in practice to ensure safe patient care.

Nurses constitute the largest group of health care providers, and their care directly influences patient outcomes (Aiken, Clarke, Cheung, Sloane, & Silber, 2003). Numerous authors writing about EBP clearly support the premise that nurses need to be knowledgeable about how to access and use research (Funk, Champagne, Wiese, & Tornquist, 1991; Olade, 2004; Parsons, Merlin, Taylor, Wilkinson, & Hiller, 2003; Pravikoff, Tanner, & Pierce, 2005; Taylor, Wilkinson, & Blue, 2001). However, a growing number of research studies (Estabrooks, Midodzi, Cummings, & Wallin, 2007;

Funk et al., 1991; Hommelstad & Cornelia, 2004; Olade, 2003; Taylor et al., 2001) have identified barriers that interfere with the ability of nurses to utilize evidence-based nursing in practice. Barriers include lack of (a) accessibility to research, (b) organizational and peer support for using research, (c) knowledge of research methods, (d) access to technology, and (e) time.

A small body of research literature has focused on nurses' attitudes and beliefs about research to explain nurses' use of evidence for practice (Melnyk et al., 2004; Morrison, 1998; Olade, 2004; Smirnoff, Ramirez, Kooplimae, Gibney, & McEvoy, 2007). An attitude is a mental position with regard to fact or state (Merriam-Webster, 2007), while a belief can be considered a conviction held in the absence of evidence (Rawnsley, 2003). Rizzuto, Bostrom, Suter, and Chenitz (1994) reported that nurses with positive attitudes and beliefs toward EBP are more likely to utilize research and incorporate it into practice than nurses whose attitudes and beliefs toward EBP are negative.

Implementing EBP is especially important in rural and remote practice, to ensure the best outcomes for populations in areas with limited health care choices and resources (Taylor et al., 2001). However, limited literature exists regarding rural nurses' access and use of research in practice (Olade, 2004; Winters et al., 2007). Professional isolation, limited access to colleagues with research backgrounds, and lack of administrative support for staff involvement in research affects rural nurses' use of research (Olade, 2003). Furthermore, limited budgets for continuing education (CE) and lack of medical libraries and technology resources place rural nurses at a disadvantage when it comes to an environment supportive of nurses' access and use of research (Olade, 2003). The further one ventures away from large urban medical centers, the less one hears about research utilization activities for EBP in nursing (Olade, 2004). Isolation from colleagues who are involved in research coupled with lack of research specific to rural nursing (Winters et al., 2007) are factors that could influence rural nurses' attitudes and beliefs about research.

PURPOSE OF THE STUDY

A gap exists between the time research findings are reported and the time they are incorporated into practice. If rural nurses are not familiar with research or how to access research, or do not value research, this gap may be exaggerated, putting patients at a disadvantage. If nursing is to be an evidence-based profession, improving the use of research findings in clinical practice must occur within urban and rural settings (Olade, 2004). The purpose of the study was to explore factors that influence rural nurses' attitudes and beliefs toward EBP. The research questions were:

1. What are rural nurses' attitudes and beliefs about research and EBP?
2. Do rural nurses find research easy to understand?
3. Do rural nurses believe the results of the research that they read?
4. Does number of years of experience as a nurse affect rural nurses' attitudes and beliefs about research?
5. Does level of education influence rural nurses' attitudes and beliefs toward research?
6. Does the size of facility that a rural nurse works in affect attitudes and beliefs toward research?
7. Does the role of a rural nurse within his or her facility affect attitudes and beliefs toward research?

THEORETICAL PERSPECTIVE

Rural nursing has been defined as the provision of health care by professional nurses to persons living in sparsely populated areas (Long & Weinert, 1989). Rural nursing is "a special variety of nursing in which the nurse must have a wide range of advanced knowledge and ability, in combination with commitment, to practice proficiently in multiple clinical areas simultaneously along the career trajectory" (Scharff, 1998, p. 37). Rural nursing theory (RNT), a descriptive middle range theory originally published by Long and Weinert, was developed so that researchers would have a framework for describing, explaining, and predicting phenomena within the rural nursing culture (Lee & McDonagh, 2006).

The theory includes three statements regarding (a) a rural person's definition of health, (b) rural health-seeking behaviors, and (c) the lack of anonymity and role diffusion experienced by rural health care providers (see Chapter 1). The third statement was specifically used to guide this study, because it is the role diffusion, coupled with the context in which rural nurses practice, that makes use of evidence so critical to rural practice.

Role diffusion may also contribute to rural nurses' attitudes and beliefs toward EBP. Rural nurses function in many roles, which may include pharmacist, dietician, respiratory therapist, and medical records clerk. Rural nurses often have to make do with what is available (Scharff, 1998), rely on information from colleagues to inform their practice (Ouzts, 2005; Winters et al., 2007), and they may not be as easily influenced by what research or evidence supports or does not support. Exploring rural nurses' attitudes and beliefs about the use of evidence in their practice will provide insight into rural nursing and direction for nursing educators, managers, and health care administrators.

METHODOLOGY

This study was a secondary analysis of data collected to explore rural nurses' access and use of research (Luparell et al., 2006a). A descriptive, cross-sectional survey design was used in the parent study to address the following research questions: To what extent are research findings available to rural nurses? What resources do rural nurses use to obtain research findings? To what extent do rural nurses find research relevant to their practice? How do rural nurses use research findings in their practice? What strategies would improve accessibility of research/information for rural nurses?

Data Collection

Participants were nurses practicing in rural settings in three northwestern states in the United States, selected from mailing lists of all registered nurses (RNs), obtained from the Board of Nursing in each state. The lists were separated into rural and nonrural areas, based on each nurse's county of residence, using the Rural–Urban Commuting Codes developed by the Economic Research Service (ERS) of the United States Department of Agriculture (USDA, 2007). For purposes of the study, counties meeting the criteria for Codes 6 to 9 were considered rural.

From the list of nurses residing in rural counties, 800 were selected at random— 300 names from each of two of the states and 200 names from the third. The cover letter describing the study and the questionnaire were mailed to each of the 800 nurses with a stamped return envelope. Nonresponders were mailed a reminder card 3 weeks after the initial mailing. There were 263 surveys returned, representing a 35.3% return rate. Overall response rates were similar for the three states. After the removal of respondents who declined to participate in the survey, provided incomplete zip code information, or lived in rural areas but commuted to urban facilities for work, 224 surveys were available for analysis.

Instrument

The questionnaire was a 9-page, 42-question survey adapted from surveys created by other researchers (Estabrooks, 1996; Funk, Tornquist, & Champagne, 1995; McKenna, Ashton, & Keeney, 2004) and modified for an American sample, based on a pilot study of 52 nurses conducted in one of the study states (Winters et al., 2006). The final survey contained questions to assess six areas of interest: (a) availability of resources, (b) sources of information, (c) access and use of the Internet, (d) use of research findings, (e) attitudes toward research-based practice, and (f) demographics. Some questions were structured to require a yes or no response, while answers to other questions were provided using a 5-point Likert-type scale (strongly agree, agree, unsure, disagree, and strongly disagree). Respondents were also given the opportunity to provide comments contributing to qualitative data. Reliability of individual items ranged from a Cronbach's alpha of 0.643 to 0.863. To decrease any potential confusion, the study tool defined "research utilization" as the use of any kind of research finding, in any kind of way, in any aspect of work as a health care practitioner. Data for the study reported here included demographic information and responses to questions related to attitudes and beliefs (see Table 18.1).

TABLE 18.1 Research Questions and Related Questionnaire Items

Research Questions	Parent Questionnaire Items
1. Do rural nurses find research easy to understand?	Q22 a, b & c. a. I feel confident in my ability to evaluate the quality of research papers. b. I find that research articles are not easily understood. c. I believe that I should take a course to help me understand research effectively.
2. Do rural nurses believe the results of the research that they read?	Q22 d & e. d. I believe the results of the research that I read. e. I would feel more confident if there was an individual experienced in research to supply me with relevant information.
3. Does number of years experience as a nurse affect rural nurses' attitudes and beliefs about research?	Q38: Total years of practice as a nurse? Q39 Total years of practice in a rural setting?
4. Does level of education influence rural nurses attitudes and beliefs toward research?	Q27 What is your basic nursing education? Q28 Year of graduation from basic nursing program. Q29 What is your highest educational achievement? Q30 Year of graduation from highest degree program.
5. Does the size of facility that a rural nurse works in affect attitudes and beliefs toward research?	Q35 What is your current, or most recent, practice setting? Q36 If applicable, number of beds in your facility.
6. Does the role of a rural nurse within their facility affect attitudes and beliefs toward research?	Q37 What is your primary position?

Source: Luparell et al. (2006b).

Data Analysis

Data were displayed using the Statistical Package for Social Sciences (SPSS, version 16, Graduate Pack) and were analyzed using descriptive statistics to determine item frequencies and measures of central tendency. Comparisons among naturally occurring groups were conducted to further explore the data. Tables and graphs were designed to visually aid in the interpretation of the survey results.

RESULTS

Sample

The majority of the 224 respondents were female (92.3%; $n = 203$), 41 to 60 years of age (62.7%; $n = 136$; $m = 50.5$), employed in health care (94.1%; $n = 207$), and worked full time (65.5%; $n = 135$). The most common place of employment was a hospital (46.4%; $n = 84$) and the most common position was that of a staff nurse (55.6%; $n = 105$). Most described their highest educational achievement as the baccalaureate degree (48.2%; $n = 105$). Sample demographics are shown in Table 18.2.

Do Rural Nurses Find Research Easy to Understand?

In response to the question, "I feel confident in my ability to evaluate the quality of research papers," the sample was divided into two nearly equal groups. In all, 48% of the nurses ($n = 108$) agreed/strongly agreed with this statement. However, just slightly more (49.4%; $n = 110$) either disagreed or were unsure of their ability to evaluate quality.

To the question, "I find that research articles are not easily understood," the sample was similarly divided. Almost one-half (49.1%; $n = 110$) of the nurses agreed/strongly agreed with the statement, and nearly an equal number disagreed/strongly disagreed or were unsure (48.6%; $n = 109$).

The participants were divided into three groups when it came to responding to the statement, "I believe that I should take a course to help me use research effectively." Just over one-third of the nurses agreed/strongly agreed with the statement, one-third disagreed/strongly disagreed, and 27.7% ($n = 62$) were unsure.

A majority of the nurses (63%; $n = 114$) indicated they would feel more confident if an individual experienced in research provided them with relevant practice information. Surprisingly, most of the nurses (58.0%; $n = 130$) were unsure if they "believed the results of the research that they read," and 12.9% ($n = 29$) reported they did not believe; only one-quarter (25.0%; $n = 56$) reported they believed the research they read.

TABLE 18.2 Sample Demographics

Category	Response	Number of Cases	% of Total Sample
Gender (n = 220)*	Female	203	92.3
	Male	17	7.7
Age (n = 217; m = 50.5 years)*	<30	17	7.8
	31–40	43	19.8
	41–50	71	32.7
	51–60	65	30.0
	>60	21	9.7
Level of Highest Educational Preparation (n = 224)	Diploma	21	9.6
	Associate degree	66	30.3
	Baccalaureate degree	105	48.2
	Master's degree	26	11.9
Employment Setting (n = 181)*	Hospital	84	46.4
	Critical access hospital	33	18.2
	Private practice	4	2.2
	Community/Public health	20	11.0
	Home health	8	4.4
	School of nursing	2	1.1
	Health clinic	14	7.7
	Nursing home	16	8.8
Primary Position (n = 189)*	Staff nurse	105	55.6
	Charge nurse	34	18.0
	Clinical nurse specialist	3	1.6
	Nurse practitioner	11	5.8
	Nurse midwife	3	1.6
	Manager	23	12.2
	Administration	5	2.6
	Education	5	2.6

*n does not equal 224 because some respondents did not answer this question.
m = mean.

Do Number of Years of Experience as a Nurse, Type of Role, or Size of Facility Affect Rural Nurses' Attitudes and Beliefs About Research?

To assess the influence of years of experience, type of role, and size of facility on rural nurses' overall attitudes toward research, it was necessary to generate composite scores for nurses' attitudes and then divide the scores into quartiles. The following labels were applied to the quartiles: (a) worst attitudes, for scores in the first quartile, (b) below average attitudes, for scores in the second quartile, (c) above average attitudes, for scores in the third quartile, and (d) best attitudes, for scores in the fourth quartile. The new composite attitude score was then analyzed, using the independent variables of total years of practice as a nurse, total years of practice in a rural setting, type of role, and size of facility.

Years of Experience

The largest portion of nurses with 1 to 5 years of experience (50%; $n = 6$) and 5 to 10 years of experience (35.5%; $n = 11$) were in the "above average" attitude group, while the largest portion of nurses with 10 to 20 years of experience (35.1%; $n = 27$) and more than 20 years of experience 29.1%; $n = 30$) were in the "best" attitude group (see Table 18.3). It is interesting to note that the second-largest segment of nurses with greater than 20 years of experience (28.2%; $n = 29$) were in the "worst" attitude group. Similar results were obtained when reviewing the data for "years of experience as a nurse in a rural setting," with one exception. Rural nurses with greater than 20 years of experience were equally divided between the "worst attitude" and the "best attitude" groups (28.2%, 29.1%, respectively; $n = 18$ in each group).

TABLE 18.3 Attitudes of Tenure Cohorts Towards Evidence-Based Practice

Attitude	Missing ($n = 1$) (%)	1 to 5 years ($n = 12$) (%)	5 to 10 years ($n = 31$) (%)	10 to 20 years ($n = 77$) (%)	More than 20 years ($n = 103$) (%)	Total ($n = 224$) (%)
Worst	100.0	0.0	22.6	19.5	28.2	23.2
Below average	0.0	25.0	22.6	23.4	23.3	23.2
Above average	0.0	50.0	35.5	22.1	19.4	24.1
Best	0.0	25.0	19.4	35.1	29.1	29.5
Total	100.0	100.0	100.0	100.0	100.0	100.0

Role

When assessing the influence of role on rural nurses' overall attitudes toward research (see Table 18.4), the largest percent of nurses in the "best" attitude group were nurse practitioners (55.0%; $n = 6$), while the greatest number in this group were staff nurses (32.0%; $n = 23$). Of the nurses falling into the "worst" attitude group, the largest percent were hospital charge nurses (38.0%; $n = 13$). The greatest number in this group were staff nurses (22.0%; $n = 23$).

Practice Setting

Similarly, the largest percent of nurses whose primary practice setting was public/community health fell into the "best" attitude group (50%; $n = 10$) and the greatest number worked in hospitals (36.9%; $n = 31$). Interestingly, the largest segment of nurses in the "worst" attitude group were also hospital based (27.4%; $n = 23$). The majority of nurses practicing in critical access hospitals (CAH) fell into the "below average" attitude group.

Does Level of Education Influence Rural Attitudes and Beliefs Toward Research?

To assess the influence of level of education on rural nurses' overall attitudes toward research, the previously described composite attitude scores were cross-tabulated with the level of education variable (see Table 18.5). The largest portion of nurses with a diploma were in the "below average" attitude group (33.3%; $n = 7$). Nurses with an associate's degree were evenly divided between the "worst" attitude group and the "best" attitude group (30.3%; $n = 20$ in each group). The largest portion of nurses with a baccalaureate degree were in the "below average" attitude group (29.5%; $n = 31$), and the largest segment of nurses with a master's degree were in the "best" attitude group (38.5%; $n = 10$).

DISCUSSION

Nearly one-half of the respondents agreed with the statement "I feel confident in my ability to evaluate the quality of research papers"; yet almost one-half reported that ". . . research articles are not easily understood." Of equal concern was the finding that nearly 71% of the participants either disbelieved or were unsure if they believed research findings. This doubt in the veracity of research findings may relate to the clarity and writing level of the research reports. It may also indicate a lack of research related to rural patients or rural nursing practice (Olade, 2004), making interpretation and application of findings difficult. If research articles are not written

TABLE 18.4 Attitudes and Role

	Staff Nurse (n = 105) (%)	Charge Nurse (n = 34) (%)	Clinical Nurse Specialist (n = 3) (%)	Nurse Practitioner (n = 11) (%)	Nurse Midwife (n = 3) (%)	Manager/ Supervisor (n = 23) (%)	Administrator Executive (n = 5) (%)	Educator/ Instructor (n = 5) (%)	Total (n = 189)* (%)
Worst	22	38	0	18	0	22	20	0	23
Below average	17	32	67	18	0	22	20	40	22
Above average	29	15	0	9	100	22	20	60	25
Best	32	15	33	55	0	35	40	0	30
Total	100	100	100	100	100	100	100	100	100

*n does not equal 224 because some respondents did not answer this question.

TABLE 18.5 Attitudes and Education

Attitudes	Diploma (n = 21) (%)	Associate Degree (n = 66) (%)	Baccalaureate Degree (n = 105) (%)	Master's Degree (n = 26) (%)	Total (n = 218)* (%)
Worst	19.0	30.3	19.0	15.4	22.0
Below average	33.3	12.1	29.5	19.2	23.4
Above average	19.0	27.3	23.8	26.9	24.8
Best	28.6	30.3	27.6	38.5	29.8
Total	100.0	100.0	100.0	100.0	100.0

*n does not equal 224 because some respondents did not answer this question.

clearly, are written above a staff nurse's level of understanding, or are on unfamiliar topics, rural nurses may find the research difficult to evaluate and therefore question their ability to believe the findings. Information literacy is the ability to (a) decide that information is needed about a subject, (b) access credible and understandable information about the subject, and (c) use the information to effectively solve a problem or make a decision (Tanner, Pierce, & Pravikoff, 2004). The lack of access to credible and understandable information is an important barrier to research utilization (Tanner et al., 2004). It is also apparent from the available literature that nurses who believe that EBP can and will enhance their practice are more likely to utilize research and incorporate it into practice than are nurses whose attitudes and beliefs about EBP are negative (Rizzuto et al., 1994). Encouraging researchers and publishers to provide research reports that are easily interpreted and are available in widely circulated practice-oriented journals may aid rural nurses' access and understanding of reports.

Positive attitudes toward research have been found to directly relate to educational levels and participation in research (Smirnoff et al., 2007). A logical implication is to design baccalaureate level research courses that focus on skills needed to access, read, interpret, and evaluate research, and include the opportunity to participate in research. However, in this study, there were nearly equal numbers of nurses who believed as disbelieved that a course could help them use research effectively. This finding may be explained by the fact that more than one-half (60.1%) of participants had at least a baccalaureate degree. Baccalaureate-prepared nurses were likely to have at least one course in research included in their curriculum. The baccalaureate-prepared nurses who believed a course would be useful may value continuing education (CE) more than the associate degree nurses or diploma-prepared nurses (Goode et al., 2001). The baccalaureate-prepared nurses who answered that they were unsure about taking a research course to help them use research effectively may have answered that way because their education was long enough ago that research was not included in their curriculum; the research course(s) taken was not adequate in helping them understand research effectively; or they believed the course was sufficient and questioned the need for further instruction. Additional research is needed to explore the relationship between completion of a research course, course design, and nurses' ability to use research findings effectively.

Most respondents indicated that they would like a research-experienced person to provide them with information. In all, 114 respondents (51%) agreed with this statement and 27 (12%) strongly agreed. Olade (2003) reported that only 20% of the nurses she surveyed considered themselves adequate in regard to research, and several investigators (Kosteniuk, D'Arcy, Stewart, & Smith, 2006; Olade, 2003; Pravikoff et al., 2005; Winters et al., 2007) reported that respondents identified nursing colleagues as the information source most used, even though professional isolation and distance can affect rural nurses' access to research knowledgeable colleagues.

Connecting rural nurses with knowledgeable research experts could be accomplished using the Internet; however, nurses who practice in rural settings are more likely to have less access to information technology than their urban counterparts (Bushy, 2002; Winters et al., 2007). Rural nurses have indicated that their computer and Internet availability is limited because of computer location, lack of overall general computer knowledge (Winters et al., 2007), and limited time to search for information (Olade, 2003; Winters et al., 2007). Lack of time may also result from the variety of roles fulfilled by rural nurses during a typical work shift.

Isolation and distance are barriers that are a constant factor in rural nursing (Long & Weinert, 1989), so asking a coworker for his or her opinion on how to perform a task may be the most efficient way to complete the task. Role modeling the use of evidence by nursing leaders has been shown to influence rural nurses' use of research (Winters et al., 2007). Hospital administrators and nursing leaders in rural and remote facilities must become proactive in encouraging the use of evidence, perhaps through practice policies and procedures, affiliation with larger institutions or universities, and assignment of research mentors or collaborators, and by making access to evidence readily available to nursing staff through professional journal subscriptions, journal clubs, and accessible technology resources.

Nurses with differing levels of experience and education were included in the study reported here. In assessing attitudes and beliefs about research based on years of *rural nursing experience*, the nurses with the "worst" attitudes in this group were the nurses with more than 20 years of experience. The "worst" attitude finding may have resulted from research not being a part of their nursing curricula or part of the culture of rural nursing. It may also reflect lack of research applicable to rural nursing, the nurses' difficulty understanding research reports, and their preference for receiving information from peers rather than from reading the literature. The "best" attitudes were found in the nurses with 1 to 5 years of experience, which may reflect their exposure to research content in their nursing programs. Further study is needed to understand the relationship between years of experience and attitudes toward research.

When measuring attitudes and beliefs, those nurses with diploma, associate, and baccalaureate degrees were found to have similar attitudes (the "worst") and nurses who were master's prepared had the "best" attitudes. This may be due to the fact that most diploma and associate degree programs have little or no research education included in their curriculum, and, although baccalaureate level programs do require at least one research course, it may not be enough for a nurse to develop an appreciation of the importance of research or to learn the skills required to understand and incorporate research into practice.

The results of this study suggest that nurses working in the direct patient care roles, such as staff nurse or charge nurse, had the "worst" attitudes about research, and those nurses whose roles were more autonomous, such as that of nurse practitioner, public health nurse, manager/supervisor, or executive, had the "best" attitudes. Perhaps nurses working in these latter roles have more access to technology, professional journals, and more time to utilize such resources. Providing access to research and a culture of expectation that practice is based on evidence is needed to move from a practice based on tradition to a one based on evolving facts. More research is needed to explore nursing roles and attributes such as autonomy and control as they relate to attitudes and beliefs about research.

Study Limitations

The statistics used for this study were descriptive. The sample size used for this secondary data analysis and the cohorts based on education, practice location, and years of experience are small, perhaps limited by the use of only one reminder to nurses complete the survey. Therefore, caution is required when drawing conclusions or generalizing the findings to all rural nurses. Because this was a secondary data analysis, no further information was obtained from participants and there was no control over the sample or how the original data were collected. More information could be gleaned from studying additional groups and cohorts. The nurses included in this study were persons living in the western United States, with the preponderance residing in Montana.

This geographical location could have influenced the results because of differing socioeconomic issues, cultural differences, and varying distances to larger cities.

CONCLUSIONS

The results of this study support the findings from others (Bushy, 2002; Kosteniuk et al., 2006; Olade, 2003), who reported that access to technology, education, and roles are factors that affect rural nurses' attitudes and beliefs toward EBP. Further research is needed to explore the role that baccalaureate education plays in determining rural nurses' attitudes and beliefs toward EBP, specifically the type and number of research courses needed in a nursing curriculum in order for a nurse to be able to properly assess and critique research information. The results also suggest that although nearly one-half of the nurses felt confident in their ability to evaluate the quality of research papers, a nearly equal number did not find research articles easy to understand and were unsure that they believed the results of the research that they read. Based on these findings, it is important for nursing educators teaching in universities and CE courses alike to include more education with respect to how to assess data for credibility and how to interpret research information.

Findings from this study support the need for research that examines the effects of length of rural and nonrural experiences and nursing position (i.e., staff nurse and charge nurse) on attitudes toward EBP. Findings from such studies will improve our understanding of rural nursing practice.

Furthermore, the results of this study support the relationship between master's education and attitudes and beliefs about EBP. These findings are in line with recommendations from the Joint Commission on Accreditation of Healthcare Organizations (JCAHO) (Elements of Performance NR.2.10.B) for CAHs and other hospitals that educational factors be considered when appointing the nurse executive (JCAHO, 2006). Requiring nurse executives to hold a master's or another postgraduate degree may significantly impact rural nurses' attitudes and beliefs about research and increase the amount of practice that is evidence based.

Nurses working in environments with a more positive culture, strong leadership, and lower rates of patient and staff adverse events report significantly more research utilization than nurses working in less positive environments (Estabrooks, Midodzi, Cummings, & Wallin, 2007). Given that nurses constitute the largest group of health care providers and their care influences patient outcomes (Aiken et al., 2003), the pressure on the nursing profession to strengthen the importance of EBP for all RNs is crucial.

REFERENCES

Aiken, L. H., Clarke, S. P., Cheung, R. B., Sloane, D. M., & Silber, J. H. (2003). Education levels of hospital nurses and surgical patient mortality. *The Journal of the American Medical Association, 290*(12), 1617–1623.

American Nurses Association (ANA). (2004) *Scope and standards for nurse administrators* (2nd ed.). Washington, DC: nursesbooks.org

American Nurses Credentialing Center (ANCC). (2005). *Magnet recognition program for recognizing excellence in nursing services: Application manual.* Washington, DC: Author.

Bushy, A. (2002). International perspectives on rural nursing: Australia, Canada, U.S.A. *Australian Journal of Rural Health, 10*, 104–111.

Case, B. (2004, April 1). *Evidence-based practice: The future of nursing.* rn.com. Retrieved September 2, 2007, from http://www.rn.com

Estabrooks, C. A. (1996). *Research utilization in nursing: Factors influencing the utilization and non-utilization of research by nurses.* Edmonton, AB: University of Alberta.

Estabrooks, C. A., Midodzi, W. K., Cummings, G. G., & Wallin, L. (2007). Predicting research use in nursing organizations: A multilevel analysis. *Nursing Research, 56*(4, Suppl. 1), S7.

Funk, S. G., Champagne, M. T., Wiese, R. A., & Tornquist, E. M. (1991). Barriers to using research findings in practice: The clinician's perspective. *Applied Nursing Research, 4*(2), 90–95.

Funk, S. G., Tornquist, E. M., & Champagne, M. T. (1995). Research utilization: Reconnecting research and practice. *AACN Clinical Issues, 6*, 105–109.

Goode, C. J., Pinkerton, S., McCausland, M. P., Southard, P., Graham, R., & Krsek, C. (2001). Documenting chief nursing officers' preference for BSN-prepared nurses. *Journal of Nursing Administration, 3*(2), 55–59.

Hommelstad, J., & Cornelia, R. (2004). Norwegian nurses' perceived barriers and facilitators to research use. *AORN Journal, 79*(3), 621–634.

Joint Commission on Accreditation of Healthcare Organizations (JCAHO). (2006, November). *Joint Commission Perspectives, 26*(11), 10–11.

Joint Commission (JC). (2008). *Accreditation programs: Hospital national patient safety goals.* Retrieved March 1, 2009, from http://www.jointcommission.org/PatientSafety/ NationalPatientSafetyGoals/09_hap_npsgs.htm

Kosteniuk, J. G., D'Arcy, C., Stewart, N., & Smith, B. (2006). Central and peripheral information source use among rural and remote registered nurses. *Journal of Advanced Nursing, 55*(1), 100–113.

Lee, H. J., & McDonagh, M. K. (2006). Examining the rural nursing theory base. In H. J. Lee & C. A. Winters (Eds.) *Rural nursing concepts, theory, and practice* (2nd ed., pp. 17–26). New York, NY: Springer Publishing.

Long, K. A., & Weinert, C. (1989). Rural nursing: Developing the theory base. *Scholarly inquiry for nursing practice: An international journal, 3*, 113–127. New York, NY: Springer Publishing.

Luparell, S., Winters, C., Lee, H., O'Lynn, C., Shreffler-Grant, J., & Hendrickx, L. (2006a). [Rural nurses' access to and use of research in practice]. Unpublished raw data.

Luparell, S., Winters, C., Lee, H., O'Lynn, C., Shreffler-Grant, J., & Hendrickx, L. (2006b). [Rural nurses' access to and use of research in practice (pp. 1–9) Questionnaire].

McKenna, H., Ashton, S., & Keeney, S. (2004). Barriers to evidence-based practice in nursing and healthcare. *Journal of Advanced Nursing, 45*(2), 178–189.

Melnyk, B. M., Fineout-Overholt, E., Feinstein, N. F., Li, H., Small, L., Wilcox, L. et al. (2004). Nurses' perceived knowledge, beliefs, skills, and needs in regarding evidence-based practice: Implications for accelerating the paradigm shifts. *World-views on Evidence-Based Nursing, 1*(3), 185–193.

Melnyk, B. M., Fineout-Overholt, E., Feinstein, N. F., Sadler, L. S., & Green-Hernandez, C. (2008). Nurse practitioner educators' perceived knowledge, beliefs, and teaching strategies regarding evidence-based practice: Implications for accelerating the integration of evidence-based practice into graduate programs. *Journal of Professional Nursing, 1*, 7–13.

Merriam-Webster. (2007). *Merriam-Webster medical dictionary*. New York, NY: Merriam-Webster.

Morrison, E. (1998). Erroneous beliefs about research held by staff nurses. *Journal of Continuing Education in Nursing, 29*(5), 196–203. Abstract retrieved July 29, 2007, from http://eric.ed.gov/ERICWebPortal/cU.S. tom/portlets/recordDetails/detailmini. jsp?_nfpb=true

Munroe, D., Duffy, P., & Fisher, C. (2006). Fostering evidence-based practice in a rural community hospital. *Journal of Nursing Administration, 36*(11), 510–512.

Olade, R. A. (2003). Attitudes and factors affecting research utilization. *Nursing Forum, 38*(4), 6–15.

Olade, R. A. (2004). Evidence-based practice and research utilization activities among rural nurses. *Clinical Scholarship, 36*(3), 220–225.

Ouzts, K. (2005). Evidence-based practice and information literacy skills in rural nurses [Abstract]. *Communicating Nursing Research, 38*(13), 287.

Parsons, J. E., Merlin, T. L., Taylor, J. E., Wilkinson, D., & Hiller, J. E. (2003). Evidence-based practice in rural and remote clinical practice: Where is the evidence? *Australian Journal of Rural Health, 11*(5), 242–248.

Pravikoff, D. S., Tanner, A. B., & Pierce, S. T. (2005). Readiness of U.S. nurses for evidence-based practice. *American Journal of Nursing, 105*(9), 40–51.

Rawnsley, M. M. (2003). Dimensions of scholarship and the advancement of nursing science: Articulating a vision. *Nursing Science Quarterly, 16*(1), 6–15.

Rizzuto, C., Bostrom, J., Suter, W. N., & Chenitz, W. C. (1994). Predictors of nurses' involvement in research activities. *Western Journal of Nursing Research, 16*(2), 193–204.

Scharff, J. E. (1998). The distinctive nature and scope of rural nursing practice: Philosophical bases. In H. J. Lee (Ed.), *Conceptual basis for rural nursing* (pp. 19–38). New York, NY: Springer Publishing.

Smirnoff, M., Ramirez, M., Kooplimae, L., Gibney, M., & McEvoy, M. (2007). Nurses' attitudes toward nursing research at a metropolitan medical center. *Applied Nursing Research, 20*(1), 24–31.

Tanner, A., Pierce, S., & Pravikoff, D. (2004). *Readiness for evidence-based practice: Information literacy needs of nurses in the United States.* MEDINFO 2004, 936–940. Retrieved August 24, 2008, from http://www.cmbi.bjmu.edu.cn/news/report/2004/; medinfo2004/pdffiles/papers/4770Tanner.pdf

Taylor, J., Wilkinson, D., & Blue, I. (2001). Towards evidence-based general practice in rural and remote Australia: An overview of key issues and a model for practice. *Rural and Remote Health, 1*(106). Retrieved October 21, 2007, from http://rrh.deakin.edu.au

United States Department of Agriculture (USDA) Economic Research Service. (2007). *Measuring rurality: Rural urban continuum codes.* Retrieved September 3, 2007, from http://www.ers.usda.gov/Briefing/Rurality/RuralUrbCon/

Winters, C. A., Lee, H. J., Besel, J., Strand, A., Echeverri, R., Jorgensen, K. P. et al. (2007). Access to and use of research by rural nurses. *Rural and Remote Health, 7*, 758. Retrieved August 24, 2008, from http://www.rrh.org.au

Winters, C. A., Lee, H. J., O'Lynn, C., Schreffler-Grant, M. J., Edge, D., McDonagh, M. et al. (2006). [Health research: Accessible, applicable and useable for rural & remote health practitioners.] Unpublished raw data.

Chapter 19

THE USE OF RURAL HOSPITALS FOR CLINICAL PLACEMENTS IN NURSING EDUCATION

Lori Hendrickx, Heidi Mennenga, and Laurie Johansen

PREDICTIONS THAT THE CURRENT NURSING shortage will continue and most likely will intensify as the demand for nurses grows have resulted in a variety of recommendations for strategies to reduce the shortage and meet the demands for additional nurses. In 2012, the U.S. Bureau of Labor Statistics reported that health care had the largest monthly increase in new job growth of any employment sector and has predicted that the size of the registered nurse workforce would need to increase by 26% by 2020 (U.S. Bureau of Labor Statistics, 2012). The need for additional nurses and these types of shortage predictions have been reported by several authors and organizations (American Association of Colleges of Nursing [AACN], 2011). Media exposure regarding the nursing shortage has increased the national awareness of the nursing shortage and has resulted in increased numbers of applicants to nursing education programs.

Despite the increased numbers of nursing school applicants, the increase has not been sufficient to meet the increased demand for registered nurses. In many cases, nursing school applicants are turned away due to shortage of faculty, inadequate numbers of clinical sites, or financial constraints. In 2009, AACN reported in the *Annual State of the Schools* that 54,991 qualified applicants were not accepted at 4-year colleges and universities (AACN, 2009), in part due to a shortage of clinical sites. Insufficient numbers of clinical sites is an issue faced by many nursing programs that primarily educate students in more urban hospital settings. These institutions often have multiple nursing programs competing for clinical time, resulting in the inability to admit more students and add additional clinical groups to facilities already saturated with students.

Opportunities for Rural Hospitals

In an effort to respond to the nursing shortage, marketing strategies have resulted in substantial increases in the numbers of entering college freshmen declaring nursing as a major. In the last 10 years, South Dakota State University (SDSU) has responded in a variety of ways to the increased demand for nursing graduates—by increasing the numbers of students accepted from 48 to 64 per semester on one campus, admitting additional students twice a year rather than once a year on another campus, adding an accelerated program with 40 students per year, and adding an additional standard program campus with 40 students per year. These changes resulted in an increase in the number of students accepted yearly from 128 to 304. Despite the large increase in students accepted, in 2011, only one-third of the qualified students applying to the South Dakota State University College of Nursing's main campus were accepted on their first application (Hendrickx, 2011). Additional expansion of the nursing program has not occurred, in part due to the lack of additional clinical placement sites.

The majority of nursing students at SDSU have traditionally received their clinical education at larger hospitals in a major city, competing with seven other nursing programs for clinical placement. Clinical experiences needed to be expanded to include evenings and weekends, and changes in the college calendar were made so that some groups could complete clinical rotations in the summer or early in January before other programs were in session. While these adjustments did result in increased availability of clinical experiences for students, another possible solution was to explore clinical opportunities in smaller, more rural health care facilities.

Implementation

SDSU has five semesters in the nursing program, with clinical experiences scheduled in all five semesters. The first semester clinical experience is in a general medical–surgical setting, with emphasis on basic nursing cares and physical assessment skills. Several years ago, the first-semester coordinator met with nursing directors in two rural hospitals to explore the possibility of placing these beginning students in their facilities for clinical. At the time, there were no other nursing programs doing clinical in these hospitals. Agreements were reached with the two rural facilities and a year-long pilot program was completed.

Nursing instructors from SDSU accompanied the students as clinical faculty for the expansion into the rural hospitals. Clinical group size was limited to eight students for one clinical instructor. After a successful implementation of the pilot program, the use of rural hospitals was expanded as the nursing program increased in size.

There were a number of considerations in the selection of appropriate rural clinical sites. The proximity to campus was considered, and all sites were within an hour's drive. The main campus of SDSU is located near the Minnesota border, so hospitals in both South Dakota and Minnesota were considered. Transportation was provided for the faculty member and the students through the campus motor pool fleet.

The size of the facility and average daily census needed to be adequate to accommodate eight students. This did not necessarily mean that there needed to be eight patients in the inpatient setting, just that there were learning opportunities for eight students. Students were usually assigned patients in the inpatient area first, and then other learning opportunities were identified. All the hospitals had active outpatient departments where students could help admit a patient for an outpatient procedure, follow the patient through the procedure, and then provide postprocedural care. Students also rotated through dialysis units and cardiac rehabilitation, and accompanied nurses on home health visits. Some of the hospitals have long-term care facilities attached, so students were rotated through the long-term care setting as well as the hospital setting.

As the number of clinical groups increased, the need for additional clinical instructors also increased. Clinical instructors were selected from the existing faculty first. Administrators in the rural hospitals were concerned that the instructor be familiar with their facility, so, initially, faculty members who had previously worked in one of the rural hospitals were approached. As additional instructors were needed, further discussion revealed that two rural hospitals had staff nurses in the educator track of SDSU's graduate program. These graduate students were then added as clinical instructors in the hospitals where they had worked as staff nurses. One additional method for recruitment of clinical instructors has semester 1 faculty members serving as preceptors for graduate students in the educator track. The graduate student spends one semester in the rural hospital setting doing clinical with a current faculty member. After graduation, these students are more comfortable doing clinical in one of the rural sites. Currently, all six rural hospitals being used for clinical have instructors who were previously employed by the hospital or assisted with clinical in a rural hospital during graduate school. This strategy has resulted in increased trust between the college and the hospital and has eased the transition for the clinical instructor and the nursing staff. Since hospitals in two states are being used, having clinical instructors who had practiced in the hospitals resulted in the instructors already holding licensure in their respective states.

Ongoing communication between the hospital and the college is maintained through two primary methods. The clinical instructor remains the primary resource for the hospital staff regarding changes in the curriculum, learning needs of the students, and responsibilities of the nursing staff in the education of the students. The semester coordinator makes yearly site visits to each site to stay in touch with the clinical instructors and the administrators at the clinical site. The semester coordinator can address any needs of the hospital staff that arise, in addition to serving as a mentor for the clinical instructors. This onsite interaction has been identified as crucial by the nursing administrators at the clinical sites.

An additional consideration was the selection of the day of the week to hold clinical. Since rural hospitals often have surgeons or specialists who are on site certain days of the week, it was found to be beneficial to hold clinical experiences on those days as much as possible. For example, patient census was often found to be higher on the day the surgeon had procedures scheduled, but typically by Friday some hospitals had discharged most of their patients.

Evaluation

Evaluation of the clinical experiences was done informally through communication among the clinical instructor, students, and semester coordinator each semester and formally through interviews with the nurse managers. Clinical instructors met with the semester coordinator to provide feedback into the type of learning experiences available, and appropriate adjustments were made. Face-to-face interviews were done with the nursing managers from the six clinical sites to determine the effectiveness of each rural hospital as a clinical site. The managers were asked to identify the benefits and challenges associated with having nursing students in their rural health care facility.

Benefits

The use of rural facilities for clinical experiences results in many benefits not only for students but also for clinical instructors, patients, staff, and administrators. The managers reported that since rural facilities often have all patients located on a single floor regardless of diagnosis, students have easy access to patients of all ages with many different health problems. A variety of experiences and exposure to other departments also await the student in a rural facility. In a single clinical day, students may be able to observe dialysis, participate in outpatient procedures, be in or other departments, in addition to caring for their primary patient. Additionally, since rural facilities do not typically have intravenous (IV) teams or lift teams, students are often able to perform these types of tasks and participate more in direct patient care.

Respondents indicated that the variety of diagnoses and experiences in one area also presents the clinical instructor with a more diverse teaching opportunity. For example, if one student is caring for a patient with pneumonia and who has crackles in the lungs, the instructor may have all the students listen to the patient's lung sounds, while another student may have a surgical patient where wound care can be completed. The clinical instructor may also choose to review the pathophysiology of the different diagnoses that students were exposed to during a single clinical day at a clinical postconference. The variety of experiences offered by a rural facility allows the clinical instructor to review a range of diagnoses and may improve student understanding of various illnesses. Nurse managers indicated that students also benefit from an increased understanding of the role of the nurse generalist and the level of autonomy that is prevalent in rural hospitals.

Students and clinical instructors are not the only benefactors of the use of rural facilities for nursing education. Respondents indicated that patients also benefit from having students in the rural facility. Since rural facilities are often underused for nursing education, patients often comment on how much they enjoy the one-on-one attention they gain from having a student care for them.

The nurse managers stated that nursing staff are also given the opportunity to mentor students, provide leadership, and share experiences. The presence of students in the clinical setting may also prompt nurses to increase their standard of care as they strive to model evidence-based practices. One nurse manager commented that her nurses "really have to be on their toes and think about what they are doing" when working with students. She commented further that nurses in a rural facility do not get much exposure to nursing students and faculty and that this is an excellent learning opportunity for the staff as well as the students.

Additionally, results indicated that administrators can use the students' exposure to rural facilities as a recruitment tool. Students often do not consider employment after graduation in a smaller facility, especially if they have never been exposed to the rural environment throughout their education. However, once exposed to the challenges and variety offered by a rural setting, students may seek employment opportunities after graduation. One respondent stated that the last three nurses hired had all been students at that rural facility during a clinical experience.

Challenges

With all the benefits that correspond to the use of rural hospitals for clinical sites, there are also challenges to overcome. As noted by Newhouse (2005), smaller patient bases, along with a variety of acuity levels, are usually experienced in rural hospital clinical sites. This can result in the rise and fall of patient census. Our interviews with nurse managers paralleled this challenge of a fluctuating census. Patient census was reported to vary from negligible to maximum census while accommodating nursing students. Utilization of a variety of nursing departments does allow facilities the capability of accommodating nursing students while experiencing a fluctuating census, in order to meet student and patient needs.

Electronic health records (EHR), as well as other technologic advances, present barriers to student opportunities as well at rural clinical sites. Rural nurse managers reported the initiation of EHR in the wake of urban facilities in the area. The rural hospital's desire to create opportunities for nursing students to use this technology during their clinical experiences is generally hindered by the inability to initiate such technology until it is being used at other urban facilities.

Constraints with space also present nurse managers with accommodation barriers for nursing students. Conference rooms, as well as locker rooms, can be modestly available, with the demand for usage extending beyond the capacity of the rural hospitals, even without considering the addition of the nursing students. Providing an environment conducive to learning in a postconference setting can take ingenuity. This ingenuity has led to postconferences being held in break rooms and unused patient rooms if conference rooms are not available.

Nurse managers noted the challenge of maintaining communication among the South Dakota State University college of nursing and the rural hospital. Visits by the semester coordinator have helped display the commitment of the South Dakota State University college of nursing to communication with the staff at rural facilities. Also, a predominant concern noted has been the familiarity of the nurse faculty member with the rural hospital. It was evident that the administration needs to feel comfortable with the level of faculty knowledge about the rural hospital. Respondents reported that utilizing instructors from the facility increased the comfort levels by assuring knowledge of the mission and vision of the facility, current policies and procedures, patient types, and staffing patterns.

Implications for Education

The use of rural hospitals for clinical placement in nursing education is an effective way to provide quality clinical education experiences to beginning nursing students while relieving some of the clinical congestion from saturated urban settings. At SDSU, the use of rural hospitals has been expanded into the second semester for medical–surgical experience and has resulted in 8 to 10 fewer clinical groups in the larger urban area. Expanding clinical education into rural hospitals has enabled the nursing program to provide additional clinical placement sites as the nursing program increases its enrollment.

Providing clinical experiences in the rural setting enables nursing students to see the importance of the generalist role of the rural nurse and to appreciate the rural nurse's greater role diffusion. Nursing students are often surprised at the variety of learning opportunities and patient care situations afforded to them in the rural hospitals. This variety of experiences allows the nursing student to appreciate the role of the rural nurse and the flexibility required to care for such a broad range of patients. Nursing practice in a rural hospital requires a specific skill set and range of knowledge that has been described as broader and involving a higher level of responsibility in comparison to urban settings (Strasser & Neusy, 2010). Several of our students who began their clinical experiences in a rural hospital asked to return to a rural setting in their final semester for their preceptorship experience, citing the variety of experiences as the predominant reason for the request.

Implications for Practice and Research

Involving nursing students in rural hospital clinical experiences provides an opportunity for rural providers to promote their facilities. Rural hospital staff have historically struggled to recruit and retain caregivers, with rural nurse vacancy rates significantly higher than vacancy rates in urban areas (LaSala, 2000; Cramer, Nienaber, Helget, & Agrawal, 2006). While many recruitment strategies have been tried, much of the research in this area suggests that exposure to rural hospitals for clinical placements is a major factor in the recruitment of health care personnel to rural settings and that students often respond positively to their rural health care experiences. Research indicates that there are three primary factors associated with students choosing to practice in rural settings: having a rural background, positive clinical experiences in a rural setting, and targeted training for rural practice (Strasser & Neusy, 2010).

Providing rural clinical experiences for undergraduate nursing students has been promoted as a recruitment strategy for rural hospitals. Neill and Taylor (2002) reported that qualitative evaluation of rural clinical placement indicated a positive student response with increased interest in rural nursing following graduation. Other studies have resulted in recommendations that rural content be included in the curriculum in order to improve recruitment and retention (Devine, 2006; Daniels, VanLiet, Skipper, Sanders, & Rhyne, 2007).

Thrall (2007) identified best practices for recruiting nurses into rural practice, which included establishing links with area colleges to provide clinical education and possibly providing funding assistance for hospital employees to attend nursing school in exchange for working at the hospital for a period of time following graduation. Rural hospitals can also develop nurse residency or internship programs for nursing students. These internship opportunities provide additional experiences in rural hospitals that are competing with urban centers that may have similar programs. In South Dakota, several rural administrators have approached the first semester coordinator at SD Rural Health Association meetings to indicate their interest in providing clinical experiences for SDSU nursing students. While some of these rural facilities are located a significant distance from the main campus, it may be possible to consider an overnight or extended experience where students could be housed locally and minimize travel time.

The rural hospitals used for clinical experiences at SDSU have all reported a positive experience with nursing students completing clinical experiences in their facilities. Clinical instructors have had similar positive experiences. While anecdotal data and clinical evaluations from students indicated a positive response to rural clinical placement, additional research is warranted to describe their perceptions of rural clinical experiences and the preparation these experiences provided for subsequent clinical rotations and eventual nursing practice.

CONCLUSION

Rural hospitals have traditionally not been selected as clinical placement sites for nursing education and are an untapped resource for nursing programs needing additional clinical resources. These facilities can provide a wide variety of opportunities for patient care and can expose the nursing student to the wealth of experiences that rural health care provides. Results from the experiences at SDSU have been positive and should encourage the exploration of rural health care facilities for nursing clinical experiences.

REFERENCES

American Association of Colleges of Nursing. (2009). *Annual state of the schools*. Retrieved June 13, 2012, from http://www.aacn.nche.edu/aacn-publications/annual-reports/AR2011.pdf

American Association of Colleges of Nursing. (2011). *Nursing shortage fact sheet*. Retrieved June 13, 2012, from www.aacn.nche.edu/Media/shortageresource.htm

Cramer, M., Nienaber, J., Helget, P., & Agrawal, S. (2006). Comparative analysis of urban and rural nursing workforce shortages in Nebraska hospitals. *Policy, Politics, & Nursing Practice, 7*(4), 248–260.

Daniels, Z. M., VanLiet, B. J., Skipper, B. J., Sanders, M. L., & Rhyne, R. L. (2007). Factors in recruiting and retaining health professionals for rural practice. *Journal of Rural Health, 23*(1), 62–71.

Devine, S. (2006). Perceptions of occupational therapists practicing in rural Australia: A graduate perspective. *Australian Occupational Health Journal, 53*(3), 205–210.

Hendrickx, L. (2011, May). *Facing a shortage of clinical sites? Rural hospitals can meet your needs*. Paper presented on May 23–24 at the Midwest Healthcare Educators' Academy, Grand Forks, ND.

Neill, J., & Taylor, K. (2002). Undergraduate nursing students' clinical experiences in rural and remote areas: Recruitment and retention. *Australian Journal of Rural Health, 10*(5), 239–243.

Newhouse, R. P. (2005). Exploring nursing issues in rural hospitals. *The Journal of Nursing Administration, 35*(7/8), 350–358.

Strasser, R., & Neusy, A. (2010). Context counts: Training health workers in and for rural and remote areas. *Bulletin of the World Health Organization, 88*(10), 777–782.

Thrall, H. (2007). Best practices for recruiting rural nurses. *Hospitals & Health Networks, 81*(12), 47–50.

U.S. Bureau of Labor Statistics (2012). *Employment projections: Occupations with the largest job growth*. Retrieved June 13, 2012 from www.bls.gov/emp/ep_table_104.htm

Chapter 20

U.S.–MEXICO BORDER: CHALLENGES AND OPPORTUNITIES IN RURAL AND BORDER HEALTH

Eva M. Moya, Guillermina Solis,
Rebeca L. Ramos, Mark W. Lusk,
and Carliene S. Quist

THE U.S.–MEXICO BORDER, "LA FRONTERA"

Borders are geopolitical and historical demarcations that separate peoples in relation to access to health care, which thereby results in wide disparities in health outcomes. Borders serve as semipermeable membranes; they limit the free movement of people, goods, and services, and limit the access to medical treatment. At the same time, diseases migrate without restriction across borders because border communities share the same physical and health environment, and human movement across borders readily permits the transmission of pathogens (Moya, Loza, & Lusk, 2012). In this chapter, we focus on the 2,000-mile U.S.–Mexico border, which Warner (1991) observes is "the bi-national border with the greatest variety in health status, entitlements, and utilization" (p. 242). We identify the health care characteristics of the region, describe the challenges of providing access to health care, and connect the challenges of border health to the goals set out in the U.S. government's document *Healthy People 2020*. We also relate the challenges of border health to the nursing profession and to its interface with other allied health professions, particularly medical social work.

The most commonly cited definition of the U.S.–Mexico border region (*La Frontera*) is spelled out in the La Paz Agreement of 1983: "100 kilometers (62.1 miles) north and south of the international boundary between the United States and Mexico" (U.S.–Mexico Border Health Commission

[USMBHC], 2003, p. 1). This expanse of land includes parts of four American states (California, Arizona, New Mexico, and Texas), 48 counties (half of which are contiguous with the international boundary (U.S.–Mexico Border Counties Coalition [USMBCC], 2006); and 26 U.S. federally recognized Native American tribes. There are 14 pairs of "sister cities," where a great deal of the binational movement occurs, both legal and illegal. The U.S.–Mexico border is the most traveled border in the world (Pan American Health Organization [PAHO], 2007, p. 733) (see Figure 20.1).

BORDER CONTEXT: GEOGRAPHY, DEMOGRAPHY, AND ENVIRONMENTAL REALITIES

Slightly more than half of the 13 million people in the border region live in the United States (PAHO, 2007). Some are permanent residents; others are "borderlanders[1] or *fronterizos and fronterizas*," and some are binational citizens or residents, including those who cross the border daily for work, school, or family visits. Many border residents rarely cross the border. Most Mexican citizens have no legal mechanism that permits them to cross, while many American citizens are afraid to cross into Mexico. Some residents are temporary, such as international migrants who may spend a few days in the border region. Others are "seasonal" migrants, such as Mexicans who work in the United States and American "snowbirds" and tourists who reside in Mexico seasonally or vacation there.

Hispanics (overwhelmingly of Mexican origin) constitute the largest ethnic group in the border region, are the largest minority group in the United States, and are the majority of the population in most of the counties along the U.S.–Mexico border (U.S. Census Bureau, 2011). In addition, the percentage of Hispanics in the U.S.–Mexico border region is increasing due to continuing immigration from Mexico and the high birth rate of border Hispanic residents (Pew Hispanic Center, 2011).

Although the Tijuana-San Ysidro and the El Paso-Ciudad Juárez metropolis are the largest international border communities in the world, most of the borderland is, in fact, rural. Just four of the 48 counties (San Diego, California; El Paso, Texas; McAllen, Texas; Brownsville, Texas) have a population density greater than 91.8 per square mile (National Rural Health Association [NRHA], 2010). Few of these rural counties, although confronted with a host of environmental problems including air, water, and human contamination from agriculture (PAHO, 2007), have public health departments, rendering them completely dependent on state health department resources for basic public health services (NRHA, 2010).

In addition, a significant border phenomenon known as *colonias* juxtaposes rural realities on the outskirts of metropolitan areas. There are approximately 2,500 *colonias* along the border (Núñez, 2012; Esparza & Donelson, 2010). They are nonincorporated communities located at the

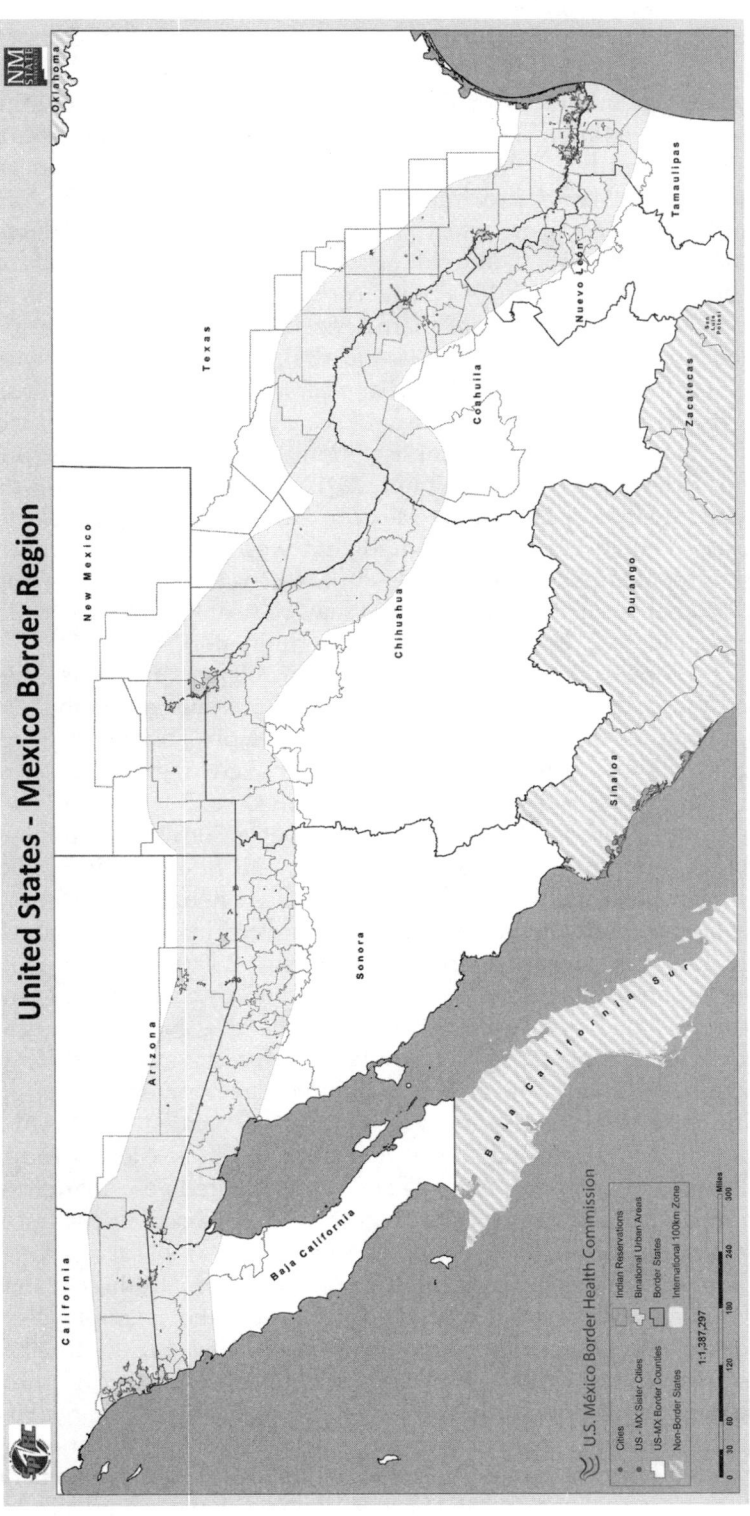

FIGURE 20.1 U.S.-Mexico Border Map. Reprinted from www.borderhealth.org by the United States–Mexico Border Health Commission in cooperation with the Department of Geography Spatial Applications Research Center (SpARC) of the New Mexico State University by permission of United States–Mexico Border Health Commission.

periphery of larger urban centers throughout the border region, providing temporary and permanent housing for residents and transnational sojourners crossing the border (Núñez, 2012). The majority of the *colonias* are located in Texas, where approximately 400,000 individuals live in 2,294 such communities (Texas Secretary of State, 2011). It is estimated that 98% of *colonia* residents are individuals of Hispanic descent, mostly of Mexican ancestry (Giusti, 2010). These communities, on the fringes of larger urban centers of power, are characterized by substandard housing, inadequate infrastructure, poor roads and drainage, substandard water and sewer facilities, lack of garbage disposal services, and dangerously high poverty. The rights and humanity of *colonia* residents are often violated by structural poverty, social isolation, political alienation, and police and federal repression (Núñez, 2012). A recent study of the health-related quality of life among Mexican Americans living in *colonias* in the Texas–Mexico border area found that women were more likely than men to report poor mental health status (Mier, Ory, Zhan, Conling, Sharkey, & Burdine, 2008). This difference may be related to domestic violence (see Staudt, 2012) and high levels of discrimination.

The U.S.–Mexico Border Counties Coalition 2006 report, *At the Crossroads: U.S.-Mexico Border Counties in Transition*, presents an analysis of several key features of the U.S.–Mexico border region. The report points out that if the 24 U.S. counties along the border were aggregated as the 51st state, they would rank 40th in per capita income, 5th in unemployment, 2nd in tuberculosis (TB), 7th in adult diabetes, 50th in health insurance coverage, 50th in high school completion, and first in poverty. For more than a decade, experts have declared that the region demands immediate attention as both the gains from doing something and the consequences of doing nothing are enormous (Shapleigh, 2009).

These disparities have multiple influences and causal factors. Many border residents had optimistic expectations that the North American Free Trade Agreement (NAFTA) would address environmental and poverty problems and bring greater economic development, including well-paying jobs. The employment opportunities created by NAFTA have tended to be low-skill and low-paying labor and service jobs. In addition, the increase of cross-border trade and the associated vehicular crossings have overwhelmed border infrastructure and increased air pollution, resulting in health and safety risks and concerns.

The border counties have unemployment rates that are higher than that for their respective states as a whole. In 2006, the unemployment rate along the U.S. side of the Texas–Mexico border was 250% to 300% higher than in the rest of the country (Moya, Loza, & Lusk, 2012). The income disparity on the border is also influenced by the region's large Hispanic population. Hispanics, on an average, earn a far lower income than non-Hispanic Whites (DeNavas-Walt, Proctor, & Smith, 2011). As unemployment has increased, the U.S. border counties have experienced a decrease in adjusted per capita income over the past 30 years. Per capita income is a core measure of community success, and the border region's income is among the lowest in the nation. A low per capita income indicates that families are struggling to earn money and break the cycle of poverty. The entire border, with the exception of the more affluent county of San Diego, has suffered from an increase in income inequality. Forty of the 48 U.S. border counties have per capita incomes lower than the state averages, ranging from 35% of the U.S. per capita income in Starr County to 97% in Kerr County. The gaps between the rich and the poor are also increasing. The rich have been getting wealthier, while the middle and lower class continue to struggle (USMBCC, 2006; Shapleigh, 2009).

In addition to growing trade between Mexico and the United States, there are cross-border networks of informal and illegal trade. There is drug trafficking along the border; El Paso, in particular, is one of the main corridors for drug smuggling into the United States. According to the U.S. Drug Enforcement Agency, 65% of the cocaine consumed in the United States enters through the Mexican border, and 99% of the heroin produced in Mexico and South America targets U.S. consumers (Good Neighbor Environmental Board, 2010).

Low levels of educational attainment and high poverty rates reflect a pervasive cycle of poverty that becomes overwhelmingly difficult to break. Increased educational attainment delivers clear economic benefits (Ewert, 2012). But, without an educational system on the U.S.–Mexico border region that delivers higher graduation rates and better education to meet the needs of the employers, lower wages will persist, and the entire border region will continue to remain poor and undeveloped.

UNIQUE HEALTH AND MEDICAL CHARACTERISTICS OF THE BORDER

Complementary Alternative Methods

Complementary and alternative methods (CAM) of health care are common among Hispanics. Recent research described the use of alternative folk medicine by Mexican American women (Lopez, 2005), the use of CAM in the largest border city (Rivera, Ortiz, Lawson, & Verma, 2002), and CAM practices within the context of binational health-care-seeking behavior and health-related quality of life among human immunodeficiency virus (HIV)-infected Latinos in the U.S.–Mexico border region (Zuñiga et al., 2011). For example, one-third of a sample of Mexican Americans living in a Texas–Mexico border community used home or "folk" remedies to augment their diabetes therapy (Brown, Garcia, Kouzekanani, & Hanis, 2002). CAM is also prevalent in the many Native American communities. At the border, CAM is an important factor for culturally competent care.

In fact, there is evidence that it enhances the efficacy of health care services (Sharp, 1998). However, it is also a concern because some CAM methods may interfere with other medical treatments, such as antiretroviral treatments (Jernewall, Zea, Reisen, & Poppen, 2005).

Promotores and *Promotoras de Salud* (Health Promoters)

In addition to CAM, *promotores* and *promotoras* (the Spanish term for community health workers [CHWs]) are part of the legacy and unique culture of the border region. The use of *promotores* has had widespread success as a low-cost, culturally appropriate prevention model in clinical settings among ethnic populations (Ramos & Ferreira-Pinto, 2006; Ramos et al., 2006). *Promotores* are "lay members of the community where they work either for pay or as volunteers" (Health Resources and Services Administration [HRSA], 2007), who, with some paraprofessional training, are able to bridge the communication gap between health care providers and communities of different cultural and ethnic backgrounds (Sánchez-Bane & Moya, 1999; Ramos & Ferreira-Pinto, 2006; Ramos, Hernandez, Ferreira-Pinto, Ortiz, & Somerville, 2006). *Promotores* have been extensively used at the U.S.–Mexico border and have proven useful, especially when there is limited access to health professionals. They serve to (1) enhance the effectiveness of the health system, particularly with regard to contraception, maternal child care, and chronic disease management, in particular diabetes (Babamoto et al., 2009), and to (2) educate communities on healthy behaviors (Joshu, Rangel, Garcia, Brownson, & O'Toole, 2007), including Mexican Americans (Lujan, Oswald, & Ortiz, 2007) and farmworkers (Ingram et al., 2007).

Cross-Border Service Utilization

Along the border, underutilization of health services in both nations is common (Macias & Morales, 2001). Many studies (Zuñiga, Blanco, Brennan, Scolari, Artamonova, & Strathdee, 2011) identified the existence of cross-border utilization of health care, including a significant number of U.S. residents who sought services in Mexico. But because few studies investigate the actual prevalence and services sought, determining the extent to which this happens is difficult—especially across the entire border region. Key factors influencing underutilization of services in Mexico are lack of insurance in the United States and limited mobility. It is critical to note, however, that although access to health care is a constitutional guarantee in the nation of Mexico (unlike in the United States), this right does not translate into equitable access to health care and resources for health-related quality of life (Moya, Loza, & Lusk, 2012; Homedes, 2012).

In addition to people, products and goods also cross the border in order to reach their markets, sometimes with adverse health consequences. In 1995, an investigation by the Texas Department of Health (TDH), ignited by the surprisingly acute mercury poisoning in a 15-year-old male in Eagle Pass, Texas, revealed that a popular Mexican "beauty cream" containing at least 6% mercuric chloride was being used throughout the border region in Texas and as far away as Houston and Chicago (Sharp, 1998). Although not on the Food and Drug Administration's approved list of imports, the cream was widely available at flea markets and ethnic grocery stores along the border. In a demonstration of both the challenges and the opportunities of the region, the TDH joined forces with federal health entities as well as state departments of health in both countries, resulting in the closure of the Mexican factory where the cream was produced as well as its removal from store shelves. Nonetheless, within 2 years, new products with similar mercury levels became widely available. Proactive and responsive collaboration among the many health entities that converge at the border is critical to mitigating the adverse effects of cross-border utilization and enhancing access to needed health services.

Protective Factors

The so-called "Hispanic or Latino health paradox" and "immigrant advantage" refers to the contradictory finding that Latinos and immigrants in the United States tend to have significantly better health and mortality outcomes than the average population, despite markedly lower socioeconomic status (SES) (Markides & Coreil, 1986; Cho, Frisbie, Rogers, 2004; Frazini & Ribbie, 2001; Hayes-Bautista et al., 2002). Findings from the Tomas Rivera Policy Institute suggest that the Latino health paradox exists for mental health issues, asthma, and high blood pressure (Tamingco, 2007). Results from this study indicated that Hispanic immigrants are healthier in terms of these three health outcomes when they first arrive in the United States; however, they become less healthy after acculturation. Studies suggest that "traditional social and cultural retention may be a protective factor for mental health of individuals of Mexican descent" (Grant et al., 2004, p. 1228). Foreign-born Mexican Americans are at significantly lower risk of *Diagnostic and Statistical Manual* (*DSM-IV*) mental disorders compared to their U.S.-born counterparts (any disorder 28.5% among foreign-born versus 47.6% among U.S.-born). However, in chronic metabolic illnesses such as diabetes, Mexican Americans residing along the border are disproportionally affected (Centers for Disease Control & Prevention [CDC], 2011).

SOCIAL DETERMINANTS, HEALTHY PEOPLE, AND HEALTH OUTCOMES

Residents of the U.S.–Mexico border envision a day when preventable death, illness, injury, and disability, as well as health disparities and inequalities, are reduced and each citizen enjoys the best health possible.

This transformation will only occur when we change our thinking about "health," examine the societal determinants (root causes), and direct more resources and interventions to address primary, causal factors that affect health. For example, health and environmental issues in the border region include air and water pollution, groundwater depletion, soil contamination, illegal outdoor burning, and infectious disease, all of which transcend national boundaries. Another factor, SES, has cumulative effects on health throughout the entire life course; reducing inequalities therein can meet numerous health objectives in the border region (Baum, Begin, Tanja, Houwelling, & Taylor, 2009). Higher income can provide better nutrition, housing, schooling, recreation, and health care (Wilkinson & Marmot, 2003). The best indicator of SES is education, as it shapes future occupational opportunities and earnings.

The *Healthy People (HP) 2020 Action Framework* (HP 2020, 2010, 2011) provides a comprehensive national strategy to control and prevent disease while addressing social determinants like those described above. *HP 2020* is the fourth iteration of a comprehensive set of 10-year national public health objectives designed to guide planning and action with the vision of ushering in a "society in which all people live long, healthy lives" (HP 2020, 2010). *HP 2020*'s objectives were informed by an interdisciplinary Federal Interagency Workgroup comprising 30 U.S. Department of Health and Human Services (DHHS) agencies and other federal partners, underscoring that health outcomes are tied to the five determinants of health (physical environment, social environment, individual behavior, biology and genetics, and health services). *HP 2020* also establishes leading health indicators (LHI), which place renewed emphasis on overcoming public health challenges and disparities, and are used to both facilitate collaboration across sectors and motivate action at all levels to improve health (HP 2020, 2011, 2010).

Healthy People is the basis for the Healthy Border (HB) program, the vehicle through which the USMBHC accomplishes two of its foundational goals: (a) identify key health issues in the border region and (b) develop programs to address these issues. A midterm review of HB 2010 was conducted in 2006. These results are included in Table 20.1. Meeting the end-of-decade targets requires the development of a coordinated effort among the many public and private health service providers. It also requires collecting detailed, uniform data for 44 (of 48) border counties spread across four states (USMBHC, 2009). Epidemiological information provides critical knowledge of what is making border residents sick and what are the primary causes of mortality on the border. This does not suggest that the border is a region of victims; the region has a remarkable history of resilience and solution-building, especially in response to rapidly growing and changing populations. We will discuss this in the "Opportunities and Innovations" section.

TABLE 20.1 The *HP2020* Leading Health Indicators and the HB2010 U.S. Objectives Detailing Epidemiological Realities of the Border Region in the First Decade of the 21st Century

Healthy People 2020 Leading Health Indicators (organized by topic)	Epidemiological and Health Determinants Data
1. Access to Health Services	
A. Persons with medical insurance	A. Combined, the 24 border counties contiguous to the border rank 50th lowest (out of 51 states) in insurance coverage for children and adults [1/A]; 22.9% of all border residents lack health insurance (44 counties); and 38% of Hispanic border residents lack health insurance [2/B]
B. Persons with a usual primary care provider	B. The percent of the border population without a place to go when they were sick (18.6%) was 36% higher than the national estimate (13.6%) [2/E]
2. Clinical Preventive Services	
C. Adults who receive a colorectal cancer screening based on the most recent guidelines	C. (No border region data)
D. Adults with hypertension whose blood pressure is under control	D. Among the border population aged 18 years or more, 20.6% (age-adjusted) had been diagnosed with high blood pressure. Of Hispanics in the border region, 22% had been diagnosed with high blood pressure, compared to 20% of non-Hispanics [2/E]
E. Adult diabetic population with an A1c value greater than 9%	E. Adult diabetic population who had two or more A1c testing in the last year (2000–2005): between 60% and 70% for all four border states, which is near national average; testing results not available [8/E] Diabetes deaths decreased significantly in New Mexico and Texas border counties and slightly in Arizona between 2000 and 2005 but increased dramatically in California border counties [4/B] Diabetes hospitalizations are significantly higher for Hispanics living in border counties [5/B]
F. Children aged 19 to 35 months who receive the recommended doses of DTaP, polio, MMR, Hib, hepatitis B, varicella, and PCV vaccines	F. The coverage rate for the 4:3:1:3 series1 was 82.4% for the United States and near 80% for each of the border states in 2005 (USMBHC, 2009)
3. Environmental Quality	
G. Air quality index (AQI) exceeding 100	G. Data not available
H. Children aged 3–11 years exposed to secondhand smoke	H. (No border data)

(continued)

TABLE 20.1 The *HP2020* Leading Health Indicators and the HB2010 U.S. Objectives Detailing Epidemiological Realities of the Border Region in the First Decade of the 21st Century *(Continued)*

Healthy People 2020 Leading Health Indicators (organized by topic)	Epidemiological and Health Determinants Data
4. Injury and Violence	
I. *Fatal injuries*	I. Total motor vehicle-related deaths in the U.S. border counties greatly outnumber deaths due to diabetes in people under 65 years and resulted in much higher numbers of "productive years lost" [7/D]
J. *Homicides*	J. Second leading cause of death among 14–24-year-olds throughout the border area and nationwide (PAHO, 2007). The homicide rate for the border counties was 4.6 per 1000 people, significantly lower than the national rate (5.9). Among border counties, those in Arizona had the highest homicide rate (8.3); the border area of Texas had by far the lowest homicide death rate (2.8). Significant differentials by sex (male:female rate = 3:1) and ethnicity (higher homicide death rate for Hispanics than non-Hispanic Whites) also existed within the border region [E]
5. Maternal, Infant, and Child Health	
K. *Infant deaths*	K. Infant mortality rate due to birth defects (per 1000 births) fell between 2000 (1.50) and 2005 (1.17) [B]
L. *Preterm births*	L. Preterm birth rate of border counties was 12.4% in 2004 but differed among the border counties in each state (California 10.7%, Texas 14%). Preterm rates were consistently higher for Hispanics (12.4%) than for non-Hispanic Whites (11%) in the border region, which mirrored the nationwide rates [E]
6. Mental Health	
M. *Suicides*	M. Suicide is the 10th leading cause of death on border (11th overall in the United States) [E] Rate of 11.2 (per 100,0000) in border counties in the year 2005 [B; National Mortality Files]
N. *Adolescents who experience major depressive episodes (MDE)*	N. Not currently being tracked
7. Nutrition, Physical Activity, and Obesity	
O. *Adults who meet current federal physical activity guidelines*	O. 50% of the Texas border county adult population does not meet the recommended level of physical activity (mirrors national average); 16% no physical activity [aerobic] [3/C]

(continued)

TABLE 20.1 The *HP2020* Leading Health Indicators and the HB2010 U.S. Objectives Detailing Epidemiological Realities of the Border Region in the First Decade of the 21st Century *(Continued)*

Healthy People 2020 Leading Health Indicators (organized by topic)	Epidemiological and Health Determinants Data
P. Adults who are obese	P. 69% of Texas border county adults are obese or overweight; 71% of Hispanics [3/C]
Q. Children and adolescents who are considered obese	Q. (Data not available for the border region)
R. Total vegetable intake for persons aged 2 years and older	R. Texas border region: 19% to 24% eat five or more servings of fruits and vegetables daily; Hispanics average 21% versus non-Hispanics 31% [3/C]
8. Oral Health	
S. Persons aged 2 years and older who used the oral health care system in the past 12 months	S. 60% in border counties; 44% among Hispanics in border counties [2/B]
9. Reproductive and Sexual Health	
T. Sexually active females aged 15 to 44 years who received reproductive health services in the past 12 months	T. (Data not available for the border region)
U. Persons living with HIV who know their serostatus	U. (Data not available for the border region)
10. Social Determinants	
V. Students who graduate with a regular diploma 4 years after starting ninth grade	V. The border counties rank as the 51st lowest state in population with high school diploma (not including San Diego County) and 50th including San Diego County) [1/A]
11. Substance Abuse	
W. Adolescents using alcohol or any illicit drugs during the past 30 days	W. (Data not available for the border region)
X. Adults engaging in binge drinking during the past 30 days	X. 16% of border residents binge drink (national average) [3/C]
12. Tobacco	
Y. Adults who are current cigarette smokers	Y. Lower prevalence in Texas border counties (17%) than state and nationwide averages. Greater for 18–29 year olds (20%) compared to 65+ (7%); need data for adolescents [3/C]
Z. Adolescents who smoked cigarettes in the past 30 days	Z. (Data not available for the border region)
Infectious Diseases 1. TB 2. HIV/AIDS	1. Border counties rank as second in the nation in prevalence [A] The U.S.–Mexico border is at high risk of elevated TB and HIV incidence and other health issues due to socioeconomic stress, rapid and dynamic population growth,

(continued)

TABLE 20.1 The *HP2020* Leading Health Indicators and the HB2010 U.S. Objectives Detailing Epidemiological Realities of the Border Region in the First Decade of the 21st Century *(Continued)*

Healthy People 2020 Leading Health Indicators (organized by topic)	Epidemiological and Health Determinants Data
	mobility and migration, and the interrelationship of cultures (Finch et al., 2001; Moya & Shedlin, 2008) and a young population (Harrison & Kennedy, 1994). TB is a subtle and complex chronic infectious disease. The extent of the disease is likely to be underreported because of mobility and migration across the border as well as the long latency of the condition after infection occurs. The incidence of TB at the border far exceeds national incidence rates in both countries 2. Aggregated prevalence rates for border counties are unavailable
Data Source	Publication Source
1. Census 2000 data	A. "At the Crossroads: U.S.–Mexico Border Communities in Transition" (USMBCC, 2006)
2. 2000–2003 National Health Interview Survey (NHIS) (NCHS/CDC)	B. HB2010 midterm report (USMBHC, 2009)
3. Data from 2007 BRFSS (15 counties contiguous to border [out of 32 total])	C. 2007 Health Risk Factors for the Texas–Mexico Border (Texas Department of State Health Services, 2007a)
4. National Mortality Data (NCHS/CDC) (Rate per 100,000)	D. Motor Vehicle Injuries: A Priority for the U.S.–Mexico Border Population (Frescas & Baker, n.d.)
5. Hospital Discharge data systems in Arizona, California, Texas (rates per 10,000)	E. "Border Lives: Health Status in the United States–Mexico Border Region" (USMBHC, 2010)
6. National Immunization Survey, data from 1998–2002	
7. CDC and Prevention Wonder Database	
8. BRFSS 2000–2005	

Note: Challenges to data collection: (a) US–Mexico Border Counties Coalition includes only counties contiguous to the border [=24]; does not go by La Paz agreement definition (100 km each way); (b) USMBHC counts data for 44 of the 48 counties that lie within the La Paz agreement border region; (c) more than half of the border counties lie only *partially* within the border zone.

The Epidemiological and Health Determinants data are followed by data sources [i.e. 1–8] and publication sources [i.e. A–E]

THE NURSING PROFESSION: CHALLENGES AND SOCIAL EPIDEMIOLOGY IN THE BORDER REGION

The U.S.–Mexico border region presents health care practitioners with great challenges due to the high prevalence of chronic illnesses such as type 2 diabetes (T2D), hypertension, increased weight, and obesity. At the same time, the region also offers great opportunities: The contributions that nurses can make are significant and may vary from provision of direct care to being drivers of health care policy. In this section, we address nursing shortage in the border region, the health state of individuals residing in the U.S.–Mexico border region, and the opportunities to utilize additional resources for provision of health care services according to the needs of the population.

The state of health and economics of residents in the U.S.–Mexico border region presents great challenges for members of the health care team and in particular nurses, who historically represent the largest number of health care professionals. Health problems are not necessarily different than they are for the rest of the country, but they are more pronounced because of barriers to accessing care, especially when dealing with chronic illnesses. The nursing shortage is greater in remote border counties such as Terrel and Hudspeth, Texas, where only one nurse practices in each county (Board of Nursing, 2010).

Nursing education is challenged to recruit and retain nurses in the U.S.–Mexico border region who can serve the population and provide innovative teaching methods that allow collaboration with other health disciplines for provision of comprehensive care. Colleges must consider recruiting at the earliest possible educational age (e.g., elementary school level) by presenting the positive and professional aspects of nursing, which may be missed in media portrayals. The University of Texas at El Paso, through its Nurse Practitioner Program "Serving the Underserved: Cultural Competence Enhancing Success" (SUCCESS) grant (2006–2009), significantly increased the number of Hispanic Spanish-speaking nurses from rural border areas by offering an online distance learning program for nurse practitioners. Additionally, clinical preceptors from rural areas were identified and students were assigned to remote clinical sites, thereby creating a greater pool of professional resources (Robinson, 2008).

There is a need for dialogue at the state policy level to address the shortage of advanced practice registered nurses (APRNs) in the border region, particularly in California and Texas. Currently, in those states, APRNs must have a supervising physician oversee their practice (Center to Champion Nursing in America, 2011), creating a limitation for mobility and independence, especially in remote geographical areas. Revising the APRN scope of practice in these states to reflect the consensus model for advanced practice would remove the barriers that prevent APRNs from working to their full level of education and competence (APRN Joint Dialogue Group, 2008).

The chronic illnesses addressed by the majority of studies conducted in the U.S.–Mexico border region have been T2D and hypertension. Both conditions are high contributors to cardiovascular disease, which is the main cause of death in the United States (CDC, 2012). The 11.8% rate of T2D among the Hispanic population in the U.S. in general has reached epidemic proportions (CDC, 2011). Moreover, along the U.S.–Mexico border, the rate of T2D is 15.7% (CDC, 2012). While T2D in the United States is listed as number six in the causes of mortality, in Texas and New Mexico, it ranks fourth as a cause of death (CDC, 2012). T2D disproportionally affects Hispanics, who comprise 85% of the population in the U.S. border counties or 7.5 million people in the U.S. border counties (CDC, 2012).

Major risk factors for T2D are obesity, body mass index (BMI) ≥ 30, and prediabetes (CDC, 2011). Prediabetes is a hyperglycemic state identified by either elevated glucose or glycosylated hemoglobin (A1c) that does not reach levels to be classified as diabetes (CDC, 2011). Both these risk factors have been identified in studies conducted in residents of the U.S.–Mexico border region (Anders et al., 2008; CDC, 2011). T2D is a complex medical condition that is highly connected to cardiovascular disease, blindness, renal disease, and changes in the nervous system, and linked to a disproportionate rate of noninjury leg amputations (CDC, 2011). Additionally, depression has emerged as a coexisting condition with this disease (Solis, 2010). Nurses and health care practitioners in the U.S.–Mexico border area are presented with an opportunity to provide services at all levels of care such as (a) exploring and conducting prevention programs to lessen the prevalence of T2D, (b) participating in screening to identify affected individuals as early as possible, and (c) providing direct care to maintain glucose control and guard against devastating complications.

Some studies conducted in the U.S.–Mexico border region highlighted the disproportionate effect of T2D in this area. Anders et al. (2008) conducted an exploratory study in a *colonia* in El Paso County to evaluate the prevalence of diabetes, access to service, and personal descriptors of the population ($N = 188$). Questions addressed were those included in the Behavioral Risk Factor Surveillance System (BRFSS) (Paso del Norte Health Foundation, 2005), which are used to gain information on factors related to chronic disease and injury. The BRFSS seeks information on health risk behaviors, disease prevention, and health care access and utilization. Of the participants reporting diabetes (15.4%), the majority (51.7%) were married women, with a mean age of 57 years, mean yearly income of $17,700, and a mean education of 6.7 years with 67.9% having received their education in Mexico. Most participants reported living in the United States for more than 10 years. Nearly half of the participants did not have health care coverage in the United States: The majority reported paying out of pocket for health services and 21% reported purchasing their diabetes medications in Mexico. Only 38% identified seeing a primary health care provider on a regular basis for the management of their diabetes.

When addressing the health state of participants with diabetes in the Anders et al. study (2008), a majority reported also having hypertension and high cholesterol. The majority (59.3%) had BMI >30, which is classified as obese (CDC, 2010). The findings by Anders et al. identified greater obesity than the Phase 1 "U.S.–Mexico Border Diabetes Prevention and Control Project" (CDC, 2012) where 38.3% of the participants were obese. The project was designed in collaboration with 10 U.S.–Mexico border states, the PAHO, several governmental agencies, and academic nonprofit organizations interested in diabetes prevention and control in the border region. Phase 1 evaluated diabetes prevalence and risk factors for the population, mainly Hispanic, residing in both sides of the border. This study identified the profile of participants with T2D much like the one conducted by the CDC (2012). The low education level, low income, and lack of consistent health care providers who assisted these individuals provide a worrisome snapshot of the challenges facing those with T2D who reside along the border. Inadequate access to health care has been identified as a root cause of health disparity; one of the ways to resolve it would be to increase the number of Spanish-speaking health care providers serving along the U.S.–Mexico border (Jones & Mulitalo, 2010).

Jones and Mulitalo (2010) examined the distribution of Hispanic physician assistants (PAs) practicing in Texas–Mexico counties (7 of 14 counties had PAs) and found that 69% of those practicing in the area were Hispanic; a positive contribution that potentially addresses the cultural needs of the border population. However, Hispanic nurses and physicians are not well represented in nonmetropolitan counties, 11 of the 14 border counties in Texas; the total number of Hispanic physicians (11.5%) and registered nurses (9.4%) in Texas are among the lowest ethnic groups represented (Texas Department of State Health Services, 2007b). According to "Texas on the Brink" (Texas Legislative Study Group, 2011), the number of physicians and nurses serving statewide are among the lowest (42nd and 44th) in the nation. A lack of health insurance and access to primary care can lead to overutilization of emergency services. Emergency departments (EDs) throughout the border region witness long waiting lines and shoulder upwards of $200 million per year in uncompensated emergency medical care (USMBCC, 2006). Registered nurses are among the largest group of health professionals; therefore, policies need to be considered to support Hispanic community residents that are interested in becoming nurses, in order to increase ethnic representation and improve service to isolated communities.

The cost of long-term treatment of T2D is astronomical; the national estimate of total medical care cost is $174 billion. Residents of the U.S.–Mexico border region are among the highest groups of uninsured; currently, 59% of Hispanics in Texas are without insurance (Texas Legislative Study Group, 2011). The economic burden of such devastating disease affects individuals, families, communities, and the nation. It is no longer an isolated problem, but one that has to be addressed collectively by all health professionals, and it has to gain the interest and commitment from policy makers at the local, state, and federal levels.

One of the ways to address the prevention, detection, and management of T2D in persons living in the U.S. border area is through the utilization of community health workers (CHWs). *Promotores* have been used successfully in other diabetes programs such a Project Dulce (Philis-Tsimikas, Fortmann, Lleva-Ocana, Walker, & Gallo, 2011), where they have been a vital part of the success of managing individuals with T2D in a culturally appropriate manner. The approach to health services for individuals suffering from chronic illnesses needs to be delivered by a group of professionals who will address the physiological needs and also consider the psychosocial and financial needs of the person. This means that an interdisciplinary team including a CHW and a health navigator (see Family Health Navigators below) may be the preferred way to provide care. The opportunities and challenges confronting health care providers call for greater exploration and will require teams of health professionals, academicians, community members, and other vested individuals to initiate dialogue and continue advocacy for lessening the disparities of access and provision of health services to residents of the U.S.–Mexico border.

OPPORTUNITIES AND INNOVATIONS

We conclude by identifying four noteworthy projects that illustrate the ways in which health care innovations have been introduced by nurses and allied health professionals. These projects have the potential for application in rural settings outside of the border region.

Photovoice: Engaging the Participation of Vulnerable Populations on the Border and Beyond

Tuberculosis (TB) morbidity and mortality are high in the U.S.–Mexico border region (CDC, 2007). Factors that contribute to an elevated incidence of TB and lower treatment adherence rates include limited access to health care services, the absence of TB education, and language barriers (CDC, 2001). Photovoice is a powerful tool to empower people affected by TB; their participation in advocacy, communication, and social mobilization is critical to addressing the high rates of deaths associated with TB among those living with HIV and acquired immunodeficiency syndrome (AIDS).

The aim of the photovoice method is to increase knowledge, awareness, and social action through photography. As such, photovoice is a method of participatory action research as well as a strategy to amplify and communicate the importance of TB–HIV/AIDS and other diseases across cultural settings from the perspective of the persons affected by the infections. Photovoice enables people to reflect personal and community concerns, to promote critical dialogue through discussions of photographs, and to reach policy makers and decision makers. Community members who are affected by a health problem receive cameras and instruction on their use and they take photographs that provide perspectives on their communities' needs and issues. Facilitators encourage dialogue using critical reflection with participants about their perspectives. The participants select images and stories as a communication strategy to advocate social action and change with leaders and decision makers (Wang, 1999). People have used photovoice to amplify their visions and experiences from the villages of rural China to a homeless shelter of Ann Arbor, Michigan; to patients affected and infected by TB in Thailand and Brazil (Amaya-Lacson Project, 2005); and in the binational project described here in El Paso, Texas/Ciudad Juarez, Mexico.

Border TB Photovoice Project

The Border TB Photovoice Project, "Voices and Images/*Voces e Imágenes*," started in 2005 through a grant awarded by the Amaya-Lacson Foundation (USMBHC, 2007). This first-ever border binational photovoice project aimed at "spreading the word, not the disease" by increasing awareness, reducing stigma associated with TB, increasing treatment adherence, expanding cross-border collaboration, and reaching policy and decision makers. The program was implemented in the sister cities of El Paso, Texas, in the United States and in Ciudad Juarez, Chihuahua, in Mexico by a collaboration[2] of governmental and nongovernmental organizations.

Outcomes demonstrate empirical support for the premise that TB and HIV are stigmatized diseases that requires empowerment in order to affect social action (De Heer, Moya, & Lacson, 2008). At a forum on the World TB Day, TB photovoice participants presented their photographs, stories, perspectives, and concerns to several influential decision makers, including a member of the U.S. Congress. Local and national (U.S. and Mexican) policy makers adhered to a "Call to Action" to eliminate TB. Countless additional leaders have signed this call to action, as the exhibit was presented to over 3,600 people on more than 25 occasions in the first year of the project. As a result, a collaboration of governmental and nongovernmental organizations backed the efforts of the project participants. The approach succeeded in enhancing awareness, promoting community advocacy, and achieving social mobilization. Notable adaptations of the initiative include:

1. Thirteen states and health jurisdictions in Mexico launched TB photovoice projects with technical assistance and training from Project Concern International (PCI).

2. PCI secured financial support from USAID Mexico to develop a three-dimensional traveling exhibit for Mexico, *"Nuestra Casa—Our House."* Stakeholders, including persons with TB and others from Tijuana, Reynosa, and Juarez, developed their vision of what it is to live with TB on the U.S.–Mexico border. The exhibit consisted of a portable representation of the home and living conditions among the most vulnerable along the border and was unveiled at the 2009 UNION Tuberculosis and Respiratory Health International Conference in Mexico.
3. *Programa Compañeros*, a community-based nongovernmental organization (NGO) in Ciudad Juarez, secured resources and funding to adapt and utilize the photovoice method to combat prejudice against people affected by HIV/AIDS, as well as those afflicted by an addiction.

In all of its manifestations, photovoice calls for practitioners and decision makers and policy makers to take action to eliminate the threat of TB. Committing to a more visible presence of individuals affected by TB–HIV/AIDS and their inclusion in program development and policy formulation is needed, notably as the policies affect rural communities and farm workers.

Global Experience with Community Health Workers of Project Concern International (PCI)

PCI is a nonprofit health and development organization founded in 1961 and headquartered in San Diego, California. PCI currently works in 15 developing countries around the world, as well as in the U.S.–Mexico border region. Over its 50-year history, PCI has focused primarily on family-centered, community-driven, integrated health and development programming. At the core of almost every one of PCI's programs over the past half century are CHWs. Typically, the CHW is a woman from the local community who has been selected based on leadership, educational level, commitment and willingness to volunteer, and a willingness to serve as a volunteer promoter of health in her local village or neighborhood.

Drawing on more than 25 years of identifying, training, and supporting *promotores* in the border city of Tijuana, Mexico, PCI has been able to creatively adapt and build upon the roles that CHWs can play in the unique U.S.–Mexico border region.

Case Management for Maternal and Child Health: HEAL

Emphasizing a life cycle approach, PCI has enhanced the CHW's case management role by adding several critical elements designed to address major barriers to health for both mothers and babies. One of these is maternal mental health. CHWs are able to support vulnerable women using PCI's

HEAL (Health Education and Action for Latinas) approach, which addresses postpartum depression, gender-based violence, and other mental health threats using a gender perspective and group support process specifically tailored for Latina women. PCI's community-oriented adaptation of the doula model provides the CHWs with yet another tool to support women and ensure healthy birth outcomes for both mother and infant.

Family Health Navigators: Building Bridges Between Families and Health Care Systems and Services

Supported by the DHHS/HRSA, the Family Health Navigator Resource Center (FHNRC) program enhances and expands the basic functions of CHWs for maximum impact. FHNRC serves the community by housing a well-trained, culturally competent, multiethnic group of FHNs who partner with the existing outreach system to deliver sensitive, high-quality, intensive, and coordinated services to families within the catchment area. Family health navigators (FHNs) help build bridges among the health care system, social service programs, and the client and his or her family to improve the utilization of services and access to high-quality care, with the end goal of improving health outcomes for persons with chronic diseases from the target populations. FHNs are able to interpret the medical culture for those who are unfamiliar with it, are knowledgeable about the county's health care system, are skilled at communicating with health care providers and institutions, and speak the same language and have a similar cultural background as the target populations. All family members (men, women, children, and elders) are included as part of the total caseload. Owing to the close family system culture of the targeted ethnic minorities, the reach often includes individuals in the extended family, such as grandparents, uncles, aunts, and cousins.

Addressing the Challenge of Sustainability

One of the most critical and universal challenges related to CHWs has been the issue of sustainability, including motivation and compensation for CHWs (Mathauer & Imhoff, 2006). On the one hand, pure volunteerism, if it lasts, is more sustainable as no additional external source of financial support would be needed. On the other hand, it does not adequately compensate an essential member of the health care team and it thereby undervalues the nonclinical aspects of health care, which include attitude and behavior change, mental/emotional support, social support, and coordination of services.

PCI has utilized several strategies designed to increase both the compensation and the sustainability of CHWs as an essential ongoing component of the health care system. Because the CHWs, including doulas, are respected and informed members of the target communities, they will continue to be viewed as a resource in the area even if funding streams for their positions diminish. The peer support system that is so key to the health education model has provided an even larger number of women in the community who are equipped with materials, knowledge, and information about perinatal and community health; it is anticipated that many of these women will continue to serve as CHWs even after the project concludes.

However, in the case of the FHNRC, PCI staff felt strongly that FHNs must be empowered to dedicate sufficient time to the project and therefore must be employees of the project rather than volunteers. While this will help ensure higher levels of accountability for the quality and consistency of their work, it is unclear how sustainable it may be in the coming years. Strategies for finding the right balance and addressing the inherent tension between adequate compensation and sustainability will continue to be sought and discussed with the CHWs and the families and communities they serve in San Diego.

The Role of *Promotoras* in Research: The Border Youth Alcohol Project

While data suggest that Mexican-origin young adults, especially those living along the border, have a high prevalence of hazardous alcohol use, alcohol-related problems, and alcohol use disorders (Wallisch & Spence, 2006), there are few studies in the published literature reporting interventions for these individuals. One study reported successful implementation of brief intervention for alcohol abuse among Mexican American primary care patients across the age spectrum (Burge et al., 1997), while another found no significant effects for alcohol use and its consequences resulting from brief motivational intervention in a primary care clinic among primarily Hispanic teens (D'Amico, Miles, Stern, & Meredith, 2008). Given that the emergency department of the hospital (ED) may be the primary source of medical care for many of these individuals (de Cosío & Boadella, 1999), as well as the potential place for brief intervention for effecting change in drinking behavior and alcohol-related problems,[3] Border Youth Alcohol Project (BYAP)[4] began by linking with emergency rooms (ERs) in El Paso, Texas.

The aims of BYAP are to (a) examine the effectiveness of the screening, brief intervention, referral, and treatment (SBIRT) model among Mexican-origin young adults (age 18–25), using a motivational intervention delivered by *promotores*, relative to standard care with and without assessment, on the reduction of heavy drinking (drinking days per week, number of drinks per day, maximum number of drinks on an occasion) and (b) to identify variables that are related to the effectiveness of the intervention and that predict successful treatment outcome.

SBIRT is based on the work of Miller (1999) and Miller and Rollnick (2002) and takes about 20 minutes to administer. This model integrates the elements of motivational interviewing and readiness to change (Prochaska & DiClemente, 1992), is patient-oriented, builds self-efficacy, and suggests specific action. SBIRT has been found useful in (a) motivating dependent drinkers to seek treatment and (b) stimulating recipients to change drinking behavior and utilize referral resources (Ballesteros, 2004). The motivational interventions tools have been translated into Spanish and adapted for the border context, which includes many recent immigrants as well as a stable population of acculturated Mexican-origin citizens.

BYAP, a randomized clinical controlled trial of brief motivational interviewing with follow-ups at 3 and 12 months, is still ongoing, but some preliminary results are positive. By mid-December 2011, the project recruited 572 patients in the ED. These patients were obtained from 2,514 potential patients screened, of which only 7% refused enrollment in the project. The study has also been successful in its ability to follow up patients, with only 4% of the 572 patients refusing to continue in the study.

The BYAP in El Paso has a different strategy than many of the previously reported similar studies of other ED populations. SBIRT in the ED has typically been administered by physicians or other health professionals (nurses, health educators, social workers, psychologists, or trained interventionists) (Sullivan, Tetrault, Braithwaite, Turner, & Fiellin, 2011), but results are mixed (Cobain et al., 2011; D'Onofrio et al., 2008). BYAP uses a participatory methodology for the data collection as well as for SBIRT, involving participants in defining their own strategies for the reduction of alcohol use and selecting the action steps inherent in brief negotiational interviewing (Bernstein, Bernstein, & Levenson, 1997), including the use of referral to agencies that can assist with alcohol reduction.

In light of the American College of Surgeons Committee on Trauma requiring Level 1 trauma centers to provide screening and brief intervention to all patients, the lessons learned from the BYAP are important as a prototype for screening, brief intervention, and referral for at-risk and dependent drinking in the ED, in this context for Mexican-origin young adults. Clinicians will benefit from exploring the role that *promotores* can have in the implementation of SBIRT in the ED in the United States to Mexican descent populations in settings where there are limited professional providers or where there are cultural competence challenges. Lessons learned from the BYAP translational research may prove especially effective in this young adult Mexican-origin population, and also may provide a better chance of ongoing implementation of SBIRT instead of or in partnership with other providers, who have limited time and other priorities.

Simulation and Standardized Patient Training for Border and Rural Practice

Increasingly, schools of nursing and colleges of health sciences have turned to simulation and training with standardized patients as mechanisms of developing and mastering patient interaction skills. These standardized patient training exercises are primarily conducted prior to the nursing and allied health students being placed in hospital or clinical settings (Nehring & Lashley, 2009). While simulation is not a new teaching technique (Harden, Stevenson, Downie, & Wilson, 1975), the evolution of high technology in digital video recording and playback has profoundly advanced the practice of simulation.

At the University of Texas at El Paso (UTEP), the School of Nursing faculty works closely with professors in the College of Health Sciences to utilize simulation and standardized patient training so as to foster a solid foundation of clinical skills and cultural competence for students of nursing and social work. These skills include communication with patients, client assessment, hand-off to physicians and other health care providers, and mastery of patient protocols that include a patient communication component. Without advanced communication skills, the student is unable to make accurate patient assessments, shape patient behaviors, enhance patient compliance with care, and assess the need for consultations by other professional such as physical therapists, social workers, and pharmacists.

The advantage of simulation in education is that by practicing, repeating, rehearsing, and mastering a patient interaction skill, the students are better prepared for working with real patients during their internships and rotations (Bogo, Regehr, Logie, Katz, Mylopoulos, & Regehr, 2011). Positive outcomes include improvements in communication skills, enhanced self-confidence and poise, better patient safety, superior interactions with other nurses and professionals, and an improved ability to deal with stress and crises (O'Sullivan, Chao, Russell, Levine, & Fabiny, 2008; Rentschler, 2007; Rushforth, 2007). Specifically, by seeing themselves on video replay, students, under the supervision of faculty, can see their strengths and pinpoint their weaknesses. This allows them to repeat the patient interaction until the professor has charted their performance as competent. In this sense, standardized patient training is built on criterion-based learning, in which a skill is demonstrated, rehearsed, practiced, and repeated until the student, professor, and standardized patient have declared the student as competent in a particular skill set.

At UTEP, simulation with standardized patients is done in four simulated hospital wards, a simulated patient apartment, and a group work laboratory. In the hospital, teams of nurses and social workers conduct examinations and assessments of patients. The nursing student conducts a physical examination consistent with the assigned diagnosis, and interviews the standardized patient, who is working from a prewritten scenario. Upon determining that the patient may face behavioral, health, substance abuse, family violence, or financial resources issues, the nurse calls for a social work consult. The masters in social work student then carries out a psychosocial assessment, writes a patient care note, and consults with the nursing student and supervisors about the treatment plan. In the patient apartment, nursing, social work, and physical therapy students do in-home simulated assessments to determine patient safety, accessibility, competency, and they carry out neglect and abuse investigations. In the group work lab, nursing and social work students practice interview techniques, group therapy skills, and patient education.

The hospital, patient apartment, and group work lab are equipped with multiple cameras and microphones, and all patient-caregiver interactions are recorded for playback. The scenarios are replayed and students review their performance with the professors and repeat the skills until competence or mastery of the skills is achieved. Students can use the recorded sessions as part of their graduate portfolio to demonstrate their skills. Standardized patient scenarios are conducted in Spanish to enhance nursing and social workers' skills in providing linguistically and culturally competent health care. Enacted scenarios include cases drawn from border and rural practice, including problems endemic to the region such as addictions, diabetes, TB, occupational injury, cardiovascular disease, and obesity-related disorders. Students consistently report that the exercises prepare them for their off-campus clinical education in a way that classroom exercises never could.

CONCLUSION

In this chapter, we described the 2,000-mile U.S.–Mexico border—a region that has a breadth of challenges with respect to health status, entitlements, and utilization. We identified the health care characteristics of the region, described the challenges of providing access to health care, and connected the challenges of border health to the goals set out in the U.S. government's framework *Healthy People 2020*. We also linked the challenges of border health to the nursing profession and its interface with other allied health professions, particularly social work in health care. We discussed how nurses practicing in the U.S.–Mexico border region have an opportunity for putting into action the theoretical preparation in rendering comprehensive care with respect and consideration to the beliefs and practices of all residents. We concluded by describing opportunities and innovations that have been developed in the border region to address the challenges of border and rural health care. These include the TB Photovoice Project, Community Health Workers of PCI, Border Youth Alcohol Project, and the University of Texas at El Paso School of Nursing's Standardized Patient Project—each of which addresses issues in health care that can easily be replicated in other rural and periurban communities.

NOTES

1. Oscar Martinez, a prominent historian and social science researcher of the border region, identifies two general types of within-the-border population. "National borderlanders" are people who have minimal or only superficial contacts with the opposite side of the border, although they are subject to foreign economic and cultural influences. "Transnational borderlanders" maintain significant ties with the neighboring nation, seeking to overcome obstacles that impede contact and taking advantage of every opportunity to visit, shop, work, study, or even live on the other side (Martinez, 1994).
2. This collaborative was led by members of the current Alliance of Border Collaboratives.
3. Recommendation from conferences sponsored by CDC and NIAAA as well as the International Conference on Alcohol and Injury: New Knowledge from Emergency Room Studies, sponsored by NIAAA, CDC, and WHO.
4. Funded by a grant from the U.S. National Institute of Alcohol Abuse and Alcoholism (Cherpitel & Woolard, 2011) and implemented by the Public Health Institute, Texas Tech Medical University, and the Alliance of Border Collaboratives. BYAP is a translational research to adapt and test screening, brief intervention, and referral to treatment (SBIRT) protocols in ED populations of Mexican descent (ages 18–35) in El Paso, Texas.

REFERENCES

Amaya-Lacson Project. 2005; posted on http://www.Photovoice.org *in November 1, 2006.*

Anders, R., Olson, T., Robinson, K., Wiebe, J., Sias, J., DiGregorio, R. et al. (2008). Diabetes prevalence and treatment adherence in residents living in a colonia located on the West Texas, US/Mexico Border. *Nursing Health Science, 10,* 195–202.

APRN Joint Dialogue Group. (2008). *Consensus model for APRN regulation: Licensure, accreditation, certification & education.* Author.

Babamoto, K. S., Sey, K. A., Camilleri, A. J., Karlan, V. J., Catalasan, J., & Morisky, D. E. (2009). Improving diabetes care and health measures among Hispanics using community health workers: Results from a randomized controlled trial. *Health Education Behavior, 36*(1), 113–126.

Ballesteros, J. (2004). Brief interventions for hazardous drinkers delivered in primary care are equally effective in men and women. *Addiction, 99,* 103–108.

Baum, F. E., Begin, M., & Houwelling, T. A. J. (2009). Changes not for the fainthearted: Reorienting health care systems toward health equity through action on the social determinants of health. *American Journal of Public Health, 99*(11), 1967–1974.

Bernstein, E., Bernstein, J., & Levenson, S. (1997). Project ASSERT: An ED-based intervention to increase access to primary care, preventive services, and the substance abuse treatment system. *Annals of Emergency Medicine, 30*, 181–189.

Board of Nursing for the State of Texas. (2010). *Currently licensed Texas RNs by county of residence*. Retrieved February 17, 2012, from http://www.bon.state.tx.us/about/stats/10-co-rn.pdf

Bogo, M., Regehr, C., Logie, C., Katz, E., Mylopoulos, M., & Regehr, G. (2011). Adapting objective structured clinical examinations to assess social work students' performance and reflections. *Journal of Social Work Education, 47*(1), 5–18. doi:10.51575/JSWE.2011.200900036.

Brown, S. A., Garcia, A. A., Kouzekanani, K., & Hanis, C. L. (2002). Culturally competent diabetes self-management education for Mexican Americans: The Starr County border health initiative. *Diabetes Care, 25*(2), 259–268.

Burge, S. K., Amodei, N., Elkin, B., Catala, S., Andrew, S. R., Lane, P. A. et al. (1997). An evaluation of two primary care interventions for alcohol abuse among Mexican-American patients. *Addiction, 92*(12), 1705–1716.

Center to Champion Nursing in America. (2011). *Consumer access and barriers to primary care physician-nurse practitioner collaboration required by state*. Retrieved February 17, 2012, from http://championnursing.org/sites/default/files/aprnmap.6.11.branded.pdf

Centers for Disease Control and Prevention. (2001, January 19). Preventing and controlling tuberculosis along the U.S.–Mexico border: Work group report. *Morbidity and Mortality Weekly Reports, 50(RR1)*, 1–12. Retrieved February 17, 2012, from http://www.cdc.gov/mmwr

Centers for Disease Control and Prevention. (2007, October 26). Reported HIV status of tuberculosis patients—United States, 1993–2005. *Morbidity and Mortality Weekly Reports, 56*(42), 1103–1106. Retrieved February 17, 2012, from http://www.cdc.gov/mmwr

Centers for Disease Control and Prevention. (2010). *Defining overweight and obesity*. Retrieved February 17, 2012, from http://www.cdc.gov/obesity/defining.html

Centers for Disease Control and Prevention. (2011). *Diabetes facts*. Retrieved February 17, 2012, from http://www.cdc.gov/diabetes/pubs/pdf/ndfs_2011.pdf

Centers for Disease Control and Prevention. (2012). *US-Mexico border diabetes prevention and control project*. Retrieved February 17, 2012, from http://www.cdc.gov/diabetes/projects/border.htm#2

Cherpitel, C. J., & Woolard, R. (2011). *Screening and brief intervention in the emergency department among Mexican-origin young adults*. National Institute on Alcohol Abuse and Alcoholism (R01 AA018119).

Cho, Y., Frisbie, W. P., & Rogers, R. G. (2004). Nativity, duration of residence, and the health of Hispanic adults in the United States. *International Migration Review, 38,* 184–211.

Cobain, K., Owens, L., Kolamunnage-Dona, R., Fitzgerald, R., Gilmore, I., & Pirmohamed, M. (2011). Brief interventions in dependent drinkers: A comparative prospective analysis in two hospitals. *Alcohol, 46*(4), 434–440.

D'Amico, E. J., Miles, J. N. V., Stern, S. A., & Meredith, L. S. (2008). Brief motivational interviewing for teens at risk of substance use consequences: A randomized pilot study in a primary care clinic. *Journal of Substance Abuse Treatment, 35*(1), 53–61.

de Cosío, F. G., & Boadella, A. (1999). Demographic factors affecting the U.S.–Mexico border health status. In M. O. Loustaunau, & M. Sánchez-Bane (Eds.), *Life, death, and in-between on the U.S.–Mexico border: Así es la vida* (pp. 1–22). Wesport, CT: Bergin & Garvey.

De Heer, H., Moya, E. M., & Lacson, R. (2008). Voices and images: Tuberculosis photovoice in a binational setting. *Cases in Public Health Communication & Marketing, 2,* 55–86. Retrieved June 11, 2012, from http://www.casesjournal.org/volume2

DeNavas-Walt, C., Proctor, B. D., & Smith, J. C. (2011). *Income, poverty, and health insurance coverage in the United States.* U.S. Census Bureau, Current Population Reports (Publication No. P60-239). Washington, DC: author. Retrieved February 17, 2012, from http://www.census.gov/prod/2011pubs/p60-239.pdf

D'Onofrio, G. D., Pantalon, M. V., Degutis, L. C., Fiellin, D. A., Busch, S. H., Chawarski, M. C. et al. (2008). Brief intervention for hazardous and harmful drinkers in the emergency department: A randomized controlled trial. *Annals of Emergency Medicine, 51*(6), 742–750.

Esparza, A., & Donelson, A. (Eds.). (2010). *The colonias reader: Economy, housing, and public health in U.S.–Mexico border colonias.* Tucson, University of Arizona Press.

Ewert, S. (2012). What its worth: Field of training and economic status in 2009. U.S. Census Bureau Current Population Reports (Publication No. P70-129). Retrieved February 17, 2012, from http://www.census.gov/prod/2012pubs/p70-129.pdf

Frazini, L., & Ribbie, J. K. (2001). Understanding the Hispanic paradox. *Ethnicity and Disease, 11*(3), 496–518.

Frescas, R., & Baker, T. (n.d.). Motor vehicle injuries: A priority for the U.S.–Mexico border population. Retrieved February 17, 2012, from http://www.borderhealth.org/files/res_1918.pdf

Giusti, C. (2010). Border communities: The case of colonias in Texas. *Development Issues, 12*(1), 21–22.

Good Neighbor Environmental Board. (2010). *A blueprint for action on the U.S.-Mexico border. Thirteenth report of the Good Neighbor Environmental Board to the President and Congress of the United States.* (EPA Publication No. 130-R-10-001). Washington, DC: Author. Retrieved February 17, 2012, from http://www.epa.gov/ofacmo/gneb/gneb_president_reports.htm

Grant, B. F., Stison, F. S., Hasin, D. S., Dawson, D. A., Chou, S. P., & Anderson, K. (2004). Immigration and lifetime prevalence of *DSM-IV* psychiatric disorders among Mexican Americans and non-Hispanic Whites in the United States: Results from the National Epidemiologic Survey on alcohol and related conditions. *Archives of General Psychiatry, 61*(12), 1226–1233.

Harden, R. M., Stevenson, M. M., Downie, W. W., & Wilson, G, M . (1975). Assessment of clinical competence using objective structured examinations. *British Medical Journal, 1,* 447–451.

Hayes-Bautista, D. E., Hsu, P., Hayes-Bautista, M., Iniguez, D., Chamberlin, C., Rico, C. et al. (2002). An anomaly within the Latino epidemiological paradox: The Latino adolescent male mortality peak. *Archives of Pediatric and Adolescent Medicine, 156,* 480–484.

Health Resources and Services Administration (HRSA). (2007). *Community health worker national workforce study.* Washington, DC: Department of Health and Human Services. Retrieved February 17, 2012, from http://bhpr.hrsa.gov/healthworkforce/reports/CHW'study2007.pdf

Healthy People 2020. (2010, July 26). *Healthy People 2020: An opportunity to address societal determinants of health in the U.S.* Washington, DC: Department of Health and Human Services. Retrieved February 17, 2012, from http://www.healthypeople.gov/2020/about/advisory/SocietalDetermi nantsHealth.pdf

Healthy People 2020. (2011). *Leading health indicators development and framework.* Washington, DC: Department of Health and Human Services. Retrieved February 17, 2012, from http://www.healthypeople.gov/2020/LHI/devel opment.aspx

Homedes, N. (2012). Achieving health equity and social justice in the U.S-Mexico border region. In M. Lusk, K. Staudt, & E. Moya, (Eds.), *Social justice in the U.S.-Mexico border region.* New York: Springer.

Ingram, M., Torres, E., Redondo, F., Bradford, G., Wang, C., & O'Toole, M. (2007). The impact of promotoras on social support and glycemic control among members of a farmworker community on the US-Mexico border. *Diabetes Educator, 33*(Supplement 6), 172S–178S.

Jernewall, N., Zea, M. C., Reisen, C. A., & Poppen, P. J. (2005). Complementary and alternative medicine and adherence to care among HIV-positive Latino gay and bisexual men. *AIDS Care, 17,* 601–609. doi:10.1080/ 09540120512331314295.

Jones, P. E., & Mulitalo, K. E. (2010). Physician assistant distribution in Texas-Mexico border counties: Public Health implications. *Journal of Environmental and Public Health, 2010*, 1–4. doi:10.1155/2010/975016.

Joshu, C. E., Rangel, L., Garcia, O., Brownson, C. A., & O'Toole, M. L. (2007). Integration of a promotora-led self-management program into a system of care. *Diabetes Educator, 33*(Supplement 6), 151S–158S.

Lopez, R. A. (2005). Use of alternative folk medicine by Mexican American women. *Journal of Immigrant Health, 7*, 23–31. doi:10.1007/s10903-005-1387-8.

Lujan, J., Oswald, S., & Ortiz, M. (2007). Promotora diabetes intervention for Mexican Americans. *Diabetes Educator, 33*(4), 660–670.

Macias, E., & Morales, L. (2001). Crossing the border for health care. *Journal of Health Care for the Poor and Underserved 12*, 77–87.

Markides, K. S., & Coreil, J. (1986). The health of Hispanics in the southwestern United States: An epidemiologic paradox. *Public Health Report, 101*, 253–265.

Martinez, O. J. (1994). *Border people: Life and society in the U.S.-Mexico borderlands.* Tuscon: University of Arizona Press.

Mathauer, I., & Imhoff, I. (2006). Health worker motivation in Africa: The role of non-financial incentives and human resource management tools. *Human Resources for Health, 4*(24).

Mier, N., Ory, M., Zhan, D., Conling, M., Sharkey, J., & Burdine, J. (2008). Health-Related quality of life among Mexican Americans living in colonias at the Texas-Mexico border. *Social Science & Medicine, 66*, 1760–1771.

Miller, W. R. (Ed.) . (1999). *Enhancing Motivation for Change in Substance Abuse.* Treatment Improvement Protocol Series #35. Rockville, MD: U.S. Department of Health and Human Services.

Miller, W. R., & Rollnick, S. (2002). *Motivational interviewing: Preparing people to change addictive behaviors.* New York: Guilford.

Moya, E., Loza, O., & Lusk, M. (2012). *Border health: Inequities, social determinants, & the case of tuberculosis and HIV.* In M. Lusk, K. Staudt, & E. Moya (Eds.), *Social justice in the U.S-Mexico Border Region.* New York: Springer.

Nehring, W. M., & Lashley, F. R. (2009). Nursing simulation: A review of the past 40 y. *Simulation & Gaming, 40*(4), 528–552.

National Rural Health Association. (2010). *Addressing the health care needs in the U.S.-Mexico border region: Policy brief.* Retrieved February 19, 2012, from http://www.raconline.org/topics/border_health.faq.php#border

Núñez, G. (2012). *Housing, colonias, and social justice in the US-Mexico border region. In* M. Lusk, K. Staudt, & E. Moya, (Eds.), *Social justice in the U.S-Mexico border region.* New York: Springer Publishing.

O'Sullivan, P., Chao, S., Russell, M., Levine, S., & Fabiny, A. (2008). Development and implementation of an objective structured clinical examination to provide formative feedback on communication and interpersonal skills in geriatric training. *Journal of the American Geriatrics Society, 56*(9), 1730–1735.

Pan American Health Organization (PAHO). (2007). United States-Mexico border area. In *Pan American Health Organization Health in the Americas: Volume II—Countries*, (pp. 733–744). Washington, DC: PAHO. Retrieved February 19, 2012, from http://new.paho.org

Paso del Norte Health Foundation. (2005, May). *How healthy are we? Border report: A status report on the health of people in El Paso County, Texas and Doña Ana County, New Mexico.* Retrieved February 19, 2012, from http://www.pdnhf.org/images/PDFs/border-reports/how-healthy-are-we.pdf

Pew Hispanic Center. (2011). *The Mexican-American boom: Births overtake immigration.* Retrieved February 19, 2012. from http://www.pewhispanic.org/files/reports/144.pdf

Philis-Tsimikas, A., Fortmann, A., Lleva-Ocana, L., Walker, C., & Gallo, L. C. (2011). Peer-led diabetes education programs in high-risk Mexican Americans improve glycemic control compared with standard approaches: A Project Dulce promotora randomized trial. *Diabetes Care, 34*(9), 1926–1931.

Prochaska, J. O., & DiClemente, C. C. (1992). Stages of change in the modification of problem behaviors. *Progress in Behavior Modification, 28*, 184–218.

Ramos, R. L., & Ferreira-Pinto, J. B. (2006). A transcultural case management model for HIV/AIDS care and prevention. *Journal of HIV/AIDS & Social Services, 5*, 139–157.

Ramos, R. L., Hernandez, A., Ferreira-Pinto, J. B., Ortiz, M., & Somerville, G. G. (2006). Promovisión: Designing a capacity-building program to strengthen and expand the role of promotores in HIV prevention. *Health Promotion Practice, 7*(4), 444–449.

Rentschler, D. D. (2007). Evaluation of undergraduate students using objective structured clinical evaluation. *Journal of Nursing Education, 46*(3), 135–139.

Rivera, J. O., Ortiz, M., Lawson, M. E., & Verma, K. M. (2002). Evaluation of the use of complementary and alternative medicine in the largest United States-Mexico border city. *Pharmacotherapy, 22*(2), 256–64.

Robinson, K. (2008). *Serving the underserved: Cultural competency enhancing success (SUCCESS) continuation project for grant #D09HP07328.* The University of Texas at El Paso.

Rushforth, H. E. (2007). Objective structured clinical examination (OSCE): Review of literature and implications for nursing education. *Nurse Education Today, 27*(5), 481–490.

Sánchez-Bane, M., & Moya, E. (1999). Community-based health promotion and community health advisors: Prevention works when they do it. In

M. O. Loustaunau, & M. Sánchez-Bane (Eds.), *Life, death, and in-between on the U.S.-Mexico border: Así es la vida*, (pp.131–154). Westport, CT: Bergin & Garvey.

Shapleigh, E. (2009). *Texas borderlands: Frontier of the future*. El Paso, Texas: Senator Eliot Shapleigh, District 29. Retrieved March 1, 2012, from http://www.epcc.edu/AboutEPCC/Documents/Texas_Borderlands.pdf

Sharp, J. (1998). *Bordering the future: Challenge and opportunity in the Texas border region*. Austin, TX: Texas Comptroller of Public Accounts. Retrieved March 1, 2012, from http://www.window.state.tx.us/border/border.html

Solis, G. (2010). *The co-existence of diabetes mellitus type 2 and depression symptoms in Mexican American adults: Its relation to glucose control, perceived stress, and physical health*. The University of Texas at El Paso). ProQuest Dissertations and Theses, Retrieved March 1, 2012, from http://search.proquest.com/docview/839313180?accountid=7121

Staudt, K. (2012). Women, gender and violence in the U.S.-Mexico border region. In M. Lusk, K Staudt, & E. Moya (Eds.), *Social justice in the U.S-Mexico border region*. New York: Springer Publishing.

Sullivan, L. E., Tetrault, J. M., Braithwaite, R. S., Turner, B. J., & Fiellin, D. A. (2011). A meta-analysis of the efficacy of nonphysician brief interventions for unhealthy alcohol use: Implications for the patient-centered medical home. *American Journal on Addictions*, 20(4), 343–356. doi:10.1111/j.1521-0391.2011.00143.x.

Tamingco, M. T. (2007). *Revisiting the Latino health paradox*. Los Angeles: Tomas Rivera Policy Center.

Texas Department of State Health Services. (2007a). Health risk factors in the Texas-Mexico border region. Retrieved March 1, 2012, from http://www.dshs.state.tx.us/borderhealth/pdf/PasoDelNorteBookletfinalstck5613186.pdf

Texas Department of State Health Services. (2007b). *Supply trends among licensed health professionals, Texas* 1980–2007 (3rd ed.). Retrieved March 1, 2012, from http://www.dshs.state.tx.us/CHS/hprc/07trends.pdf

Texas Legislative Study Group. (2011). *Texas on the brink: A report from the Texas legislative study group on the state of our state*. Retrieved October 10, 2011, from http://texaslsg.org/texasonthebrink/

Texas Secretary of State. (2011). *Texas colonias: A thumbnail sketch of conditions, issues, challenges and opportunities*. Retrieved October 10, 2011, from http://www.sos.state.tx.us/border/colonias/faqs.html

U.S. Census Bureau. (2011, May). *The Hispanic population: 2010: 2010 census briefs*. (U.S. Census Bureau Publication No. C2010BR-04). Retrieved December 13, 2010, from http://www.census.gov/prod/cen2010/briefs/c2010br-04.pdf

U.S.-Mexico Border Counties Coalition. (2006). *At the crossroads: U.S.-Mexico border counties in transition*. El Paso, Texas: USMBCC. Retrieved January 28, 2012, from www.bordercounties.org

U.S.-Mexico Border Health Commission. (2003). *Healthy Border 2010: An agenda for improving health on the United States-Mexico border*. Retrieved January 28, 2012, from http://www.borderhealth.org

U.S.-Mexico Border Health Commission. (2007, August). Photovoice project. *USMBHC Newsletter*. Retrieved January 28, 2012, from http://www.borderhealth.org/files/archived/2007/BHC_Newsletter_August07.pdf

U.S.-Mexico Border Health Commission. (2009). *Midterm review: Healthy Border 2010*. Retrieved January 28, 2012, from http://www.borderhealth.org.

U.S.-Mexico Border Health Commission. (2010). *Border lives: Health status in the United States-Mexico border region*. Retrieved January 28, 2012, from http://www.borderhealth.org.

Wallisch, L., & Spence, R. (2006). Alcohol and drug use, abuse, and dependence in urban areas and colonias of the Texas-Mexico border. *Hispanic Journal of Behavioral Sciences, 28*(2), 286–307.

Wang, C. C. (1999). Photovoice: A participatory action research strategy applied to women's health. *Journal of Women's Health,* 8(2), 185–192.

Warner, D. (1991). Health issues at the US-Mexico border. *Journal of the American Medical Association, 265,* 242–247.

Warner, D. C., & Jahnke, L. R. (2003). *U.S.-Mexico border health issues: The Texas Rio Grande Valley*. University of Texas Health Science Center at San Antonio: Regional Center for Health Workforce Studies.

Wilkinson, R., & Marmot, M. (2003). *Social Determinants of Health: The Solid Facts* (2nd ed.). Copenhagen, tDenmark: World Health Organization.

Zuñiga, M. L., Blanco, E., Brennan, J. J., Scolari, R., Artamonova, I. V., & Strathdee, S. A. (2011). Binational care-seeking behavior and health-related quality of life among HIV-infected Latinos in the U.S.-Mexico border region. *Journal of the Association of Nurses in AIDS Care, 22*(3), 162–172.

Chapter 21

REESTABLISHING NURSING EDUCATION IN HAITI: NURSES HELPING NURSES AFTER COMPLEX HUMANITARIAN EMERGENCIES

Michele V. Sare

> *Of all forms of inequity,*
> *injustice in healthcare is the most shocking and inhumane.*
> MARTIN LUTHER KING, JR. (SEBELIUS, 2012, P. 1)

> *As we would expect, the poor countries ... provide crudely obvious*
> *illustrations of severe deprivation, but the phenomenon is present*
> *even in the richest countries. Indeed, the deprived groups in the*
> *"First World" live, in many ways, in the "Third."*
> (FARMER, 2005, PP. XI–XII)

IN A DISCUSSION ON RURAL nursing and the concepts that are germane to nursing in rural—often resource-poor—settings, we must include communities in developed, industrialized, and *developing* countries if we are to address the full spectrum of challenges facing nursing in rural locales. There are communities in the United States where health data mirror developing countries. In one county in South Dakota, the life expectancy is only 64 years—only 2 years older than in Haiti. According to the Robert Wood Johnson Foundation's recently released County Health Rankings (2011), Mississippi experiences 10,811 years of potential life lost as compared to Montana at 7,403; the percent of live births with a low birth weight is 11.8% in Mississippi and just 7.1% in Montana. Lessons learned across borders can help strengthen nursing practice in an array of rural settings.

FROM MONTANA TO HAITI

On January 12, 2010, at about 4:00 p.m., I arrived in Haiti for the first time. My purpose for traveling to Haiti had been to visit a school of nursing to assess what it would take to teach a public health nursing course in a country where little public health infrastructure existed. The city that I would visit was Léogâne, Haiti, located along the coast and just 20 miles to the west of Haiti's capital city of Port au Prince.

Léogâne is in the Quest Department (department is a designation similar to "state" in the United States) (Figure 21.1). The population of Léogâne was approximately 135,000 (with a catchment area of approximately 300,000) and had one baccalaureate nursing program that had graduated just one class in its 5 years of existence. Until that time, the school had not offered community health nursing (CHN) nor public health nursing (PHN) theory and practice in its curriculum. My association with the School of Nursing began in 2009 when I volunteered to design a CHN and PHN course based on U.S. standards, guidelines, and ethics to be presented for the nursing school's consideration. Once they approved the course, I worked for approximately 1 year with the school's U.S.-based board of directors and the dean to arrange a time to work in Haiti in order to culturally and practically align the syllabus with the Haitian culture. I arrived in Haiti just 40 minutes before the devastating earthquake in January 2010.

My medical–surgical nursing skills were immediately put to the test, but the most important and desperately needed skills were leadership, management, and principles of public health nursing. It was the nurses

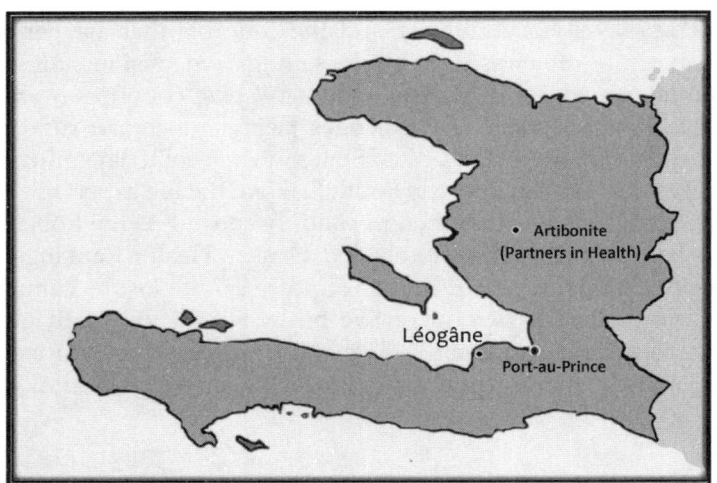

FIGURE 21.1 Léogâne, Haiti.

who had the skills, knowledge, and attributes to lead the only emergency health care available in Léogâne—where 80% to 90% of the community was destroyed by the earthquake (UNifeed, 2010). The United Nations (U.N.) found that Léogâne was the worst-affected area, and the U.S. military estimated that 20,000 to 30,000 persons were killed in Léogâne as a result of the earthquake and the 52 aftershocks occurring over the next 18 days (ABC News, 2010). The number killed is equivalent to 15% to 22% of the population and 80% to 90% destruction of U.S. cities such as Montgomery, Alabama; Des Moines, Iowa; Albany, New York; or Madison, Wisconsin. The scope, breadth, and scale of loss, suffering, and disability that the people of Léogâne and the catchment area suffered were staggering. Outside aid would not reach Léogâne, the quake's epicenter, for almost a week. While international aid poured into Port au Prince, the world did not learn of the extreme suffering and loss in Léogâne until film crews from CNN, ABC, and others stumbled across the devastation. The world had believed that the epicenter had been Port au Prince. This is an essential lesson on the need for emergency preparedness and redundant communication systems everywhere.

I and a small group of young Haitian student nurses, three newly graduated nurses, and people from the community banded together to care for thousands of injured during the 6 terribly long days without outside aid. "I want the world to know the truth of Haiti—to know who the real heroes were through those dark days—who continue to be everyday heroes" (Sare, 2011, p. 13).

In Léogâne, with 80% to 90% destruction of the community—and little food, few medical supplies, nearly continuous aftershocks, threats of tsunamis, scarce potable water supplies, little personal protective equipment, and hundreds of dying and severely injured babies, children, men, and women—it was nurses who went to work. The student nurses and newly graduated nurses would ask me "how and why, Michele" and together, we splinted multiple complex fractures; sutured and dressed gaping wounds with makeshift dressings; managed fluids and electrolytes; diligently tried to manage and control infection; assessed and treated multiple trauma victims; taught family and friends how to care for the injured; taught one another; prescribed whatever antibiotics and pain medication could be found; comforted and held the dying; amputated crushed hands and fingers; and went from patient-to-patient while kneeling on the lawn that was masquerading as a trauma center for as long as daylight and the flashlights would allow ... too afraid to go inside the buildings that were still standing. This was nursing in the most extreme conditions imaginable, and it was nursing that gave the only hope to the people of Léogâne, Haiti. Nurses saved lives.

The young students and new nurses were very skilled at several techniques—such as inserting an intravenous catheter or even suturing a deep wound. What they lacked were critical thinking skills and an understanding of the principles of what was needed; they had never heard the term "evidence-based practice." Without textbooks, computer labs, and anatomy, biology, and microbiology labs, or faculty trained and educated in pedagogy and andragogy, their learning had been rote; listen to a lecture for several hours, take notes when possible—if paper and writing utensils were available—and then repeat the content when tested. Occasional visiting faculty might bring in some innovative teaching techniques, but the majority of the course content was delivered by one U.S. educated, associate degree prepared, registered nurse (RN) and one or two Haitian physicians who taught anatomy and physiology.

Some of the students and young nurses could only function within the tight confines of what the Institute of Medicine has termed "functional doers" (technique-driven persons who respond to orders (Institute of Medicine [IOM], 2011, p. 223). There were however, one amazing young Haitian student and three newly graduated nurses who asked, watched, and learned how to take on leadership roles for the many patients and their family members, and served as mentors for their peers.

On January 13, 2010 at about 4:30 a.m., I found myself stepping over bodies, people, and makeshift stretchers—all on the ground—in the pitch-black of the first morning after the quake. The smells, sounds, and the dread were suffocating, but then a voice whispered, "It is so hard. I will go with you." One of the students was at my elbow and we did indeed "go together." It was harder than anything that I can imagine but together we saved hundreds. If I can offer one lesson in how we can and must help Haiti—or anyplace and any people—after a humanitarian emergency—it is this lesson that nurses need to learn—"it is so hard—let's go together."

> Global health is the goal of improving health for all people in all nations. (IOM, 2009, p. 18)

HAITI'S DEMOGRAPHICS AND HEALTH DATA: IMPACTS ON HEALTH CARE

Haiti is a developing country with a low standard of living (gross national income [GNI] of $1123 per capita in U.S. dollars [USD]) and a low human development index (HDI) (indication of life expectancy, level of education, and income) (United Nations Development Program [UNDP], 2011, 2012). Of the 187 nations rated by the UNDP, Haiti is ranked 158th in human development. Haiti has an underdeveloped industrial and agricultural base and mass urbanization (3 million of Haiti's 9 million persons live in Port au Prince—a city with a population of less than 800,000 in the

1980s). The tremendous humanitarian emergency in Haiti in 2010 was more the result of social injustice, inequality, and disparity than simply the tragic result of a seismic event. Haiti suffers from poverty levels of 54% to 78% (The World Bank, 2006), a lack of public utilities (such as water, septic, and electricity), lack of a functioning health care system, lack of a political infrastructure, a nursing ratio of 1:10,000 (Bailey, 2010), and, prior to the 2010 quake, only 46% of Haitians had access to health care (World Health Organization [WHO], 2011).

By every measure Léogâne is a resource-poor setting. If not for the large population, the U.S. designation of frontier would also apply. According to the Rural Assistance Center (2012), frontier areas are the most rural of settled places along the rural–urban continuum. While the term *frontier* is sometimes defined simplistically as places having a population density of six or fewer people per square mile, other important factors that may isolate a community need to be considered. "Therefore, preferred definitions are more complex and address isolation by considering distance in miles and travel time in minutes to services" (p. 1).

Today, 5% of Haiti's population are Taíno or White—often of mixed blood and referred to as "mulattos." The remaining 95% are of African heritage. Over 80% of the population is Roman Catholic; 16% are Protestant; and roughly half of the population practices voodoo (Central Intelligence Agency [CIA], 2012, p. 1). According to the CIA World Factbook (2010), the average age in Haiti is 20.2 years; the average life expectancy is 62 years; and the maternal and infant mortality rates are the highest in the Western Hemisphere. Humanitarian emergencies are a daily occurrence in Haiti.

CONCEPTS OF POPULATION-BASED NURSING PRACTICE AND THE SOCIAL DETERMINANTS OF HEALTH (SDH): CHALLENGES FACING HAITIAN NURSES AND NURSE EDUCATORS

To understand how nursing before, during, and after humanitarian emergencies might optimally function, it is essential that nurses understand the broader social context within which natural disasters—or other disasters—occur. In 2005, the WHO established the Commission on Social Determinants of Health (CSDH) to study the variables that affect health. These variables or determining factors, such as schooling, poverty, food insecurity, environmental conditions, policies and politics, and access to quality health care relate to the universal declaration of human rights (United Nations, 1948) and directly affect health, disease, and mortality rates (WHO, 2008) (see Box 21.1). In 2005, the CSDH set strategies to define and address these determinants.

> **BOX 21.1 ARTICLE 25 OF THE UNIVERSAL DECLARATION OF HUMAN RIGHTS (UN GENERAL ASSEMBLY, DECEMBER 10, 1948)**
>
> "Everyone has the right to a standard of living adequate for the health and well-being of himself and of his family, including food, clothing, housing, and medical care and necessary social services, and the right to security in the event of unemployment, sickness, disability, widowhood, old age or other lack of livelihood in circumstances beyond his control" (United Nations, 1948).

Determinant 1: Environment: Built and Natural (Water, Sanitation, Housing, Agriculture, and Food Production)

Haiti has a land mass of 10,714 square miles—about the size of the state of Maryland in the United States—with just 0.7% covered in water. Over 97% of Haiti has been deforested (Renaud B., & Renaud C., 2010). Much of the forests—durable and precious woods like teak—were used by colonial Europeans and early Americans to build fine furniture, ships, and buildings. Sugarcane did so well in the Caribbean climate that many acres of land were deforested to grow sugarcane.

Those living in poverty continue to deforest Haiti as they rely on the meager $0.10 USD per bucket of charcoal, made from the small remaining trees, to trade for rice to feed their family. Erosion, water shortages, a lack of cooking fuel, and the effects of changed climate patterns resulting from the significantly altered vegetation patterns have contributed to Haiti's poor and inadequate food production, susceptibility to hurricanes (as land-water temperatures have changed), and even destroyed fishing beds, as the silts from eroded runoff reach the coastal areas. These are the environmental conditions that hold Haiti in the grasp of poverty.

Haiti has two rainy seasons, April–June and October–November, and a hurricane season between July and September. The annual rainfall, however, is sporadic and leaves much of Haiti in drought conditions for several months each year. The intimate ties between health and environment are profoundly evident in Haiti—challenging nurses to understand their role in creating and sustaining healthy natural environments.

Haiti's built environment is predominately constructed of cinder blocks and poor grade cement or mud. Building practices are neither regulated nor standardized and do not meet even the most fundamental safe building codes. As was evident in the 2010 earthquake, most structures were not able to withstand seismic activity. Even today, after the influx of international aid, pre-quake building practices continue as Haitians have scrambled to rebuild their lives and to find shelter for their families. With an absence of indoor plumbing, potable water supplies, trash/sanitation services, and a lack of power grids to supply in-home electricity equitably across the population, the built environment also poses a serious challenge for nursing's ability to affect a healthy built environments for Haitians.

Determinant 2: Genetics and Historical Factors

Haiti's written history began in 1492 when Columbus happened to land upon the island—claiming it for Spain and renaming it Hispaniola. The native people of Hispaniola, the Taíno, are all but gone—lost to disease imported from Europe, genocide, and the slavery trade of colonial times (Corbett, 1999). As an unwitting player in the conflicts in Europe, Haiti eventually became a French Colony in 1697. Once known as an agricultural gem, Haiti became a human commodity resource for the French and the American slave trade.

After suffering many violent abuses at the hands of slave owners, in 1804 Haiti threw off its oppressors and became the first and only sovereign nation to gain its independence through a Black slave revolution. The dominant world (White) countries did not recognize Haiti's independence until almost 25 years later—and Haiti did not repay the debt levied by France until the early 1900s. Haiti has never risen from the poverty thus inflicted; add corruption, an uneven international trade position, and excessive exports, and it is clear that Haiti's current poverty remains tied to global drivers. As a Black nation, Haiti was economically and politically ostracized by the industrialized countries that had built their economies on the backs of slavery. The stage had been set for decades of embargos and inequitable trade agreements (Public Broadcasting System [PBS], 2004). While genetics do impact the health of this predominately African-Haitian population with biological risk factors for high blood pressure, stroke, and diabetes, these are not the sole indicators of health related to familial traits. In Haiti, the deep ties to the political and social institution of slavery, and the kidnapping and displacement of millions of Africans during the 300-year slave-trade practice, have proven to be powerful determinants of health. Washington (2002) first coined the term *cultural trauma and collective memory* in relation to how descendants of slavery reconfigured collective memories of the meaning of slavery. From this cultural trauma, Washington hypothesized that descendants of slaves have adopted a type of learned hopelessness, with dreams of citizenship, cultural integration, and respect going unmet (2002). For Haiti, this became a type of national identity that is expressed by the author's Haitian friends even today.

In 2008, Hurricane Gustav decimated Haiti. A U.S. embargo kept essential food supplies from those most in need, so—instead of just losing people to drowning or being swept out to sea or epidemics of dysentery from the contaminated water supplies—countless hundreds also died of starvation (United States Institute of Peace, 2008). A short 2 years later, the quake destroyed lives—killing over 350,000 (Haitian estimates and, having been there, I know that even this number is low). Add these environmental onslaughts to political corruption and tyranny, and mass urbanization, and environmental factors become unreasonable determinants of health that require nurses to work across disciplines to understand and collaborate. Haiti's next big humanitarian emergency is just around the corner.

> When it is a matter of telling the truth and serving the victims, let unwelcome truths be told. (Farmer, 2005, p. 22)

Determinant 3: Economy

It is ironic that the poverty that engulfs Haiti was a key factor in the 2010 loss of life, injury, and disability as a result of the earthquake. While the world had the capability and capacity to respond with millions of dollars in aid and tremendous resources, the trail of aid greatly diminished in less than 2 years after the quake—returning Haiti to its nearly pre-2010 economic state. The difficult day-to-day work of problem solving and maintenance in Haiti is often no match for the more exciting stages of trauma and drama.

In total, 75% of the population is unemployed; 50% live in abject (or absolute) poverty, defined by the World Bank as living on less than $2.00 USD per day or a GNI of $670 USD (World Bank, 2010). As a whole, 78% of the population lives in poverty (about $3.00 USD per day or a GNI of $1123 USD) (World Bank, 2010). Poverty is the inability to make choices and have opportunities. Access to nutritious foods, quality health care, transportation, education, and the ability to self-determine are all based on a person's income. How can the largest health care workforce in the world—with 35 million nurses and midwives (WHO, 2009)—participate in addressing the economy, a cardinal determinant of health? Of the complex variables that plague Haiti's ability to achieve higher levels of national health, barriers hindering the acquisition and retention of necessary funds and knowledge of and systems necessary to handle funds appropriately remain the largest roadblocks. In an informal survey of six prominent deans of Haitian schools of nursing, I found that none taught business skills or theory. In another informal survey (Sare, 2010), 21 senior nursing students were asked if they had a bank account and if they knew how to create a simple budget: 14% said that they had a bank account and none could describe a budget. In another informal survey (Sare, 2011) of 42 university students, none could explain a budget, and a prominent banking leader in Haiti explained that money was spent once he received it and that he could not save any or make future plans for upcoming expenses.

Determinant 4: Education

Currently, no formal standards for nursing practice exist in Haiti. There are approximately 10 schools of nursing that are recognized by the Ministry of Public Health and Population (MSPP) (comparable to a Ministry of Health), but this is not a formal designation. There are potentially hundreds of schools of nursing in Haiti, but they are not regulated; there is no formal oversight of curricula, or faculty qualifications. Because of the extreme nursing shortage in Haiti—one nurse for every 10,000 persons—opportunists take advantage of the lack of oversight and set up "schools of nursing." As one Haitian explained, "If the cleaning lady watches a nurse start an IV, then practices a little by stealing supplies to do so, and then approaches the hospital administrator and says "I am a nurse, see, I can start an IV," there is a good chance that the cleaning lady will be hired as a nurse" (personal communication, senior nursing student, Léogâne, Haiti, January 15, 2010). The student went on to explain that nurses are disrespected—even being spat-upon—and that wages are low compared to other professions—so much so that nurses cannot make enough to provide for basic needs.

Curriculum is often based on foreign models, if it exists at all. In Léogâne's School of Nursing, no curriculum existed, rather, syllabi from U.S. faculty who were willing to share it were used to teach classes. Text books are rare in Haiti and libraries are virtually nonexistent. While some nurses and students have access to computers and the Internet in Port au Prince, students and nurses in rural areas (where 6 million Haitians—or two-thirds of the population—live) find these necessities in sparse supply and primarily reliant on solar power.

Skills labs—if they exist—often have used/broken mannequins and donated supplies. Skills labs are generally too small and inadequately equipped—often with as many as 80 students having access to two mannequins and one indwelling urinary catheter kit. Faculty members do not have any specific training as clinical instructors and many teach as they were taught. Without access to the Internet and current texts, instruction lags behind evidence-based practice guidelines.

Without a course of study for nursing educators—andragogy, curriculum design, implementation, and evaluation—many nursing courses are taught via lecture and focus on rote memory; a learning style and paradigm that does not develop critical thinking skills or attributes. There are no processes to establish, assess, or assure faculty competence. Many Haitian nursing students—as a cultural norm—cannot or may not formally evaluate their teachers.

Professional development and continuous education for the nursing workforce does not exist in Haiti. With the many non government organizations (NGOs) in-country since 2010, there have been some private efforts to improve the quality of nursing practice. As mentioned previously, employers desperate to hire a "nurse" may hire unqualified personnel who may lack even a secondary school education. Health care agencies of all kinds play a key role to understanding why quality and standards in nursing practice in Haiti remain so challenging; if the very industry that employs nurses does not adhere to standard-based nursing practice, then it is very difficult for regulatory agencies—such as the Ministry of Public Health and Population (MSPP) to regulate nursing practice.

Determinant 5: Health Care Services

Health care in Haiti (by an informal report from 10 Haitian nurses working in various health care settings in different locales in Haiti) has improved since 2010 with the influx of NGOs and fiscal resources. Health care tends to be focused in and around Port au Prince. Including Port au Prince, there are seven main cores of health care in Haiti—all as a result of NGOs or international partners having focused on that area. These areas are the Central Plateau (Partners in Health [PIH]), Northern Haiti (in and around Cap Haitian—various NGOs), Jérémie (Haiti Health Foundation), Jacmel (multiple NGOs), St. Marc's (PIH and schools such as Harvard), and Léogâne (multiple NGOs since the January 12, 2010 quake). Outlying areas—from these seven cores—depend on mobile clinics, sporadic NGO involvement, and on the types of volunteers and supplies that are available to help. Some Haitians have never been seen by any type of health care provider, while others may wait with a fractured pelvis for 2 months and have to be carried in a wheelbarrow by friends or family to a mobile clinic 2 days' travel by foot (or, in this case, wheelbarrow) for care. One young man had waited several weeks after a motor-vehicle accident to have his fractured jaw wired with a sterilized coat hanger. Access to quality health care is indeed a tremendous barrier—determinant—to the health and well-being of Haitians.

> If access to health care is considered a human right, who is considered human enough to have that right? (Farmer, 2005, p. 206)

Medications—often donated through NGOs—are not supplied through a dependable needs-based system. Many medications are sold on the black market and are often outdated or have been improperly stored. Visiting any local roadside market, one can find antibiotics, analgesics, an assortment of disease-specific medications, and many alternative therapies as well.

While there are many aspects to consider when assessing health services as a determinant of health, it is not possible to offer more than a cursory overview here. At the heart of Haiti's health care chasms are poverty, lack of education (health literacy), cultural beliefs and practices, and an absolute lack of standards, guidelines, and ethics governing practice and practice settings. Truly, in this regard, Haiti is an NGO Health Care Republic. The opportunities for nurses to leverage their knowledge and skills are without bounds. The leading causes of death in Haiti are nearly all preventable (see Table 21.1) (World Life Expectancy, 2012).

Determinant 6: Policy and Politics—Social Structures

According to a brief prepared by Kristoff and Panarelli (2010) for the U.S. Institute of Peace, there are over 3,000 NGOs working in Haiti (with some estimates as high as 12,000). Many are concerned that Haiti has become a Republic of NGOs—a system that runs parallel to the Haitian government and cannot be regulated. In the early months after the 2010 disaster, many hoped that the Clinton Haiti Foundation would facilitate the registry and coordination of the hundreds of NGOs entering Haiti on a weekly basis, but for a myriad of reasons, NGOs did not cooperate. While concerns about the role of NGOs in Haiti's development have been expressed for decades, these issues have gained increasing prominence following the January 12, 2010 earthquake. "Historically, funneling aid through NGOs has perpetuated a situation of limited government capacity and weak institutions. Haiti looks to NGOs rather than their government for basic public services" (Kristoff & Panarelli, 2010, p. 1).

Thousands of nurses have traveled to Haiti to work in trauma centers, in public health, in maternal–child clinics, with large aid organizations, in local hospitals, and to teach in schools of nursing. Nursing students have traveled there to complete cultural immersion studies, and countless hundreds more dream of going to Haiti to be of service. There is the potential for significant mutual benefit as cultural concepts, ideas, learning, and knowledge are equally exchanged. Given the risk of dependence

TABLE 21.1 Leading Causes of Death (in %)

1. Influenza	10.75
2. HIV/AIDS	10.56
3. Stroke	10.39
4. Diarrheal diseases	7.82
5. Hypertension	5.43
6. Diabetes mellitus	4.37
7. Tuberculosis	4.28
8. Coronary heart disease	3.91
9. Anemia	3.37
10. Meningitis	3.27

and an undermined sociopolitical system resulting from NGO models, nursing must heed the lessons learned from others and continually work to create their own obsolescence as outsiders seeking to solve Haiti's challenges.

With a relatively new president, a new prime minister, many new members of the legislative branch of the government, and many new ministers for the departments within Haiti's government, the challenges of rebuilding Haiti while building systems and infrastructure for health care are staggering. A unique and difficult dilemma that is faced by Haiti's nursing workforce is the mass exodus of nurses and other professionals since the destructive years of the Duvalier rule, the years of political corruption, and extreme poverty. Some estimates place the Haitian diaspora at over 2 million—just since the 1960s. Some refer to this as Haiti's 11th department (recalling that a department is similar to a U.S. state). According to the National Council Licensure Examination for Registered Nurses (NCLEX®) Passers by Region for 2001 to 2005, 2% of 34,000 foreign-trained nurses testing for their U.S. nursing license, or 680 nurses, came from the Caribbean (NCLEX, 2012). It is unknown how many were Haitian, as these data are not recorded in the United States. Recall that with a ratio of just one nurse to 10,000 persons in Haiti, if Haitians made up 10% of this diaspora, this exodus would represent a significant proportion of Haiti's nursing workforce. Haitian nurses also migrate to the United Kingdom and France. Without sound research and a monitoring of nurse migration, the international nursing community cannot help to address this conundrum.

Facing difficult work environments, disrespect, few supplies, poor wages, and an absence of standards, guidelines, and ethics for education and health care, many of Haiti's nurses have chosen and will continue to choose to migrate. Improving working conditions within Haiti is an ethical and economic predicament that has wide-reaching implications for health in Haiti and for Haiti's nurses.

Determinant 7: Individual Lifestyle

Of notable concern is the discernable increase in cars, motos (motorcycles), semi-trucks, heavy equipment, and buses in Haiti. Prior to the 2010 earthquake, major Haitian highways were no more than wide two-lane roads without lane markings. An apt description for driving on Haiti's busy roadways had been "just-in-time"—meaning that the cars, pedestrians that out-number the cars, and even the chickens seemed able to get out of the way of oncoming or passing traffic "just in time." But this is no longer the case.

Few wear seatbelts, if they exist, and there are no regulations, driving schools, or testing necessary to obtain a license. Drivers in Haiti are skilled, but did not drive especially safely prior to January 12, 2010. Over the past

2 years of traveling in Haiti, it is apparent that the roads are congested with many imported vehicles, and no changes were made to the systems and culture of driving to accommodate the increased congestion. Many roads remain damaged from the sink-holes and upheavals from the 2010 earthquake, and improvements have not been made to handle the excessive traffic loads. Motor vehicle accidents have become an endemic problem with no emergency medical system established to respond—and—if one could—congested roadways would most likely block access in an emergency (U.S. Department of State [USDS], 2011).

Indoor air quality is compromised with the burning of charcoal and kerosene. Only about 25% of Haitians have access to toilets or latrines, and public urinating is a common practice. Spitting is also common. Haitians do not wash their hands after handling meat products, after toileting, or after handling other bio-contaminants. Water and soaps are rarely available as they are scarce and precious commodities. Toilet paper is a Western luxury. Haitians are, however, fastidious in their appearance, often wearing clothes that are very clean and ironed. Dental hygiene and bathing are practiced daily during the rainy seasons by using buckets of water.

Anecdotally, tobacco use and alcohol consumption appear to be common. Rum is a major product of Haiti, but somewhat of a luxury item (recall that the average income is less than $2 USD per day). Neither cigarettes nor alcohol are consumed in large quantities by the majority of the population on a regular basis. These are commodities that the wealthy or addictive personalities seek, but no data exist to verify frequency or general use by the population.

The video *Unnatural Causes* (2008), reveals that researchers discovered that the greatest barrier to health and well-being is the lack of self-determination as a result of poverty and unequal access to education. The chronic stressors of not knowing how a family will afford food or pay for school are determinants of health, excess death, and disability, and pose barriers to the education of a competent Haitian nursing workforce. If the determinants of health are not addressed and remedied, then preparing a nursing workforce to assist better, prevent, and mitigate another humanitarian emergency in Haiti may be futile.

RURAL NURSING CONCEPTS: HELPING NURSES IN HAITI TO APPLY THEORY TO PRACTICE

Rural nursing theory, originally published by Long and Weinert in 1989 (see Chapter 1), presents three theoretical statements to describe rural persons' health beliefs and behaviors and the practice of nurses who care for them. Lee and McDonagh (see Chapter 2) provide an update to the rural nursing theory base by recommending the inclusion of six new concepts. The theoretical statements and new concepts are listed in Table 21.2 along with observations of relevance to rural Haitians.

TABLE 21.2 Rural Nursing Theory and Relevance to Haiti

Literature Review: Long and Weinert (chapter 1) *Rural Nursing: Developing the Theory Base*	Observations of Relevance to Haitian Rural Dwellers
"#1 Rural dwellers define health as an ability to work, to be productive, to do usual tasks"	Large percentages of Haitians across urban and rural settings live in poverty; ability to maintain work to feed themselves and family might best explain how health is defined.
"#2 Rural dwellers are self-reliant and resist accepting help or services from those seen as 'outsiders' or from agencies seen as national or regional 'welfare' programs"	Over two-thirds of Haitians do not have access to health care. Persons will walk for miles and wait for hours to access health care. While Haitians are very self-reliant, with the high poverty levels, they embrace any available health care, and philanthropic health care may be all they can afford. No national insurance or safety-net exists.
"#3 Health care providers in rural areas must deal with a lack of anonymity and greater role diffusion . . ."	Anonymity cannot be translated in the same cultural context, but "role diffusion" is especially relevant, as is evidenced by the examples from this chapter.
Lee and McDonagh (chapter 2) Updating the rural nursing theory base.	Observations of relevance to Haitian rural dwellers
New concept #1 ". . . distance . . ." (seeing health care as inaccessible)	Distance is a complex variable in Haiti; transportation may be via foot and take several weeks to reach a destination, a few days by horse or donkey. Others have access to motorized transportation. Distance may not be a relevant cultural context that can be compared, but rural dwellers do feel that all services are centralized in the capital and that the government fails to meet their health care needs.
New concept #2 ". . . resources . . ." (availability of)	Resources are a significant variable impacting health. Equitable deployment of health workers, equitable distribution of health facilities, availability of funds and equipment is a challenge in developed countries, but staggering in developing countries like Haiti.
New concept #3 ". . . health-seeking behavior . . ."	Theories have long supported that health-seeking behaviors are grounded in culture and situational realities. Each culture has unique health-seeking

(continued)

TABLE 21.2 Rural Nursing Theory and Relevance to Haiti (Continued)

Lee and McDonagh (chapter 2) Updating the rural nursing theory base.	Observations of relevance to Haitian rural dwellers
	behaviors that lead to its interpretation of how best to promote healthy relationships in all areas on one's life (spiritual, physical, mental). Health literacy, superstitions founded in folk practices (some Voodoo) and religious beliefs (Haiti is 80% Roman Catholic) affect practices such as birth control and mistrust of health care providers (one corrupt dictator was a physician).
New concept #4 "... choice (to live in a rural community and to choose a health care provider) ..."	Making a conscious decision to live in a rural community is not an option for most Haitians. Those who are place-bound in rural settings are there for economic reasons. Mass urbanization in Haiti is the result of excessive poverty and attempts by persons to make a better life. Rural Haiti is not seen in the same 'return to the land' or retirement attraction as it is in the United States. Choice is not often a viable option. Being trained in urban settings, health care workers rarely export to rural settings (much like the United States)
New avenue #5 "... environmental context ..."	Environmental context is an important theme across borders. Resources needed are specific to a setting. In Haiti, droughts, limited access to potable water, land erosion, hurricanes, poor roads/access, geological instability, and even vector-borne disease are issues that nurses must learn to address.
New concept #6 "... social capital ..."	Social capital is a strength that leads many outsiders to describe Haitians with adjectives such as resilient, hardy, strong, survivors, etc. Health care workers in rural settings across borders must be integrated into the community to build trust and to be effective working with stakeholders and decision makers, e.g., building social capital, support systems, and networks.

NURSES COMING TO THE AID OF NURSES AFTER THE 2010 EARTHQUAKE

There are several nursing organizations outside of Haiti that have worked to help rebuild and build anew the nursing education infrastructure. However, there is not a single organized structure through which nurses can directly assist nurses in Haiti. Many aid organizations (NGOs, the

UN, WHO, and some governmental agencies—like USAID) accept nurses for long-and short-term positions. Some pay for air travel, or in-country transportation, accommodations, food, and security while others require that nurses cover their own expenses. The Haitian MPSS is neither well staffed nor equipped to organize and monitor the influx and origin of nurses who enter the country. Nor are they able to hire consultants or foreign nurses within their ministry. The MSPP is housed in a large Quonset-type hut (a large plastic dome-shaped facility) and is very crowded—with all the offices of the Ministry in one common space—in three rows of desks. It is not the most ideal work environment.

The National Association of Nurses Licensed in Haiti (NANIH) (comparable to the U.S. National State Board of Nursing) is rebuilding their facilities and infrastructure following the earthquake (International Council of Nursing [ICN], 2011). The ICN, with headquarters in Geneva, Switzerland, serves as consultant and advisor to NANIH and has assisted with construction costs. They are also assisting with the rebuilding of the academic structures and system of the National University in Port au Prince, the country's largest college of nursing. The ICN also convened in Haiti in 2011 to assist in planning the infrastructure for the NANIH.

In the United States, Regis College School of Nursing, Science, and Health Professions, located in Massachusetts, is partnering with the National University and the Ministry of Public Health and Population to build a master's in nursing program with a focus on education. Their work has been ongoing since 2007. Many other foreign colleges of nursing have expressed interest in Haiti, but the commitment is expensive and requires a long-term dedication of resources and a champion to carry the project through to completion.

One of the many terrible casualties of the 2010 earthquake was that many leaders and future leaders in Haiti perished in their schools, classrooms, and while at work. Three of Haiti's feminist thinkers, Myriam Merlet, Magalie Marcelin, and Ann Marie Coriolan also perished. Merlet, founder of Enfofamn, sought to raise awareness of women and their issues through the news media; Marcelin helped to establish Kay Fanm (Woman's House), which provided services and shelter to women affected by domestic violence; and Coriolan founded the group Solidarité Fanm Ayisyen (Solidarity With Haitian Women) and advocated for women's issues in the political and social arenas (Deibert, 2010).

The College of Nursing at the National University in Port au Prince lost over 100 student nurses and most of their nursing faculty. How have they carried on? How have they not succumbed to grief and helplessness? The school's dean was at the First International Symposium for Nursing in Haiti, pleading for help to rebuild her school. Her grief was deep and her words came with great difficulty, but she was resolute to help Haiti through nursing; she was resolute that her dear students and colleagues had not died in vain, but would be honored by coming back stronger and better.

As mentioned previously (see Determinant 6), there has been no way to regulate who, what, and when resources reach Haiti. International partners brought a mobile French–English electronic library to Port au Prince, one of eight to be deployed in hospitals, clinics, and nursing schools. The libraries have been donated by the Swiss Nurses Association (ASI), the Geneva University Hospitals (HUG), the University Hospital Centre Vaud (CHUV), and Elsevier USA (ICN, 2011). Unfortunately, most Haitians speak Creole. French is the language of the wealthy, and many schools of nursing are without electricity or even a safe place to house the small library. WHO would like to avoid the supply of inappropriate medicines and equipment to Haiti and ensure that essential medical supplies are identified and provided in order to best support the health relief efforts underway in the country (ICN, 2011).

In the aftermath of the 2010 Haitian earthquake, we had little personal protective equipment, were exposed to every type of human body fluid imaginable, and had no way to wash between patients. I asked my dear colleague if she had had her vaccinations. When she stood and said "No Michele, we are Haitians, we are not worthy of vaccine," I began to work with Direct Relief International (DRI) in Santa Barbara, California, who in turn worked with Merck Pharmaceuticals—to provide basic immunizations for student nurses in Haiti. DRI and Merck were remarkable in their commitment to help nurses.

Many organizations and individuals continue to help Haiti to heal and prosper. It is important to note that most Haitians—and the Creole language—do not have a word that means "empowerment." My Haitian friends and colleagues are most grateful for "speaking goodness into their lives." Perhaps this is the greatest need for every Haitian?

DISCUSSION

As might be imagined, my life forever changed in those fateful days in January 2010. I returned in the summer of 2010 to teach the public health nursing course. The students and I conducted a focused community health assessment (CHA) on water and sanitation and two of the students presented these findings at a UN Health Cluster meeting. From that meeting, a team was formed that began working to drain standing water (thereby decreasing mosquito populations), install more latrines, and educate people living in densely crowded tent cities about gray water and excrement. Cattle, pigs, and goats were kept from children's play areas and common paths, and engineers and their crews were directed to repair broken water pipes. The UN team was very impressed by the nursing students and as one student asked, "Michele, you mean that we can do something about this?" I am not sure more rewarding words could ever be spoken to a teacher!

As a nurse who chose to live in a rural community and work in many rural and frontier communities domestically and internationally, I can confidently assert that those marginalized populations are the very populations that suffer the greatest health care injustices. They are the ones who make up the 2 billion persons who suffer excess death, decreased quality of life, lost work days, and who experience unreasonable suffering and disability. Nowhere have I met so many people who I am honored to know, who are courageous, kind, and generous, than in those dark days during and immediately following the January 12, 2010, earthquake in Haiti. Persons that I have had the privilege to work beside in developing countries have more to give in life skills and lessons than many of us in developed countries may ever have to offer.

It is so hard, I will go with you.

It is one thing to bear witness to, to spout data from, or to offer ideas for reforms and solutions to the challenges facing nurses in Haiti and quite another to walk along side Haiti's nurses; to work with them, help them to design and strengthen their standards, guidelines, ethics, and systems; and to empower Haiti's nurses to address and solve their own challenges. It would seem that the world's largest health care workforce, whose domain is care, might be able to do just that. This is what informs my work, is the purpose of *Nurses for Nurses International*, and what will sustain my jagged journey with Haiti.

REFERENCES

ABC News. (January 17, 2010). *Tens of thousands isolated at quake epicenter North America correspondent Lisa Millar and wires.* Updated January 18, 2010, 00:56:00; Retrieved April 7, 2012, from http://www.abc.net.au/news/2010-01-17/tens-of-thousands-isolated-at-quake-epicentre/1211748

Bailey, L. (January 19, 2010). *Nursing foundation leader discusses health care challenges in Haiti;* Record Update; University of Michigan; Retrieved April 7, 2012, from http://www.ur.umich.edu/update/archives/100119/haitinurse

California Newsreel. (2008). *Unnatural causes.* Retrieved April 10, 2010, from http://www.unnaturalcauses.org/

Central Intelligence Agency (CIA). (2012). *CIA world fact-book-Haiti.* Retrieved April 10, 2012, from https://www.cia.gov/library/publications/the-world-factbook/geos/ha.html

Corbett, R. (1999). *Pre-Columbian Hispaniola—Arawak/Taino Native Americans.* Retrieved April 22, 2012, from http://www.webster.edu/~corbetre/haiti/history/precolumbian/tainover.htm

Deibert, M. (January 25, 2010). *Death and devastation Haunt Haiti's Universities. The Chronicle of Higher Education.* Retrieved April 11, 2012, from http://chronicle.com/article/DeathDevastation-Haunt/63725/

Farmer, P. (2005). *Pathologies of power health, human rights, and the new war on the poor.* Berkeley and Los Angeles, CA: University of California Press.

Institute of Medicine (IOM). (2009). *The U.S. commitment to global health recommendations for the public and private sectors.* Washington, DC: National Academies Press. International Council of Nursing (ICN) (2011). *Rebuilding nursing in Haiti.* Retrieved April 11, 2012, from http://www.icn. http://www.icn.ch/news/whats-new-archives/rebuilding-nursing-in-haiti-1307.html

Institute of Medicine (IOM). (2011). *The future of nursing leading change, advancing health.* Washington, DC: The National Academies Press.

International Council of Nursing (ICN). (2011). *Objectives.* Retrieved April 11, 2012, from http://www.icn.ch/news/objectives/

Kristoff, M., & Panarelli, L. (April 2010) . *Peace brief: Haiti. A republic of NGOs?* United States Institute for Peace. Retrieved April 8, 2012, from http://www.usip.org/publications/haiti-republic-ngos

NCLEX. (2012). *NCLEX examinations.* Retrieved June 16, 2012, from http://www.ncsbn.org/nclex.htm

Public Broadcasting System (PBS) (Compiled by Harper, E.). (2004). *Online NewsHour, Haiti in turmoil.* Retrieved April 22, 2012, from http://www.pbs.org/newshour/bb/latin_america/haiti/history.html

Renaud, B., & Renaud, C. (2010). *World: Haiti's legacy of environmental disaster. New York Times Video.* Retrieved April 8, 2012, from http://www.youtube.com/watch?v=kLmpFHSsGD0

Robert Wood Johnson Foundation (RWJF). (2011). *County health rankings & roadmaps: A healthier nation, county-by-county.* Retrieved April 10, 2012, from http://www.countyhealthrankings.org/app/mississippi/2012/measures/outcomes/37/map

Rural Assistance Center (RAC). (2012). *Frontier.* Health and Human Services Information for Rural America. Retrieved April 9, 2012, from http://www.raconline.org/topics/frontier/

Sare, M. V. (2010). *Informal survey of nursing and healthcare in Haiti.* Hall, MT: Nurses for Nurses International.

Sare, M. V. (2011). *Today, Léogâne.* Hall, MT: NFNI Publishing.

Sebelius, Secretary. (2012). *Statement from Secretary Sebelius for Martin Luther King, Jr. Day—Jan. 2012*. Retrieved May 4, 2012, from http://www.hhs.gov/news/press/2012pres/01/20120113a.html

UNifeed. (January 18, 2010). *Haiti/Léogâne Destruction*. United Nations News and Media. Retrieved April 9, 2012, from http://www.unmultimedia.org/tv/unifeed/d/14325.html

United Nations Development Program (UNDP). (2012). *Human development index*. UNDP. Retrieved April 8, 2012, from http://hdr.undp.org/en/statistics/hdi/

United Nations Drafting Committee (1948). *Article 25, The universal declaration of human rights*. Retrieved December 13, 2012, from http://www.un.org/en/documents/udhr/index.shtmlUN

United States Department of State (USDS). (August 8, 2011). *Travel warning U.S. Department of State, Haiti*. Retrieved June 15, 2012, from http://travel.state.gov/travel/cis_pa_tw/tw/tw_5541.html

United States Institute of Peace (USIP). (2008). *Haiti after the storms: Weather and conflict*. Retrieved May 4, 2012, from http://www.usip.org/publications/haiti-after-the-storms-weather-and-conflict

Washington, E. R. (2002). Cultural trauma: Slavery and the formation of the African-American identity. *American Journal of Sociology, 108*(3), 689–691.

World Bank, The. (October 8, 2006). *Haiti at a glance*. Retrieved April 7, 2012, from http://siteresources.worldbank.org/INTHAITI/Resources/Haiti.AAG.pdf

World Bank, The. (2010). *Haiti data and statistics*. Retrieved April 7, 2012, from http://web.worldbank.org/WBSITE/EXTERNAL/COUNTRIES/LACEXT/HAITIEXTN/0,,menuPK:338204~pagePK:141132~piPK:141109~theSitePK:338165,00.htm

World Health Organization (WHO). (2008). *Introduction to social determinants of health (SDH) and political strategies for action*. Retrieved April 7, 2012, from http://www.who.int/social_determinants/en/

World Health Organization (WHO). (March 2011). *Haitian health care: A follow-up*. Retrieved April 7, 2012, from http://www.who.int/features/2011/haiti/en/index.html

World Life Expectancy. (2012). *World health rankings Haiti*. Retrieved June 16, 2012, from http://www.worldlifeexpectancy.com/country-health-profile/haiti

FURTHER READING

Encyclopedia of the Nations. (2012). *Climate—Haiti—average, annual*. Retrieved April 11, 2012, from http://www.nationsencyclopedia.com/Americas/Haiti-CLIMATE.html#b#ixzz1rTROzabS

OxFam. (2009). *Haiti, a gathering storm.* Retrieved April 9, 2012, from http://www.oxfam.org/sites/www.oxfam.org/files/haiti-gathering-storm-en-0911.pdf

Padgett, T. (November 19, 2010) *Underneath Haiti, another big quake waiting to occur. TIME World.* Retrieved April 7, 2012, from http://www.time.com/time/world/article/0,8599,2031863,00.html#ixzz1rQBZLncI)

United Nations Development Program (UNDP). (2011). *Human development index and its components.* UNDP. Retrieved April 8, 2012, from http://hdr.undp.org/en/media/HDR_2011_EN_Table1.pdf

Winters, C. A., & Lee, H. L. (Eds.). (2006). *Rural nursing concepts, theory and practice* (2nd ed.) New York, NY: Springer Publishing.

Winters, C. A., & Lee, H. L. (Eds.) (2010). *Rural nursing concepts, theory and practice* (3rd ed.) New York, NY: Springer Publishing.

Chapter 22
ENVIRONMENTAL RISK REDUCTION FOR RURAL CHILDREN
Wade G. Hill and Patricia Butterfield

RURAL LIVING IS OFTEN PORTRAYED as inherently healthy and wholesome, with children enjoying the benefits of fresh air and clean water. The idealized view of rural life is perpetuated by what some have referred to as the "agrarian myth," in which youngsters thrive on living away from the artificiality and materialism of cities (Kelsey, 1994, p. 1171). However, the realities of rural living and their requisite patterns of environmental exposure are complex, dynamic, and multidimensional. Exposure risks to children vary by place, by time, and by age. The risks also vary by parents' occupations, seasonal changes, and jurisdictional policies addressing the use and disposal of local toxicants. Each of these factors, plus many more, creates a complicated web of exposures that influence current and future risks of disease. Exposure patterns in children are so multifaceted that it is not unusual to see very different measures of exposure among three or four children living under the same roof. Such are the challenges in understanding environmental health risks to children living in rural communities.

However, the challenges inherent in assessing complex exposures in children are, in many ways, dwarfed by the ability of the current health care system to document patterns of exposure in groups at risk. Neither exposures to biological and chemical agents nor their potential health consequences (e.g., asthma, neurodegenerative diseases) are recorded systematically in medical databases. Health providers have a superficial understanding of only the most prevalent exposures (e.g., lead) and are typically at a loss to answer clients' questions about other common exposure risks (e.g., pesticides, solvents, metals).

For more than 200 years, rural areas have been considered the "dumping ground" of a production-based economy. Items (e.g., nuclear waste, antiquated military supplies) and activities (e.g., mining, smelting) considered dangerous, distasteful, or requiring large plots of land have been preferentially located in remote parts of the country. Contaminants from such historic activities have left a legacy of risks for local residents. Since the contamination is not routinely discovered until decades later, the culpable group often can no longer be located; the community must rely on federal resources for cleanup and remediation resources. Typically, rural municipalities lack both the financial, technical, and scientific expertise (e.g., laboratories, behavioral researchers) to understand local exposures and their commensurate health risks. Small county and regional health departments in the United States, which have been understaffed and over-mandated since September 11, 2001, often field questions about environmental risks in their area, but lack the time and money to fully pursue investigative efforts. Rural families who live in unincorporated areas may live adjacent to agricultural (e.g., combined animal feeding operations) and industrial facilities, but may be unaware of risks associated with such facilities.

Despite risk patterns that may pose a threat to young children, contaminant patterns in rural communities are understudied and rural citizens are often underrepresented in environmental health research (Malcoe, Lynch, Keger, & Skaggs, 2002). Research in rural communities has focused almost exclusively on the sequelae from a specific agent (e.g., mercury, arsenic) or contaminant site (e.g., Environmental Protection Agency [EPA] Superfund site). Such research has provided an important foundation about the health consequences of living adjacent to a mine, railroad yard, or waste disposal site. However, examining environmental health risks from a single-agent perspective provides a myopic view of risks to a family or community, rather than providing families with answers about their overall health risks and what they can do to minimize such risks.

Requirements of rural nursing practice necessarily follow trends in the health status of populations, demographic changes, and the dynamic nature of the determinants of health, illness, and safety. From a population view, perhaps no segment of our society requires more attention in promoting health than young children. It is known that the most rapid mental growth occurs during early childhood and that the early years are critical in the development of intelligence, personality, and social behavior (Bellamy, 2002). Equally important is an understanding that children are particularly susceptible to environmental exposures, as the exploratory behaviors of childhood are the principal ways that children learn (Moya, Bearer, & Etzel, 2004).

Rural nurses have a unique opportunity to identify and intervene in cases where environmental exposures to children exist. Despite commonly held notions that rural environments offer isolation from environmental contaminants, many rural areas offer the most potent environmental exposures in the United States. For example, the state of Montana currently has 11 sites of industrial contamination listed on the National Priority List (Superfund), and ranks 14th among the states in land releases of toxic contaminants (Scorecard.org, 2012). Although rural childhood environmental exposures may result from effluents of extractive industries or other industrial sites, many chronic environmental exposures occur within the home, where caregivers and nurses have significant capacity for intervention. By making common-sense, low-cost changes to behaviors, caregivers of young children can prevent environmental exposures that may manifest in negative health outcomes.

ENVIRONMENTAL RISK REDUCTION THROUGH NURSING INTERVENTION AND EDUCATION

The Environmental Risk Reduction through Nursing Intervention and Education (ERRNIE) study was a 6-year project designed primarily to (a) determine the prevalence of multiple environmental exposures among rural children; and (b) deliver and evaluate environmental risk-reduction education to rural households by public health nurses through a randomized controlled trial. Because nurses generally feel unprepared to manage environmental health issues (Van Dongen, 2002), the ERRNIE project also evaluated the capacity and needs of public health nurses to integrate environmental health into their practice. The ERRNIE project capitalizes on the existing public health infrastructure that currently accesses at-risk populations through programs such as Women, Infants, and Children (WIC), immunization clinics, and the Head Start program, among others. Childhood exposures of interest in the ERRNIE study are those that occur in or around homes and include environmental tobacco smoke (ETS), radon, carbon monoxide (CO), lead, impurities in well water, and in-wall moisture as a marker for potential mold growth. In the discussion that follows we focus on the second objective of the ERRNIE study, to deliver and evaluate environmental risk-reduction education to rural households by public health nurses through a randomized controlled trial. Specifically, improvements in self-efficacy and precaution adoption among participants will be discussed. Full study findings have been published by Butterfield, Hill, Postma, Butterfield, and Odom-Maryon (2011).

The conceptual basis for the ERRNIE project is the Translational Environmental Research in Rural Areas (TERRA) model (Figure 22.1) which posits that environmental risk-reduction (ERR) interventions have the ability to change both environmental risks, as well as family members perceptions of risk. Following positive changes in actual and perceived risks, health and behavioral outcomes are related to both proximal and distal outcomes (Butterfield & Postma, 2009).

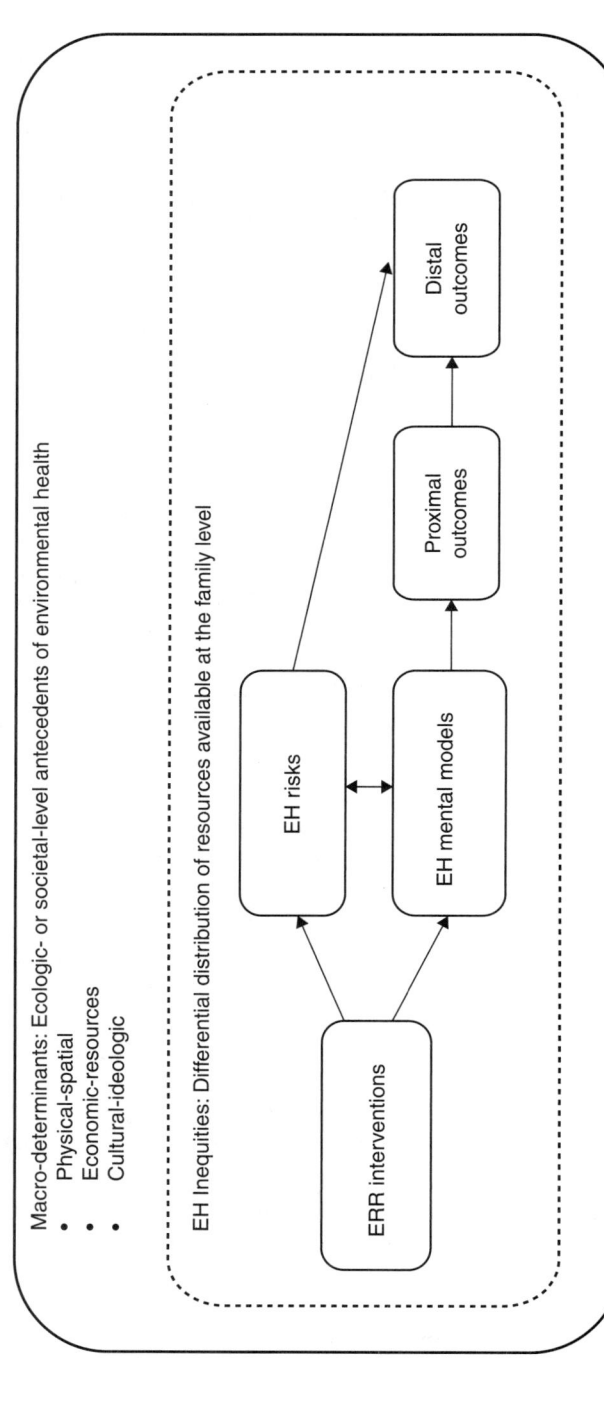

FIGURE 22.1 TERRA framework: Key concepts and relationships. EH = environmental health. ERR = environmental risk reduction.

METHODS

Design

Participants in the randomized controlled trial resided in either Gallatin County, Montana, or Whatcom County, Washington. Performance sites were selected based on similar demographic profiles and added geographic diversity. All participants were recruited from county public health departments, community contacts, and similar community social service agencies. Eligibility criteria included (a) live outside of city limits, (b) household income at or less than 250% of the federal poverty level, (c) a child in the home aged 7 years or younger, (d) English literacy, and (e) use of a nonmunicipal water source. After random assignment, data on self-efficacy and risk-reduction behaviors associated with household environmental risks (radon, carbon monoxide, lead, water contaminants, in-wall humidity, environmental tobacco smoke) were collected at baseline and again at 3 months for both intervention and control groups. The intervention consisted of four home visits over a 4- to 6-week period, each lasting approximately 1 hour and containing tailored information about risks present within the home, determined by baseline testing. Public health nurses offered precautionary information to participants of the intervention group, intended to effectively address the risk in question and to offer no-cost or low-cost solutions. Participants in the control group received a letter containing their baseline testing results, threshold values, and referral to the local public health agency.

Measurement

Standard demographic and socioeconomic questions were asked, in addition to measurements that addressed study aims; questions were focused on self-efficacy for environmental risk reduction and precaution adoption. Self-efficacy is defined as one's belief in his or her ability to carry out a specific behavior; it was measured in two ways. First, a general self-efficacy scale was constructed, according to Bandura's Guide for Constructing Self-Efficacy Scales (Bandura, 2001), containing 11 items. Likewise, a second set of 18 risk items in six subscales was developed to address specific actions related to each environmental risk of interest. The instrument was circulated among environmental health experts to assess content validity and pilot-tested to evaluate reliability (all Cronbach's alpha ≥ 0.80).

Precaution adoption for environmental risks was measured according to Weinstein's Precaution Adoption Process Model (Weinstein & Sandman, 2002). This model observes that precaution adoption may occur in five steps including:

1. Unaware of issue
2. Unengaged by issue

3. Decided not to act
4. Decided to act
5. Action taken

For this study, precaution adoption was measured both by a sum of positive steps toward action for all agents included in the study and for each individual agent (six risks).

FINDINGS

Sample Description

Participants included 235 adults, randomized by household into the treatment group ($n = 119$) and control group ($n = 116$). Over 90% of primary adults enrolled were female and non-Hispanic Whites. The average age of participants was between 30 and 35 years, and about 80% of participants were married. As expected, household incomes were low, with more than half reporting annual incomes between $25,000 and $50,000. No significant differences were found between intervention and control groups on demographic or socioeconomic factors.

Self-Efficacy and Precaution Adoption

The analysis examined the improvement in self-efficacy and precaution adoption, comparing the treatment and control groups from baseline to 3 months. Treatment effects were examined using both linear and logistic regression modeling through the use of generalized estimating equation (GEE) models. Overall, at 3 months, the intervention group had significantly higher scores on general environmental self-efficacy, on all six subscales of risk-specific self-efficacy, on general precaution adoption, and on five of six subscales of risk-specific precaution adoption.

For general self-efficacy, the intervention appeared to increase scores by about 10 points (100-point scale) ($b = 9.5$; 95% CI = 6.5, 12.5). The greatest impact of the intervention appeared for risk-specific self-efficacy for radon (intervention = 86.2 ± 22.1; control 69.7 ± 27.7; $p < .001$) and lead (intervention = 89.2 ± 15.6; control 76.6 ± 22.2; $p < .001$). The smallest increase in self-efficacy was found for environmental tobacco smoke (intervention = 94.6 ± 9.8; control 90.3 ± 14.0; $p < .002$) although significant differences were still present.

Participants of the intervention also showed significant improvements in precaution adoption relative to the control group. About 70% of the intervention group reported some improvement in precaution adoption compared to only 30% of the control group (OR = 3.9; 95% CI = 2.2, 6.7; $p < .001$). Although the intervention had minimal impact on precautions taken for environmental tobacco smoke, significant differences existed between treatment and controls for precautions about lead, carbon monoxide, radon, in-wall humidity, and well-water contaminants.

DISCUSSION

Data from the ERRNIE project support the efficacy of environmental risk-reduction interventions among rural populations that receive public health services. These data indicate that risks to rural families can be modified with nursing intervention within the home. Although each exposure carries unique risk of health consequences, exposures that occur in or around the home may be prevented with simple low-cost solutions.

Behaviors aimed at reducing environmental health risks for children focusing in or around the home have been organized into four main categories: (a) environmental modification; (b) caretaker vigilance; (c) food; (d) home and personal hygiene; (e) and behavioral modification (Schneider & Freeman, 2000). Many of the behaviors within these categories require little to no resources and have the potential to yield significant benefits in risk reduction from exposure to environmental contaminants. Environmental modification includes actions such as placing doormats at home entry areas to collect potential contaminants, designating places isolated from living areas where dirty clothes and shoes are stored, and keeping household chemicals out of reach of children. Caretaker vigilance requires adults who are responsible for children to consider issues such as the hygiene and food preparation practices of day care services and not allowing anyone to smoke in the presence of their children. Food, home, and personal hygiene simply directs adults to wash foods well, maintain safe food cooking and storage practices, and teach children the importance of hand washing. Finally, important aspects of behavioral modification with respect to children's environmental health include enforcing the use of utensils for eating and running tap water for a period of time before drinking.

Changing household-centered environmental risks among rural families requires focus on behavioral determinants such as self-efficacy and precaution adoption. Although low-cost solutions exist for predominant household environmental risks, families with young children must have the tools to understand risk and must feel confident taking action when risks are present. As with many behavioral changes, it is useful to consider action itself as a series of steps; precautions leading to risk abatement are not discrete outcomes but rather a series of decisions about commitment to taking action. The ERRNIE was strengthened by this approach to behavioral change. Future studies will need to evaluate whether self-efficacy and precaution adoption can modify actual exposures, by using long-term follow-up with objective measures such as household testing and biomarkers.

CONCLUSIONS AND IMPLICATIONS FOR RURAL NURSING

Although many environmental health problems are necessarily addressed on a population level through policy and regulation, changes in health protection can be slow and may often be at odds with other forces in the social milieu, such as economics. Although policy may be ideal for broad-based reform to prevent childhood exposures to environmental contaminants, nurses working at the household level have a significant capacity to assist families in understanding and identifying health risks and risk-avoidance strategies.

Families and communities often look to nurses for guidance on health risks, especially those associated with hazards at home or work (National Environmental Education & Training Foundation, 2002). Rural areas provide a context for increased risk of environmental exposures for children, risks that may have both acute and long-term health consequences. Lack of resources, regulatory fragmentation, and the inadequacy of data and data systems contribute to this context (Center for Rural Health Practice, 2004), and rural nurses should become increasingly aware of how they can improve the environmental health of their communities.

ACKNOWLEDGMENT

This research was financially supported by National Institutes of Health (NIH) Grant No. 1 P20 RR17670-01, Center for Environmental Health Faculty; 1K01NR009984; 1 R01 NR009239-01A1.

REFERENCES

Bandura, A. (2001). *A guide for constructing self-efficacy scales*. Palo Alto, CA: Stanford University.

Bellamy, C. (2002). Child health. In R. Detels, J. McEwen, R. Beaglehole, & H. Tanaka (Eds.), *Oxford textbook of public health* (4th ed., pp. 1603–1622). Oxford, UK: Oxford University Press.

Butterfield, P. G., Hill, W. G., Postma, J., Butterfield, P. W., & Odom-Maryon, T. (2011). Effectiveness of a household environmental health intervention delivered by rural public health nurses. *American Journal of Public Health*, *101*(S1), S262–S270.

Butterfield, P. G., & Postma, J. (2009). The TERRA framework: Conceptualizing rural environmental health inequities through an environmental justice lens. *Advances in Nursing Science, 32*(2), 107–117.

Center for Rural Health Practice. (2004). *Bridging the health divide: The rural public health research agenda.* Pittsburgh, PA: University of Pittsburgh.

Kelsey, T. W. (1994). The agrarian myth and policy responses to farm safety. *American Journal of Public Health, 84,* 1171–1177.

Malcoe, L. H., Lynch, R. A., Keger, M. C., & Skaggs, V. J. (2002). Lead sources, behaviors, and socioeconomic factors in relation to blood lead of Native American and White children: A community-based assessment of a former mining area. *Environmental Health Perspectives, 110*(Suppl. 2), 221–231.

Moya, J., Bearer, C. F., & Etzel, R. A. (2004). Children's behavior and physiology and how it affects exposure to environmental contaminants. *Pediatrics, 113*(Suppl. 3), 996–1006.

National Center for Environmental Health. (2003). *Second National Report on Human Exposure to environmental chemicals.* Retrieved July 28, 2004, from http://www.cdc.gov/exposurereport/2nd/pdf/secondner.pdf

National Environmental Education & Training Foundation. (2002). Nurses and environmental health: Success through action. In *Agency for toxic substances and disease registry* (Ed.), Washington, DC: Author.

Needleman, H. L., Schell, A., Bellinger, D., Leviton, A., & Allred, E. N. (1990). The long-term effects of exposure to low doses of lead in childhood. An 11-year follow-up report. *New England Journal of Medicine, 322,* 83–88.

Pirkle, J. L., Flegal, K. M., Bernert, J. T., Brody, D. J., Etzel, R. A., & Maurer, K. R. (1996). Exposure of the US population to ETS: The Third National Health and Nutrition Examination Survey, 1988 to 1991. *Journal of the American Medical Association, 275,* 1233–1240.

Schneider, D., & Freeman, N. (2000). *Childrens environmental health: Reducing risk in a dangerous world.* Washington, DC: American Public Health Association.

Scorecard.org. (2012). *Land contamination report: Montana.* Retrieved July 30, 2012, from http://scorecard.goodguide.com/env-releases/state-choose-issue.tcl?usps_abbrev=MT

Van Dongen, C. J. (2002). Environmental health and nursing practice: A survey of registered nurses. *Applied Nursing Research, 15*(2), 67–73.

Weinstein, N. D., & Sandman, P. M. (2002). *The precaution adoption process model.* San Francisco, CA: Jossey-Bass.

Chapter 23

THE CULTURE OF RURAL COMMUNITIES: AN EXAMINATION OF RURAL NURSING CONCEPTS AT THE COMMUNITY LEVEL

Nancy E. Findholt

IN THE LATE 1970S, FACULTY members and graduate students at Montana State University-Bozeman College of Nursing initiated a 6-year ethnographic study to explore the health beliefs and practices of rural Montana residents (Long & Weinert, 1989; Weinert & Long, 1987). Several of the concepts that emerged from this research were later validated by a quantitative survey and became the foundation for a theory of rural nursing. These concepts included work beliefs and health beliefs, isolation and distance, self-reliance, lack of anonymity, outsider or insider, and old-timer or newcomer. My purpose in this chapter is to describe how these concepts were manifested over 2 decades later and at the community level in three rural communities in Oregon.

The findings that I present here represent a portion of the results I obtained from a study (Findholt, 2004) examining the influence of rurality on community participation in a community health development initiative. Although many researchers have sought to identify the factors that influence community participation, most previous studies have focused on the characteristics of people who participate and those who do not, the reasons people choose to participate, or the characteristics of organizations that facilitate or hinder participation (Wandersman & Florin, 2000). Very few investigators have explored how community characteristics affect participation, yet these characteristics may have a significant effect on the forms or levels of participation that are possible, as well as on the outcomes of participation that can be achieved. This study of rural community participation was guided by a conceptual framework that posited that the ability of a rural community to participate in health development is both facilitated and hindered by factors in the culture, physical setting, and social structure of the community. Among the cultural factors included in the conceptual framework were three that were derived from the Montana State University-Bozeman research. These were (a) the priority given to health, (b) perceived efficacy of collective action, and (c) insider or outsider differentiation.

PRIORITY GIVEN TO HEALTH

Priority given to health was defined as the priority assigned to health programs as compared to economic programs at the community level. It corresponded to the concept of "work beliefs and health beliefs." The Montana State University-Bozeman study found that rural residents assessed their health needs in relation to work roles and work activities (Weinert & Long, 1987). Being productive in their role was of primary importance to these individuals, and health problems were often ignored unless they interfered with the ability to work. On the basis of these findings, I proposed in the current study that rural communities would place a higher value on economic development than on health development.

PERCEIVED EFFICACY OF COLLECTIVE ACTION

Perceived efficacy of collective action referred to the belief of community members in their ability to work together to solve problems. This cultural variable corresponded to the concept of "self-reliance." The Montana State University-Bozeman findings revealed that rural people were self-reliant in coping with personal and family health problems and preferred self-care, or care provided by family and friends, over professional care (Weinert & Long, 1987). Thus, in the current study I proposed that rural residents, as a whole, would have confidence in their collective ability to solve problems, including problems related to health.

INSIDER OR OUTSIDER DIFFERENTIATION

Finally, insider or outsider differentiation was a phrase chosen to refer to the degree to which community members, as a group, accepted and trusted individuals based upon their tenure in the community. It was derived from the concepts of "insider or outsider" and "old-timer or newcomer." The ethnographic data collected in Montana suggested that rural people organized their social environment around these concepts and determined who to accept and who to trust based upon variables such as length of residence, family history, and type of occupation (Weinert & Long, 1987).

Therefore, I anticipated that in a rural community a health development leader who was well-known to residents and perceived as an insider would be more likely accepted than a leader who was viewed as an outsider.

I did not include the concepts of "isolation and distance" and "lack of anonymity" in the conceptual framework for this study and, therefore, they were not among the cultural factors that I intentionally explored. However, as described in this chapter, some of the qualitative findings did provide insight into the presence of these characteristics in the rural communities.

METHODS

This research employed a multiple-case study design featuring three communities that were engaged in the Community Health Improvement Partnership, a health development initiative offered by the Office of Rural Health (ORH) (2003) in Oregon. Besides being selected for their involvement in the health development effort, the communities chosen as cases were required to meet specific criteria for rurality that were established using the Rural–Urban Commuting Area (RUCA) scale. The RUCA scale classifies census tracts based upon size and daily commuting patterns (Rural Health Research Center, 2002). Communities participating in this study were required to have a main town of no more than 9,999 people, no primary or secondary commuting flow greater than 5% to an urban area, and no secondary flow greater than 30% to a large town. I used these criteria to restrict the sample to communities with small populations that were unlikely to be influenced by urban culture. I labeled the three communities chosen for the sample Communities A, B, and C.

I collected data reported in this chapter through key informant interviews and focus groups with community members. The key informants were health professionals or members of local health boards. The focus group participants included school administrators, small business owners, retirees, employees of social service organizations, and others from the nonhealth sectors of the community. All of the respondents were participants in the health development planning team. I conducted 21 key informant interviews and six focus groups.

I designed the interview questions to solicit the respondents' perceptions of their community and of community members' views, rather than their personal opinions. To assess the priority given to health, I asked the respondents how their community ranked health in comparison with other concerns, such as the economy, environment, or infrastructure. I assessed perceived efficacy of collective action by asking the respondents whether most residents believed that by working together they could bring about general improvements in the community, and whether residents believed they had the collective ability to improve the community's health. I assessed insider or outsider differentiation by asking whether the leader of the health development initiative was perceived by residents as an insider and whether this perception had an effect on their acceptance of the leader.

I used semi-structured interviews to facilitate comparability of the data across communities; however, I also encouraged the respondents to describe other community characteristics they believed had influenced participation in the health development initiative. It was through these opportunities that the comments concerning isolation and lack of anonymity emerged.

Data analysis occurred concurrently with data collection and consisted of three interwoven processes, described by Miles and Huberman (1994). These were data reduction, data display, and conclusion drawing and verification. Data reduction involved simplifying and abstracting the raw data through a process of writing summaries, coding, and writing memos. Data display occurred as I compressed the data and organized it into matrices. I developed within-case displays first, and later "stacked" these to create cross-case displays. I accomplished conclusion drawing and verification by making contrasts and comparisons across different communities and different data sources, looking for evidence of patterns and examining exceptions to patterns, following up on surprises, and looking for negative evidence.

DESCRIPTION OF THE COMMUNITIES

The communities that participated in this study were not towns, but were regions with boundaries that corresponded to the service area of the local hospital. The service area boundaries were delineated by the Office of Rural Health (2003) when the communities were chosen to participate in the health development initiative. Table 23.1 shows demographics of Communities A, B, and C.

Community A was, in many respects, the neediest and most rural of the three communities. It was a sparsely populated and isolated coastal region, 72 miles by winding roads from the county seat, with the oldest and poorest residents and an economy that was floundering. The traditional industries of forestry and fishing had declined significantly in recent years, forcing many families to leave the area. An effort was being made to attract tourists and to recruit new businesses, but at the time of this study, the economy remained depressed.

Community B encompassed a large portion of a county located in the ranch and farm lands of eastern Oregon. Of the three communities included in the study, Community B was the farthest from a metropolitan area of 50,000 or more residents. However, its main town was over twice as large as Community A's, and a major interstate highway traversed the community. Besides agriculture, which was a large component of the economy,

TABLE 23.1 Selected Demographic Characteristics of Study Communities as Compared with Oregon

Community characteristic	Community A	Community B	Community C	Oregon
Size	7,641 residents with one main town, population 4,230	14,266 residents with one main town, population 9,840	44,479 residents with two main towns, population 9,532 and 5,903	N/A
Median age	47.3	45	44	40
% White race	91.7	94.3	90.6	82.7
% below poverty	15.8	14.4	13.9	11.6
% Population age 25+ without high school diploma	19.6	20	15.1	14.9

Note: From *Demographic-Socioeconomic, and Health Status Report*, by Office of Rural Health, 2003, Oregon Health Sciences University, Portland, and from *Oregon Population Report*, by Portland State University, Population Research Center, 2002, Portland State University, Oregon.

many people were employed in human services (health care, education, and social services) or in wood products manufacturing, an industry that had been developed to replace the loss of jobs in forestry. Demographic statistics for this region revealed a community that was older and poorer than the state as a whole, yet was younger and less poor than Community A.

Community C was the largest, least rural, and least needy of the study communities. This community was an entire county located on the coast in western Oregon. There were two main towns in the county, both of which were less than 60 miles from a major metropolitan corridor. The region was popular as a weekend and vacation retreat and as a retirement destination, and had an economy based on tourism. Residents described the community as having two populations: (a) the retirees, who were generally well educated and financially comfortable, and (b) the people who struggled to make ends meet by working in the tourist industry. Both groups were quite transient; the community had few long-term residents. Overall, the population was poorer, older, and less educated than the state as a whole, but was closer to the state demographic averages than either Communities A or B.

RESULTS

Priority Given to Health

The case study data revealed that the priority given to health matters, in comparison with the economy, was relatively high in these communities.

Although some of the respondents believed that economic development or issues such as infrastructure improvement and education were more important to their community than health development, approximately half of the people from each study site said that health was one of their community's top concerns.

One reason that was cited for the high priority given to health was the change in the communities' demographics. Respondents explained that as the percentage of residents who were poor or old had increased, there had been a corresponding increase in the need for health care services, which in turn had placed a burden on the community, resulting in greater attention being given to health issues. In Communities A and C, the influx of retirees was also cited as a reason for the high priority given to health. It was noted that the retirees expected adequate health care services. Furthermore, respondents in all of the study sites observed that health had become a higher priority in their communities as local leaders learned that to recruit business and to attract newcomers they needed to have a strong health care system.

Perceived Efficacy of Collective Action

The degree to which residents had confidence in their collective ability to improve the community varied across the study sites. Most of the respondents in Community A reported that residents believed that by working together they could achieve positive change. Similarly, in Community B it was noted that some, and possibly most, of the residents had confidence in collective action. However, in Community C over half of the people I interviewed stated that a large segment of the population was pessimistic or negative about community efforts.

In contrast to the varying degrees of confidence concerning general community improvement, the findings show that residents in all of the communities were quite skeptical about their ability to resolve community health problems. A primary reason given for the skepticism was that the complexity and magnitude of the rural health care crisis made the problems seem overwhelming. However, lack of experience in making health improvements and the failure of other social programs were also cited as factors that contributed to residents' skepticism.

Insider or Outsider Differentiation

In Communities A and C two people in each community were identified as being leaders of the health development initiative. One of these was viewed as a community insider and the other as an outsider. In Community B only one person was identified as the leader. She was well-known among members of the agricultural sector, but was unknown to other residents.

Whether leaders were perceived as insiders or outsiders appeared to have little effect on how they were accepted by residents in any of the study sites. Although a few respondents said that familiarity was essential in establishing credibility and trust, most thought that the leader's skills and personality were more important. It is interesting that one theme that emerged across the communities was that having a leader who was unknown was beneficial to the health development effort in that it allowed the process to be perceived as unbiased and impartial. Respondents explained that in a small community where residents know the leaders' opinions on issues, they are apt to assume that planning projects led by a known leader will be slanted in favor of that leader's agenda.

Although the concepts of insider versus outsider and old-timer versus newcomer had little relevance in terms of the communities' acceptance of the health development leader, these concepts did emerge as factors that defined, and in some cases divided, the residents in two of the study sites. In Communities A and B, individuals who had resided in these communities for as long as 24 years were described by themselves or by others as newcomers, a finding that suggests that they were not fully integrated into the community. In addition, many of the respondents in Community A reported that tension existed among the newcomers, who were interested in changing the community, and the old-timers, who wanted things to remain the same. On the other hand, in Community C several respondents commented that the concepts of old-timer and newcomer had little meaning because there were so many newcomers. As one person stated, "We're so used to different people.... It's not something that divides the community at all."

Lack of Anonymity

Lack of anonymity was mentioned only in Community A. Respondents there noted that one of the challenges of serving on a health planning team in a small community was that team members knew each other well and interacted often, thus they were reluctant to be confrontational or to express opinions that conflicted with others in the group. This had the effect of reducing openness during discussions. One person observed, "That's the thing that I think is the hardest part about this process in a small community, is the inability to ... be frank about things."

Isolation and Distance

The comments concerning isolation and distance emerged during discussions of collective efficacy. Because of the distances that separated the study communities from larger communities, respondents perceived that they were isolated. For example, one individual from Community A observed that the next largest community was 70 miles away and "may as well be on the moon."

Some of the respondents believed that their community's isolation was a positive factor in that residents realized they needed to work together to solve problems. As one person explained,

> We're just not sitting there, looking for someone else to solve the problems because, you know, we're out here in all this ground and there ain't no cavalry. There's no cavalry. We've just got to figure out what to do.

However, it was also noted that isolation and distance contributed to a sense of collective depression, a sense of skepticism about whether positive change was possible, and a feeling of being disenfranchised. Furthermore, isolation made it difficult for rural communities to solve problems because their access to resources was very limited.

DISCUSSION

The discovery that health development was a rather high priority in these communities was unexpected in light of the earlier findings from Montana. One explanation for the inconsistency between this study's findings and those reported by Montana State University-Bozeman researchers might be that many of the Montana subjects were people who were still working, whereas the participants in the current study were from aging communities with many residents who were no longer working. Just as it is logical to assume that an individual's interest in health would increase with age, so too might a community's interest in health increase as its population ages. It is important to note, however, that one of the reasons cited for the high priority given to health in the Oregon communities was that health services were necessary for economic development. This perspective of health as a means to an economic end was very similar to the Montana observations.

The high level of skepticism among residents concerning their collective ability to resolve community health problems was also unexpected, given that Weinert and Long (1987) had found that rural people had confidence in their ability to manage personal and family health problems. It is possible that Oregon residents had less confidence in their ability to address health concerns than Montana residents had. However, it is also likely that solving community health problems was perceived by rural people as different, and perhaps more complex, than solving problems pertaining to their own health or the health of family members.

Another finding that was unanticipated was that the communities' acceptance of the health development leader was not, for the most part, influenced by residents' perceptions of the leader as an insider or an outsider. I had assumed that if the concepts of insider and outsider divided the community, which was clearly the case in Community A, then insider status would be a critical element in assuring that the leader was accepted. However, the respondents' comments suggested that in a small community where people know the local leaders and are aware of their opinions, familiarity might actually hinder residents' acceptance of the leader. This finding relates to lack of anonymity, which is discussed next.

The case study data pertaining to lack of anonymity were consistent with those obtained by Weinert and Long (1987). The comments made by respondents in Community A concerning the difficulties of serving on a planning team with people they knew well were very similar to remarks made by rural nurses who were part of the Montana sample. These nurses had reported that because their patients were often also their neighbors, friends, or family members, it was difficult for them to separate their professional and personal roles (Long & Weinert, 1989).

The findings pertaining to the residents' perception of their isolation were inconsistent with Weinert and Long's (1987) results. Although the Oregon respondents described their communities as isolated, Montana residents who lived outside of town and traveled more than 50 miles to receive routine health care did not view themselves as isolated (Long & Weinert, 1989).

In summary, only one of the concepts that were identified in the early Montana research was evident in the community level data collected in Oregon. This concept was lack of anonymity, a characteristic pertaining more to the small size of a community than to rurality per se.

CONCLUSION

These findings, drawn from a study of rural community participation in a health development initiative, provide insight into the culture of rural communities and serve to extend rural nursing theory by revealing how the concepts identified in the initial theory work were manifested at the community level in Oregon. The many inconsistencies between this study's findings and those of the early Montana research may be due to several factors, but one likely cause is that the culture of rural communities has changed in the 30-plus years since the initial data were collected. Given the loss of jobs in traditional rural industries, advances in telecommunications and transportation, relocation of retirees to rural areas, and other major social changes that have impacted rural communities, it follows that rural culture has been altered.

The results of this study have relevance to all nurses who have an interest in improving rural health, and especially to those who practice in a rural setting. The health of rural Americans is closely linked to factors in the culture, economy, demography, and geography of rural places (Ricketts, 1999). Thus, to successfully impact the health of rural people, nurses need to have an understanding of rural communities. Furthermore, for nurses interested in community-based practice in a rural setting, it is important to understand community-level perspectives of health as well as community-level influences on health decision making.

The findings from this study were limited by several factors, including the small size and limited diversity of the sample, the potential for bias in the use of health development committee members as representatives of their community, and the lack of an urban comparison group. Further research is needed to explore whether the characteristics identified in this research are unique to rural communities and to confirm their applicability in other rural settings.

REFERENCES

Findholt, N. E. (2004). *The influence of rurality on community participation in a community health development initiative*. Unpublished doctoral dissertation, Oregon Health and Science University, Portland.

Long, K. A., & Weinert, C. (1989). Rural nursing: Developing the theory base. *Scholarly Inquiry for Nursing Practice, 3*(2), 113–127.

Miles, M. B., & Huberman, A. M. (1994). *Qualitative data analysis* (2nd ed.). Thousand Oaks, CA: Sage.

Office of Rural Health (ORH). (2003). *Demographic, socioeconomic, and health status report*. Portland, OR: Oregon Health and Science University.

Portland State University (PSU). Population Research Center. (2002). *Oregon population report*. Retrieved February 19, 2003, from http://www.upa.pdx.edu/CPRC/

Ricketts, T. C. (1999). Introduction. In T. C. Ricketts, III (Ed.), *Rural health in the United States* (pp. 1–6). New York, NY: Oxford University Press.

Rural Health Research Center. (2002). *Rural–urban commuting area codes (RUCAs)*. Retrieved February 3, 2003, from http://wwww.fammed.washington.edu/wwamirhrc/rucas/rucas.html

Wandersman, A., & Florin, P. (2000). Citizen participation and community organizations. In J. Rappaport, & E. Seidman (Eds.), *Handbook of community psychology* (pp. 247–272). New York, NY: Kluwer Academic/Plenum.

Weinert, C., & Long, K. A. (1987). Understanding the health care needs of rural families. *Family Relations, 36,* 450–455.

Chapter 24

COMMUNITY RESILIENCY AND RURAL NURSING: CANADIAN AND AUSTRALIAN PERSPECTIVES

Judith C. Kulig, Desley Hegney, and Dana S. Edge

Resiliency is [a] community that's willing to pick up an issue, work with it, and decide what they want to do about it ... without blowing the place apart.
COMMUNITY RESIDENT

In the last several years, considerable discussion about the applicability of resiliency to understand and augment community functioning has occurred. Community resiliency is a process that describes change, provides an opportunity to focus on strengths, and offers opportunities for residents to be involved. Agencies such as the Red Cross have found that through the development of social capital and cross-sectoral coalitions in communities that have experienced disasters, resiliency is enhanced (J. Walter, 2005). In this chapter, examples of Canadian-led and Australian-led research on community resiliency in Canada, Australia, and the United States illustrate how rural communities have dealt with adversity. The rural communities in the Canadian-led research discussed here were all under 10,000 in population size, which matches the rural and small town definition commonly used to describe communities of that size outside the commuting zones of large urban centers (du Plessis, Beshiri, Bollman, & Clemenson, 2001). Communities serve to satisfy their members' needs (MacMillan & Chavis, 1986) and are places where interactions and social relationships are tantamount (Bellah, Madsen, Sullivan, Swidler, & Tipton, 1996; Hawe, 1994). The community-based research exemplars suggest how rural registered nurses (RNs) can enhance community resiliency and ultimately improve the health status of rural residents and the sustainability of rural communities.

BACKGROUND TO RESILIENCY RESEARCH

Historically, resilience has been studied among individuals, particularly young children, who were living in challenging circumstances. Numerous scholars have used "resilience" to describe a trait held by individuals as a result of dealing with adversity. However, since the 1990s, resiliency has also been used to describe the "process" communities undergo when dealing with adversity. This process also refers to the ability of a community to strengthen and change despite the adversity encountered (Brown & Kulig, 1996/1997; Kulig, 1999, 2000; Kulig & Hanson, 1996). Various factors are important within the community resiliency process, including community infrastructure, such as health and social service departments and social capital, represented by neighborhood networks and associations (Breton, 2001). Events such as public fairs and festivals add to a sense of self, place, and community while also enhancing viability and vitality that contribute to the resiliency of communities (Porter, 2000).

There is no definitive answer about the relationship between individual and community resiliency. Although we speculate that "you can't have one without the other," it remains unclear if there are a certain number of resilient individuals required to ensure that community resiliency occurs or if there is a specific type of relationship between individual and community resiliency. Additional research is needed among a variety of rural communities in order to further our understanding of this and other issues related to community resiliency.

OVERVIEW OF RESEARCH STUDIES ON COMMUNITY RESILIENCY

A series of studies on community resiliency based on Canadian, U.S., and Australian rural communities have been conducted in order to understand the concept. This brief overview provides highlights from the qualitative and focus-group interviews conducted within the case studies. Interviews and analyses occurred simultaneously, with interviews continuing until data saturation occurred in each investigation. Trustworthiness was established through member checking, independent audit of themes, and presentation of preliminary findings to residents (Creswell, 2007; Streubert, Speziale, & Carpenter, 2007). Principles of community development guided the conduct of the studies, with community consultation prior to study commencement, establishment of community advisory teams, employment and training of local research assistants, and dissemination of findings back to community members (Labonte, 1993). Table 24.1 provides a visual presentation of the specific studies and their accompanying sample sizes.

TABLE 24.1 Summary of Resiliency Studies in Canadian, U.S., and Australian Communities

Community Studied	Year	# Qualitative Interviews n	# Focus Group Interviews n
Crowsnest Pass, AB, Canada	1995	40	74
Southeastern Kentucky, USA	1997	23	
Crowsnest Pass, AB, Canada	1998	22	
Hinton, AB, Canada	2003	25	
Riverside Meadows, AB, Canada	2003	27	
Hardisty, AB, Canada	2003	30	
Crowsnest Pass, AB, Canada	2006–2007	30	
Barriere, BC, Canada	2007–2008	30	
La Ronge, SK, Canada	2007–2008	27	
Stanthorpe, Australia	2007–2008	11 (phase 1)	
		74 (phase 2)	20
TOTAL		339	94
		GRAND TOTAL	n = 433

Canadian and U.S. Exemplars

The initial studies on community resiliency (Brown & Kulig, 1996/1997; Kulig, 1999) were conducted in an amalgamated community, the Crowsnest Pass, in southern Alberta, Canada, with an approximate population of 6,000 (Statistics Canada, 2006). Before 1979, the amalgamated community had been a series of former coal-mining towns, hamlets, and improvement districts. In total, three studies that focused on resiliency have been conducted in this community.

The "Pass," as it is often referred to, has experienced a number of challenging events: (a) the Frank Slide, a well-known mountain slide that partially buried one of the hamlets in 1903, killing over 75 people; (b) the worst mine disaster in Canadian history, which led to the death of 189 miners and left 400 children fatherless in 1914; (c) community strife related to the coal industry, including strikes and lockouts; and (d) the resultant economic decline from the loss of underground coal mining in the late 1970s. Natural disasters continue to be common with severe windstorms leading to extensive damage to homes and businesses. Two recent natural disasters include the Lost Creek Fire in 2003 and the ice storm in 2005 that left numerous residents without power for up to 5 days.

The first study in the Pass dealt with the general history of the area and the participants' perspectives about how the aforementioned historical events shaped their community and contributed to its resiliency (Brown & Kulig, 1996/1997; Kulig & Hanson, 1996). The second study focused on the attempts to create a community health center and how this process actually damaged the community's resiliency (Kulig & Waldner, 1999). The third study addressed the community's response to the Lost Creek Fire, the worst wildfire experienced by the community, which led to evacuations and the loss of 21,000 hectares (51,800 acres) of land (Kulig et al., 2007). In each study, regardless of the issue being addressed by the community, the individuals were interviewed about their perspectives regarding the functioning of the Pass, how the community faced the many challenges it had encountered, and their understanding of community resiliency.

Between the first and second investigations in the Pass, the first author conducted an interrelated study examining how community-based workers enhanced community resiliency in southeastern Kentucky in the United States (Kulig, 1999, 2000). The setting was chosen for study because of the similarities to the Pass, including a coal mining history with strikes and community unrest. The area in Kentucky was rural in nature with the towns having a few hundred to a few thousand residents in each. The findings from the studies conducted in the Pass and in Kentucky led to the beginnings of a community resiliency model in 1995, which has since been revised, and will be described in a subsequent section. Building upon the emerging community resiliency model, a pilot study explored whether community resiliency could be linked to health status in several resource-reliant central Alberta communities. Agricultural-based rural communities have experienced a number of economic and social challenges, including a decline in the number of family farms (Bollman & Rothwell, 2002), with a simultaneous increase in intensive livestock operations (ILOs) (Cole, Todd, & Wing, 2000; Wing & Wolf, 2000). Community tensions arise when plans are proposed to locate ILOs in farming communities. Conflicts can result as rural residents typically value family farm ownership over corporate ownership, and rural beliefs of mutual respect and reciprocal exchange may not be respected (Schiffman, Miller, Suggs, & Graham, 1995; Thu et al., 1997). Similarly, natural resource communities, such as mining towns, experience competing interests of generating economic opportunities for residents and minimizing mining extraction environmental concerns.

Two rural communities in central Alberta were chosen for the pilot study. The agricultural-based community of Hardisty and surrounding communities successfully prevented the establishment of an ILO in their community. The second rural community was the mining community of Hinton, which dealt with a coal mining closure (Kulig, Edge, & Joyce, 2008a, 2008b). The urban neighborhood of Riverside Meadows was also included. This community was originally a French Canadian village, and at the time of the study was dealing with identity issues. These three communities were chosen because of the challenges that they were addressing.

Understanding Resiliency Through Disaster Research

Finally, the most recent and current studies on community resiliency focus on the relationship between the phenomenon and disasters (Kulig et al., 2007). Given the increased number of disasters worldwide and the impact of wildfire on residents in rural communities (Public Safety & Emergency Preparedness Canada, 2005), the current ongoing study is examining two communities that experienced wildfires that led to evacuations and property losses (Kulig et al., 2011).

The communities Barriere (British Columbia, population 2,500) and La Ronge (Saskatchewan, population 5,700) are rural and remote communities, respectively (Statistics Canada, 2006). Both study sites are isolated from larger cities, with Barriere economically struggling while La Ronge has experienced a shortage of skilled workers for their currently booming mining industry. Both communities include aboriginal residents who participate in all sectors of community life. The fire in Barriere burned 26,420 hectares (65,257 acres), led to the evacuation of the entire community, and destroyed over 80 homes and businesses. In La Ronge, the fire burned over 8 kilometers, a partial evacuation of the community occurred, and eight homes were destroyed. In each community, the wildfire disaster was seen as a potential stimulus for the community's resiliency.

Australian Case Studies

Between 2005 and 2007, a study was undertaken in the Australian town of Stanthorpe. The aim of the study was to work collaboratively with members of this rural community to develop, implement, and evaluate a model that enhances resilience in rural people and communities. Stanthorpe is located in southeast Queensland, and at the time of the study, the town and its satellite communities had an area of 2,699 square kilometers and a population of 10,124 (Australian Bureau of Statistics, 2007). The main industries included fruit and vegetable production, wineries, and tourism. At the time of the study, the area was experiencing a protracted drought, and in the previous 2 years, it had also experienced "black" frosts, hailstorms, and bushfires. The area was rated as highly disadvantaged on the National Index of Social and Economic Disadvantage (Australian Bureau of Statistics, 2006), with almost 60% of the population in the lowest 20th percentile.

The study was carried out in three phases. Phase 1 of the study involved face-to-face interviews with 11 people identified as being resilient. It was designed to explore key informants' conceptions of resilience, both as an individual and as a community characteristic (Hegney et al., 2007). Phase 2 used a modified convergent interviewing technique (Dick, 1990) to interview six groups (service providers, those with special needs, youth, farmers, the commercial sector, and those "resilient" individuals identified from phase 1 of the study). A total of 74 people participated in the face-to-face interviews. Following data analysis of phase 1 and 2 data, resilient concepts were identified. These concepts were then evaluated using a modified photovoice exercise and a focus group of community members. The final product was 11 concepts that were seen to be linked to individual, group, or community resilience: (1) social networks and support, (2) positive outlook, (3) learning, (4) early experience, (5) environment and lifestyle, (6) infrastructure and support services, (7) sense of purpose, (8) diverse and innovative economy, (9) embracing differences, (10) beliefs, and (11) leadership. One of the products of the study was the development of a "toolkit," which explained each of the 11 concepts and gave examples of how the concept could be assessed and programs introduced to enhance the concept.

DEVELOPING THEORY ABOUT COMMUNITY RESILIENCY

The initial study in 1995 focused on community resiliency in the Pass and led to the development of a model that illustrated that when specific variables combined and interacted, resiliency was the result (see Figure 24.1) (Kulig, 2000). These variables, which emphasize social interactions and relationships, include (a) the ability to cope with divisions, (b) leadership, (c) community togetherness, and (d) networks. In this version of the model, resiliency is seen as constantly fluctuating, depending upon the situation that was being addressed. However, it was also crucial that community cohesiveness be present, otherwise resiliency would not occur.

The subsequent study, conducted in Kentucky (Kulig, 1998) and supported by the second study in the Pass (Kulig, 1999), led to the revision of

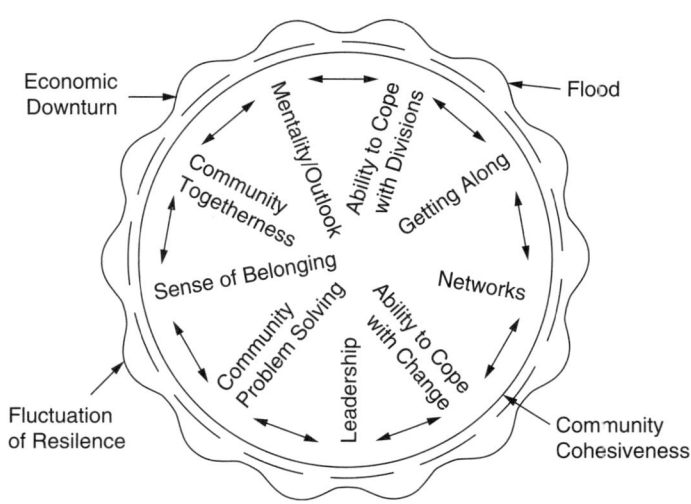

FIGURE 24.1 Original community resiliency model.

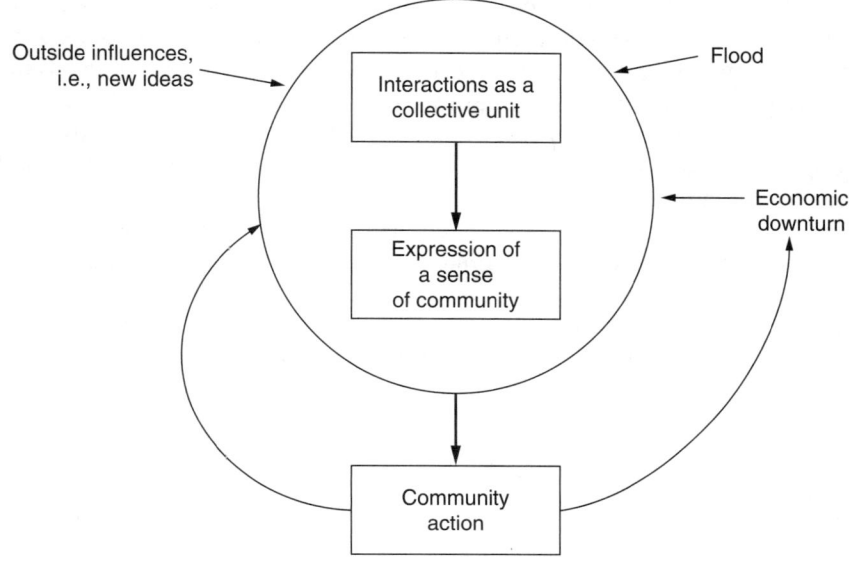

FIGURE 24.2 Revised resiliency model.

the original model (see Figure 24.2). The findings from these studies also confirmed that resiliency is a process that is influenced by variables such as the presence of community leadership, proactive members, and the ability to use a community problem-solving process. These variables contributed to the development of community cohesiveness, an important precursor to community resiliency. Community resiliency therefore implies three processes: (1) the community experiencing interactions as a collective unit, including "getting along" and "a sense of belonging"; (2) the development of a "sense of community," demonstrated by a mentality and outlook and community togetherness; and (3) community action, shown by the coping with divisions, dealing with change in a positive way, the accompaniment of visionary leadership, and the surfacing of community problem solving. In order for community resiliency to develop, these internal processes are required, as well as the consideration and incorporation of new ideas from the outside.

Varying levels of resiliency were displayed by communities in the previous studies. For community-based workers, the findings suggest that there are different times when they can intervene to potentially enhance a community's resiliency. Being proactive was found to be very important to resiliency, as proactiveness signals a community's flexibility and openness to change and to new ideas. Finally, a sense of hope and community pride was noted as tantamount for resiliency to occur.

The central Alberta pilot study focused on the relationships between health status and community resiliency, not only with interviews, but also by the examination of health databases (Kulig, Edge, & Joyce,

2008a). Residents in the urban neighborhood scored lowest on sense of belonging on the household survey, compared to their rural counterparts in Hardisty and Hinton. This finding, along with the interview data, raised questions about the degree of resiliency present in the neighborhood, as a sense of community is associated with community resiliency. In addition, Riverside Meadows had higher proportions of self-reported physician-diagnosed depression and a corresponding increase in health care utilization for mental diseases. These results represent the first time that quantitative evidence has linked health status and community resiliency. Consequently, the community resiliency model was again revised (see Figure 24.3). In the latest revision, sense of belonging and community pride are results of a sense of community rather than the other way around.

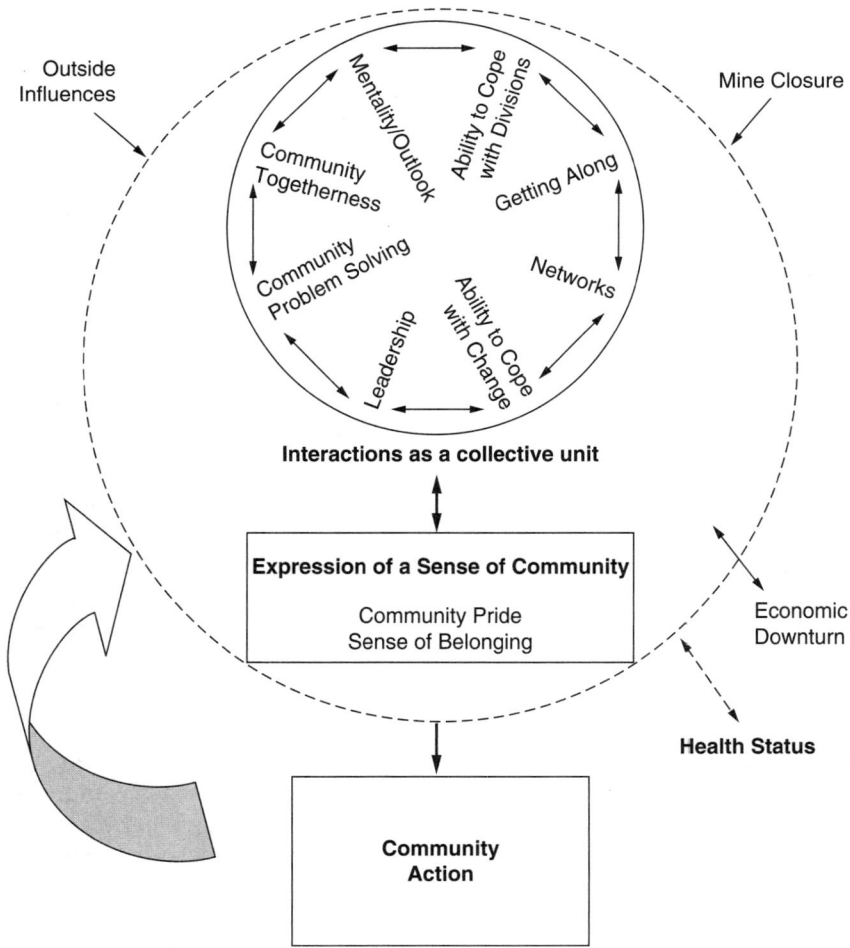

FIGURE 24.3 Updated resiliency model.

The characteristics of and barriers to community resiliency were further clarified in the central Alberta pilot study (Kulig et al., 2007). Community resiliency includes the following five characteristics: (a) positive infrastructure, such as a diverse economy and gathering places; (b) intact social infrastructure (i.e., residents honoring history); (c) constructive people characteristics, exemplified by core leadership and people participating; (d) problem-solving processes that are transparent and collective in nature; and (e) helpful conceptual characteristics, such as being proactive, community pride, and "stick-to-itiveness." Barriers to resiliency consist of (a) challenging events, such as the community dealing with a series of successive adverse events or dealing with a natural disaster; (b) negative infrastructure characteristics, for example, an economic downturn or poor access to services; (c) harmful social infrastructure, such as a high crime rate and a lack of community spirit; (d) limited people infrastructure, including a lack of knowledge and education, a lack of participation, and a lack of leadership; (e) compromised conceptual infrastructure, for instance, a failure to be proactive; and (f) attitudinal characteristics like complacency, rigidity, and individualism.

The most recent study conducted in the Pass focused on the impact of the Lost Creek Fire on community resiliency (Kulig et al., 2007) but did not lead to any additional changes in the model. With a focus on perceptions of risk, vulnerability, and community resiliency in a disaster, findings from the Lost Creek Fire investigation imply that vulnerability, at the individual and community level, tests resiliency and affects the community response to adversity. The challenge will be to examine the association between perceived vulnerability and community resiliency.

The study in Barriere and La Ronge has confirmed the importance of resiliency in explaining how these communities have dealt with the wildfires (Kulig et al., 2011). The data analysis has noted a deeper understanding of resiliency within rural communities (Kulig et al., in press).

In summary, community resiliency is a theoretical model that describes processes that rural communities undergo when dealing with adversity. It requires, at a minimum, informal leadership, community togetherness, and a positive proactive community outlook. Resiliency naturally fluctuates but can be positively influenced by residents and community-based workers. Given the threats to rural sustainability, it is vitally important to consider how rural RNs can assist in this process to positively influence the health of rural residents.

ROLE OF RURAL REGISTERED NURSES IN ENHANCING COMMUNITY RESILIENCY

Rural RNs assume a generalist role in their practice with rural communities (Kulig, MacLeod, Stewart, & Pitblado, 2008). By using the community resiliency model, rural nurses can collectively attend to the overall needs of the community while also supporting the health of rural residents. In practical terms, this is achieved by focusing on the model's separate components (see Figure 24.3).

Interactions as a Collective Unit

It is very clear that the threats to rural sustainability focus on the loss of infrastructure and the subsequent losses of opportunities for interactions and networking. This first aspect of the community resiliency model can be considered a "building phase" that requires the work of many to be successful.

Rural RNs assist in this process of strengthening infrastructure by enhancing networks that foster feelings of "getting along," and a sense of belonging through their professional roles and as community residents. At multiple levels of interchanges (C. Walter, 2005), rural nurses use a holistic approach that fosters interactions and exchanges between all community members, regardless of gender, age, economic, religious, or ethnic backgrounds. In short, rural nursing requires working across sectors, with a variety of people. Rural nurses are typically very good at being "inclusive." Nurses in rural settings care for their neighbors, friends, and family members, as their personal and professional roles are inseparable. Their worldview extends beyond the walls of the health care facilities or institutions where they practice and acknowledges the social and political dynamics of their community. All of this means that rural nurses can assist in enhancing community members' sense of belonging and networking. Using a holistic approach that incorporates community input and involvement, rural nurses can plan programs, activities, and initiatives that naturally result in increased community resiliency.

The negative effect of threats to rural sustainability can be mediated via rural nurses by working with community members to identify individual and community assets. This is the first step in addressing community need while also providing opportunities for engagement at the individual resident level. Working from a whole-community approach to health promotion, nurses can assist in creating partnerships and in fostering community champions. These actions can lead to an overall increase in a community's capacity. However, none of these steps will be effective unless the community is willing to be involved. Community involvement is not "expected" and requires time, trust, and mutual regard between rural RNs, rural residents, and other stakeholders within the community. Without community buy-in, planned initiatives will stall or fail.

Developing a Sense of Community

Frequently, rural nurses are at the front lines, making decisions that influence the community in its entirety. Opportunities for visionary ideas and the action toward those goals require that nurses work with community residents. This activity alone is a positive step in the development of community togetherness and cohesion. Positive community spirit and hopefulness can be encouraged within the community in other ways. If the community has had success in developing interactions as a collective unit, then their sense of community will begin to expand. It can be further fostered by implementing activities that will augment community pride. For example, even a simple activity such as naming a "yard of the month" during summer when gardens are at their height can increase pride in one's physical community. This example demonstrates the importance of the link between community resiliency and a community's overall health.

Community Action

Being proactive is key to community resiliency. Given their professional presence in a rural community, nurses, along with others, can advocate for changes in public policy (Kulig, Nahachewsky, Thomlinson, MacLeod, & Curran, 2004). Local knowledge and skill in policy development among the nursing collective can be used to support rural residents in efforts to effect change. As interpreters of health information for the public, rural nurses have a responsibility to provide accurate information about local health issues. For example, rural RNs can help decipher information about potential environmental threats from ILOs on rural residents' health, and can use their connections to bring experts to the community to share their knowledge on specific topics. Community processes can be employed to ensure that community residents' opinions are heard and are used in determining which specific actions need to be taken. One example is a community profile process that includes local individuals and community members at large being involved in the planning and generation of solutions for identified issues (University of New Hampshire, n.d.).

RECOMMENDATIONS FOR NURSING EDUCATION

In the past two decades, the relationship between social determinants of health and the well-being of communities has received renewed interest and exploration (Kawachi & Berkman, 2003). In undergraduate nursing programs, the examination of societal forces that influence health have typically been discussed in community health nursing courses (Vollman, Anderson, & McFarlane, 2008). Relatively new models, such as the population health promotion model, provide visual representations of the interconnections between the social determinants of health, the various populations to serve (e.g., individual, family, community, society), and components of the Ottawa charter (Hamilton & Bhatti, 1996). In particular, the five components of the Ottawa charter—(1) strengthen community action, (2) build public health policy, (3) create supportive environments, (4) develop personal skills, and (5) reorient health services—should lead to enhanced community resiliency if enacted. The different components of the resiliency model allow for connections with the population health promotion model and provide further rationale for the link between community resiliency and health status. Educators can use the revised model of community resiliency as a starting point for student discussion about the underlying reasons why rural communities and urban neighborhoods may vary in how they deal with adversity.

RECOMMENDATIONS FOR FUTURE RESEARCH

Several recommendations for future research in community resiliency arise in this discussion. Suggestions include (a) focusing on communities that have dealt with different kinds of natural disasters (i.e., floods, hurricanes, tornadoes) in order to provide comparative data; (b) conducting mixed method studies to identify the components of resiliency; (c) establishing international studies to allow for further examination and comparison of the concept; (d) performing a systematic review to compare resiliency, empowerment, and social capital; and, (e) carrying out a metasynthesis of community resiliency studies.

CONCLUSION

Community resiliency is the ability of communities to "bounce back" and deal with adverse situations that they face. When communities demonstrate resiliency, they also display adaptability and the capacity to move forward. Communities with resiliency also reveal that they can maintain themselves as strong, functioning, collective units. Given that rural sustainability is a growing concern, resiliency gives hope to rural communities that are struggling. It also demonstrates an important role that rural RNs play in enhancing resiliency, and thereby potentially improving the health of all rural residents.

REFERENCES

Australian Bureau of Statistics. (2006). *Socio-economic index for areas*. Canberra: Commonwealth of Australia.

Australian Bureau of Statistics. (2007). *Australian Bureau of Statistics 2006 Census*. Canberra: Commonwealth of Australia.

Bellah, R., Madsen, R., Sullivan, W., Swidler, A., & Tipton, S. (1996). *Habits of the heart: Individualism and commitment in American life.* Los Angeles: University of California Press.

Bollman, R. D., & Rothwell, N. (2002). *Key features of Canadian agriculture. Presentation to the Workshop of "Structural Change in the Agribusiness Sector" organized by the Cooperative Program in Agricultural Marketing and Business.* Edmonton: University of Alberta.

Breton, M. (2001). Neighborhood resiliency. *Journal of Community Practice, 9*(1), 21–36.

Brown, D., & Kulig, J. (1996/1997). The concept of resiliency: Theoretical lessons from community research. *Health & Canadian Society, 4*(1), 29–50.

Cole, D., Todd, L., & Wing, S. (2000). Concentrated swine feeding operations and public health: A review of occupational and community health effects. *Environmental Health Perspectives, 108*(8), 685–699.

Creswell, J. W. (2007). *Qualitative inquiry & research design: Choosing among five approaches* (2nd ed.). Thousand Oaks, CA: Sage.

Dick, B. (1990). *Convergent interviewing.* Brisbane: Interchange.

du Plessis, V., Beshiri, R., Bollman, R., & Clemenson, H. (2001). Definitions of rural. *Rural and Small Town Analysis Bulletin, 3*(3), Catalogue #21 006 XIE. Ottawa: Statistics Canada.

Hamilton, N., & Bhatti, T. (1996). *Population health promotion: An integrated model of population health and health promotion.* Ottawa, ON: Health Promotion Development Division, Health Canada.

Hawe, P. (1994). Capturing the meaning of "community" in community intervention evaluation. *Health Promotion International, 9*(3), 199–210. doi: 10.1093/heapro/9.3.199

Hegney, D., Buikstra, E., Baker, P., Rogers-Clark, C., Pearce, S., Ross, H. et al. (2007). Individual resilience in rural people, a Queensland study, Australia. *Rural and Remote Health, 7,* 620. http://www.rrh.org.au/articles/subviewnew.asp?ArticleID=620

Kawachi, I., & Berkman, L. F. (Eds.). (2003). *Neighbourhoods and health.* Oxford, UK: Oxford University Press.

Kulig, J. (1998). *The enhancement of community resiliency by community-based workers in Central Appalachia.* Lethbridge, AB: University of Lethbridge, Regional Centre for Health Promotion and Community Studies.

Kulig, J. (1999). Sensing collectivity and building skills: Rural communities and community resiliency. In W. Ramp, J. Kulig, I. Townshend, & V. McGowan (Eds.), *Health in rural settings: Contexts for action* (pp. 223–244). Lethbridge, AB: University of Lethbridge.

Kulig, J. (2000). Community resiliency: The potential for community health nursing theory development. *Public Health Nursing, 17*(5), 374–385.

Kulig, J., Edge, D., & Joyce, B. (2008a). Community resiliency as a measure of collective health status: Perspectives from rural communities. *Canadian Journal of Nursing Research, 40*(4), 92–110.

Kulig, J., Edge, D., & Joyce, B. (2008b). Understanding community resiliency in rural communities through multi-method research. *Journal of Rural and Community Development, 3*(3). http://www.jrcd.ca/viewarticle.php?id=181&layout=abstract

Kulig, J., Edge, D., Townshend, I., Lightfoot, N., & Reimer, W. (in press). Community Resiliency: Emerging Theoretical Insights. *Journal of Community Psychology*.

Kulig, J., & Hanson, L. (1996). *Discussion and expansion of the concept of resiliency: Summary of a think tank*. University of Lethbridge: Final Report.

Kulig, J., MacLeod, M., Stewart, N., & Pitblado, R. (2008). Clients in rural areas. In L. Stamler, & L. Yui (Eds.), *Community health nursing: A Canadian perspective* (2nd ed., pp. 301–310). Toronto, ON: Pearson.

Kulig, J., Nahachewsky, D., Thomlinson, E., MacLeod, M., & Curran, F. (2004). Maximizing the involvement of rural nurses in policy. *The Canadian Journal of Nursing Leadership, 17*(1), 88–96.

Kulig, J., Reimer, W., Townshend, I., Edge, D., & Lightfoot, N. (2011). *Understanding links between wildfires and community resiliency: Lessons learned for disaster preparation and mitigation*. Lethbridge, Alberta, Canada: University of Lethbridge.

Kulig, J., Reimer, W., Townshend, I., Edge, D., Neves-Graca, K., Lightfoot, N. et al. (2007). *Understanding resiliency and risk: A final report of the Lost Creek Fire pilot study*. Lethbridge, Alberta, Canada: University of Lethbridge.

Kulig, J., & Waldner, M. (1999). Lessons in community development: Attempting to create a community wellness centre. *Journal of Community Development Society, 30*(1), 29–47.

Labonte, R. (1993). Community-based, community development programming. In *Health promotion and empowerment:Practice frameworks* (pp. 32–34). Toronto, ON: Centre for Health Promotion and ParticipACTION.

MacMillan, D. W., & Chavis, D. M. (1986). Sense of community: A definition and theory. *Journal of Community Psychology, 14*, 6–23.

Porter, M. K. (2000). Integrating resilient young into strong communities through festivals, fairs, and feasts. In S. Danish, & T. Gullota (Eds.), *Developing competent youth and strong communities through after-school programming*. Annapolis, MD: CWLA Press.

Public Safety and Emergency Preparedness Canada. Fact sheets: National disaster mitigation strategy (NDMS). (2005). Retrieved June 21, 2005, from http://www.ocipep. gc.ca/info_pro/fact_sheets/general/P_NDMS_e.asp

Schiffman, S. S., Miller, E. A. S., Suggs, M. S., & Graham, B. G. (1995). The effects of environmental odours emanating from commercial swine operations on the mood of nearby residents. *Brain Research Bulletin, 37*(4), 369–375.

Statistics Canada. (2006). Community profiles. Retrieved March 3, 2009, from www.statcan.gc.ca

Streubert Speziale, H. J., & Carpenter, D. R. (2007). *Qualitative research in nursing: Advancing the humanistic imperative* (4th ed.). Philadelphia: Lippincott Williams & Wilkins.

Thu, K., Donham, K., Ziegenhorn, R., Reynolds, S., Thorne, P. S., Subramanian, P. et al. (1997). A control study of the physical and mental health of residents living near a large-scale swine operation. *Journal of Agricultural Safety and Health, 3*(1), 13–26.

University of New Hampshire Cooperative Extension. (n.d.). *Community profiles*. Retrieved August 15, 1999 from http://extension.unh.edu/CommDev/CommProf.htm

Vollman, A. R., Anderson, E. T., & McFarlane, J. (2008). *Canadian community as partner: Theory & multidisciplinary practice* (2nd ed.). Philadelphia: Lippincott Williams & Wilkins.

Walter, C. (2005). Community building practice: A conceptual framework. In M. Minkler (Ed.), *Community building and community organizing for health* (2nd ed., pp. 66–81). New Brunswick, NJ: Rutgers University Press.

Walter, J. (2005). *World disasters report 2004: Focus on community resilience*. Geneva: International Federation of Red Cross and Red Cross Societies.

Wing, S., & Wolf, S. (2000). Intensive livestock operation, health and quality of life among eastern North Carolina residents. *Environmental Health Perspectives, 108*(3), 233–238.

Chapter 25

INFLUENCE OF THE RURAL ENVIRONMENT ON CHILDREN'S PHYSICAL ACTIVITY AND EATING BEHAVIORS

Nancy E. Findholt, Linda J. Jerofke,
Yvonne L. Michael, and
Victoria W. Brogoitti

SINCE THE 1980s, THE PREVALENCE of childhood obesity has tripled, making it one of the most serious public health threats in the United States (Ogden et al., 2006). Rural populations appear to be especially vulnerable to obesity. Several studies have identified higher rates of obesity among rural children and adolescents than among their urban or suburban counterparts (Joens-Matre et al., 2008; Lewis et al., 2006; Lutfiyya, Lipsky, Wisdom-Behounek, & Inpanbutr-Martinkus, 2007).

Why obesity prevalence is higher among rural youth is not completely clear at this time, but some evidence suggests that the rural environment presents challenges to obtaining physical activity and healthy foods. One recent study found that a dispersed residential layout, lack of an attractive town center, threats to personal safety (e.g., fear of drug dealers or child molesters), and lack of accessible open spaces were barriers to physical activity for children in some rural communities (Yousefian, Ziller, Swartz, & Hartley, 2008). A second study found that rural schools and schools with many low-income students were less likely than urban or wealthier schools to have policies that promoted physical activity and healthful nutrition—a characteristic that could impede the establishment of healthy behaviors among students in these schools (Nanney, Bohner, & Friedrichs, 2008). Also, research involving adults has shed light on factors within the rural environment that may be hindrances to physical activity and healthy eating habits among children. Previous studies have found that rural adults perceived fewer places available to them for exercise than urban or suburban adults (Parks, Housemann, & Brownson, 2003; Wilcox, Castro, King, Housemann, & Brownson, 2000). Also, rural adult women were more likely than urban women to report street-related hazards, such as absence of sidewalks and unattended dogs, as impediments to walking (Wilcox et al., 2000). Furthermore, Liese, Weis, Pluto, Smith, and Lawson (2007) identified many barriers to obtaining healthful and inexpensive foods in rural areas, including a preponderance of convenience stores as compared to large grocery stores.

Identifying the factors within rural schools and communities that affect children's physical activity and eating patterns is imperative for the development of interventions that are likely to be effective in preventing obesity among rural children. In this chapter, we present the findings of a study that explored the perceptions of rural children concerning environmental influences on their physical activity and food choices.

METHODS

This research was an exploratory study using qualitative methods. Data were collected through focus groups with rural children. The study setting was Union County, Oregon, a sparsely populated agricultural region in the northeast part of the state with a predominately Caucasian population (94.3%). The sample was drawn from fifth-grade classes in four (out of eight total) public elementary schools in Union County. These schools were selected because they represented the variability in size and socioeconomic status that existed among schools in the county. Total school enrollment ranged from 102 to 467, and the percentage of students eligible for free or reduced-price lunches ranged from 39% to 77%. Two of the schools were located in Union County's largest community (population 12,540) and two were located in communities of 1,670 and 490 residents, respectively.

Two focus groups, segregated by gender, were conducted in each of the four schools. Of the 41 children who participated, 22 were girls and 93% were Caucasian. Discussion topics included: (a) the adequacy of physical activity resources in the school and community; (b) the ease or difficulty of being active during and outside of school; (c) satisfaction with school meals and the mealtime experience; (d) access to and utilization of convenience markets and fast-food outlets; and (e) adult influences on children's physical activity and food choices. Each focus group lasted approximately 1 hour and was audiotaped and transcribed verbatim. The transcripts were analyzed using a modified version of focused coding and grounded theory methods (Miles & Huberman, 1994; Strauss & Corbin, 1990). Study procedures were approved by the Institutional Review Boards at Oregon Health & Science University and Eastern Oregon University.

RESULTS

The data analysis revealed several barriers to physical activity and healthy food choices within the rural schools and communities. However, factors that promoted healthy behaviors were identified as well. The following represents the major themes and insights gained from the focus groups.

Barriers to Physical Activity

Unsafe streets emerged as a major hindrance to walking or bicycling to school or for pleasure. Several students commented on the lack of bike lanes and expressed concern about bicycling on the streets. Others reported that the speed of traffic kept them from using the streets. For example, one student said, "[My street] is really dangerous because cars go really fast. But our neighbors have a big driveway, so I just go up and down that." Long distances between home and school and adverse weather conditions were also cited as impediments to walking or bicycling to school.

Inadequate facilities for exercise and play were identified as a barrier to physical activity within the schools. Problems included insufficient gym space (i.e., too many classes sharing a gym and/or gyms that also served as the school cafeteria); limited playground equipment; and a shortage of balls and jump ropes. Similarly, inadequate facilities and equipment were an impediment to physical activity outside of school, especially in the smallest community. Students in this town said that there was just one small park with almost no playground equipment. Students living in Union County's largest community were generally satisfied with the city parks, although some said that there should be more resources, such as ice skating rinks and skateboard facilities.

Several students expressed concern about the quality and quantity of physical education (PE). Approximately half indicated that they received PE only twice per week, and some noted that PE classes were not vigorous. One girl stated, "I think that [PE] is ... too easy. We don't get a whole lot of exercise because ... people just sit around and stuff." Furthermore, many students reported that denial of recess was commonly used as a disciplinary measure: "Sometimes, if you get in trouble or you don't bring your homework back, you don't get to go to recess. ... Or, if you go to the bathroom during class." ["Then you don't get to go to recess?"] "Yeah, because you are wasting your class time."

Factors That Supported Physical Activity

The availability of noncurricular sports programs emerged as a facilitator of physical activity outside of school. A variety of team sports were offered to children of both genders, and participation in sports appeared to be common, particularly among boys. The male students told us that they and their peers were involved in many sports. One said that he participated in at least five sports per year, and another stated, "I get about two hours of activity every day almost. I'm in wrestling and other things." The female students mentioned participating in sports less often than did the male students, which may indicate that fewer girls participated.

Union County's natural environment (e.g., the mountains, forests, and open spaces) was also commonly cited as a factor that supported physical activity. One student explained, "I believe the environment we live in around here ... you know, we have great ski mountains and camping areas. Since we live in an area like [this], it makes it easier to get to a place where you can get good exercise but still have fun with it." Many students reported activities such as hiking, hunting, skiing, playing in creeks, and climbing trees. The community's sociocultural norms also appeared to support outdoor activity, as evidenced by this quote: "There are many ranchers here and people that go hunting, and being outdoors is really important to this community."

Adults were generally perceived as a good influence in regard to physical activity. Several students reported that their teachers and other adults were active (e.g., walked, bicycled, or skied), and that many coached or attended children's sports events. Others said that their parents and teachers urged them to play outdoors, participate in sports, or both, and that teachers played with them during recess and PE. A few students, however, did not believe that physical activity was important to adults in their community, and noted that many adults were overweight and sedentary.

Barriers to Healthy Food Choices

Poor quality school meals, specifically the entrées, emerged as a primary impediment to a healthy diet. Students reported that most of the entrées were prepackaged rather than homemade, and that the food tasted "artificial" and was salty and greasy. This comment was typical: "[S]ometimes [the school food] is really gross. They say it is healthy, but some chicken ... you can open it and you can see all the grease. ..." It was also noted that fast-food choices were served frequently. One student said, "Sometimes they have pizza and then that week they make just stuff out of pizza, like pizza sticks and then maybe pizza again. ... Sometimes they have breakfast pizza that is basically leftover pizza that they put meat on it with eggs."

Limited cafeteria space and an unpleasant cafeteria environment were also reported as hindrances to healthy eating. Many students said that lunchtime was rushed because a large number of classes had to be accommodated in a small cafeteria. Others said that cooks or other school personnel often scolded them for talking during lunch or for not finishing their meal, and that the cafeteria was very noisy. Students further noted that teachers often did not model healthy eating habits. One said, "[T]hey are always putting ... brownies and cookies in the teachers' lounge." Others observed that teachers "drink soda right at their desk" even though students were not permitted to have soda.

The presence of convenience stores near many elementary schools emerged as a barrier to healthy food choices outside of school. The students reported that they and their peers frequently purchased snacks from these stores. Common snack items included energy drinks, pop, beef jerky, cheese sticks, candy, chips, and deep-fried deli foods.

Factors That Supported Healthy Food Choices

Gardening appeared to be a social norm that promoted healthy diets. Many students said that their families had gardens, fruit trees, or both, and most said that they commonly ate fresh fruits and vegetables when these were in season. For example, when asked how often he ate fresh fruit, one student said, "Every time I can get to the tree. I like going down to my tree and getting a plum off of it." However, it appeared that most family gardens were small and that preserving produce was an uncommon practice.

Hunting also emerged as a community norm that may support healthful eating, and fishing was common as well. Many students reported eating game regularly, and some stated that all of their meat was obtained through hunting or fishing.

Despite the comments about teachers drinking soda and eating sweets, most of the students said that nutrition was important to adults in their school. Several noted that teachers and food service personnel encouraged them to select fruits and vegetables from the salad bar, and that the teachers often ate salads themselves. Some also observed that the school staff had removed the soda machine and had stopped giving out candy in the classroom. Others said that their teachers had invited nutritionists to speak in their classes.

Finally, it was reported that salad bars were available in the school cafeterias. However, the type and quality of the foods offered appeared to be variable. Some students said that their school's salad bar included a variety of fresh fruits and vegetables, such as broccoli, carrots, beets, cauliflower, apples, and oranges. Others, however, observed that foods such as Jell-O and desserts were available. In addition, several students said that the vegetables were often soft or otherwise unappealing. One stated, "The salad bar has beets [but they are] gross and heavily salted. [The lettuce] is iceberg lettuce, so there is no nutritional value to it."

DISCUSSION

The results of this study provide insight into conditions within rural schools and communities that negatively affect children's physical activity and eating habits and may contribute to the high rates of childhood obesity in rural populations. Addressing these conditions is essential, but this will not be an easy task. Just as characteristics of the rural environment create obstacles to healthy behaviors, so too do rural characteristics (such as transportation barriers, limited access to grant funding, low public funding levels for services and programs, and difficulties recruiting staff) present challenges for the delivery of health promotion programs (Phillips & McLeroy, 2004). On the other hand, there are strengths within rural communities upon which health promotion programs might be built. Our study findings suggest several environmental characteristics that could be enhanced or expanded to provide children with increased opportunities to obtain physical activity and healthy foods.

Organized after-school sports may be one resource for promoting physical activity. Similar to other studies (Bilinski, Semchuk, & Chad, 2005; Davis et al., 2008), we found that involvement in sports is a way that many rural children obtain physical activity, although participation in sports appeared to be more common among boys than girls. Attention should be given to developing after-school activities that appeal to girls. Also, because many traditional sports, such as football and wrestling, are not lifelong activities, offering alternatives, such as dance, would be beneficial.

Another resource that may be especially important in promoting physical activity among rural children is access to the natural environment. A growing body of evidence has documented numerous benefits for children that are associated with spending time outdoors in natural settings, including increased physical activity and improved mental health and cognition (Kuo & Taylor, 2004; Sallis, Prochaska, & Taylor, 2000; Wells & Evans, 2003). Rural communities are fortunate in having ample open spaces. However, efforts may need to be made to improve access and to ensure that children can travel to these areas safely. Also, enhancements to the outdoor spaces, such as trail development, might stimulate increased use.

The culture of gardening and hunting that was identified in this study is an asset that could be further developed to promote healthy eating habits. Potential strategies include developing school gardens, farmers' markets, and venues for sharing produce in churches or community centers; providing information and resources (e.g., pressure canners, community freezers) to families to encourage food preservation; and developing farm-to-school programs, which link farmers with school cafeterias to increase the use of locally grown, fresh produce in the schools.

This study was limited by the use of self-report data, which are subject to error, and by the inclusion of only one rural county. The barriers and assets that we identified might not be the same as those found in other rural areas. For this reason, we recommend that nurses who are interested in developing an obesity prevention program in a rural community begin by conducting a thorough assessment to identify the barriers and strengths that exist in that community. We also recommend that replication of this study be done using a larger and more diverse sample. Finally, the use of objective measures of physical activity and eating patterns would enhance the qualitative findings. Addressing these issues may aid in developing interventions that will be effective in preventing obesity among rural children.

ACKNOWLEDGMENT

This study was funded with a grant from the Northwest Health Foundation, Portland, Oregon.

REFERENCES

Bilinski, H., Semchuk, K. M., & Chad, K. (2005). Understanding physical activity patterns of rural Canadian children. *Online Journal of Rural Nursing and Health Care, 5*, 73–82.

Davis, A. M., Boles, R. E., James, R. L., Sullivan, D. K., Donnelly, J. E., Swirczynski, D. L. et al. (2008). Health behaviors and weight status among urban and rural children. *Rural and Remote Health* (Online), *8*, 1–11. Available at www.rrh.org.au/articles/subviewnew.asp?ArticleID=810

Joens-Matre, R. R., Welk, G. J., Calabro, M. A., Russel, D. W., Nicklay, E., & Hensley, L. D. (2008). Rural–urban differences in physical activity, physical fitness, and over-weight prevalence of children. *Journal of Rural Health, 24*, 49–54.

Kuo, F. E., & Taylor, A. F. (2004). A potential natural treatment for attention-deficit/ hyperactivity disorder: Evidence from a national study. *American Journal of Public Health, 94*, 1580–1586.

Lewis, R. C., Meyer, M. C., Lehman, S. C., Trowbridge, F. L., Bason, J. J., Yurman, K. H. et al. (2006). Prevalence and degree of childhood and adolescent overweight in rural, urban, and suburban Georgia. *Journal of School Health, 76*, 126–132.

Liese, A. D., Weis, K. E., Pluto, D., Smith, E., & Lawson, A. (2007). Food store types, availability, and cost of foods in a rural environment. *Journal of the American Dietetic Association, 107*, 1916–1923.

Lutfiyya, M. N., Lipsky, M. S., Wisdom-Behounek, J., & Inpanbutr-Martinkus, M. (2007). Is rural residency a risk factor for overweight and obesity for U.S. children? *Obesity, 15*, 2348–2356.

Miles, M. B., & Huberman, A. M. (1994). *Qualitative data analysis* (2nd ed.). Thousand Oaks, CA: Sage.

Nanney, M. S., Bohner, C., & Friedrichs, M. (2008). Poverty-related factors associated with obesity prevention policies in Utah secondary schools. *Journal of the American Dietetic Association, 108*, 1210–1215.

Ogden, C. L., Carrol, M. D., Curtin, L. R., McDowell, M. A., Tabak, C. J., & Flegal, K. M. (2006). Prevalence of overweight and obesity in the United States, 1999–2004. *Journal of the American Medical Association, 295,* 1549–1555.

Parks, S. E., Housemann, R., & Brownson, R. C. (2003). Differential correlates of physical activity in urban and rural adults of various socioeconomic backgrounds in the United States. *Journal of Epidemiology & Community Health, 57,* 29–35.

Phillips, C. D., & McLeroy, K. R. (2004). Tailoring programs and services to meet rural needs. *American Journal of Public Health, 94,* 1662–1663.

Sallis, J. F., Prochaska, J. J., & Taylor, W. C. (2000). A review of correlates of physical activity of children and adolescents. *Medicine & Science in Sports & Exercise, 32,* 963–975.

Strauss, A., & Corbin, J. (1990). *Basics of qualitative research: Grounded theory procedures and techniques.* Newbury Park, CA: Sage.

Wells, N. M., & Evans, G. W. (2003). Nearby nature: A buffer of life stress among rural children. *Environment and Behavior, 35,* 311–330.

Wilcox, S., Castro, C., King, A. C., Housemann, R., & Brownson, R. C. (2000). Determinants of leisure time physical activity in rural compared with urban older and ethnically diverse women in the United States. *Journal of Epidemiology & Community Health, 54,* 667–672.

Yousefian, A., Ziller, E., Swartz, J., & Hartley, D. (2008). *Active living for rural youth.* Portland, ME: University of Southern Maine, Maine Rural Health Research Center.

Chapter 26

PUBLIC HEALTH ACCREDITATION IN RURAL AND FRONTIER COUNTIES: A MONTANA PERSPECTIVE

Michele V. Sare

> *Over the past 20 years, several large scale efforts have significantly influenced public health practice and initiated a movement toward national accreditation of public health.*
> (BIALEK, DUFFY, & MORAN, 2009, P. 113)

> *The social, cultural, and global contexts of the nation's health are also undergoing rapid and dramatic change.*
> (INSTITUTE OF MEDICINE, 2002, P. 1)

IN 2007, I RETURNED TO PUBLIC HEALTH (PH) after 6 years in academia to act as the administrator and head of the Public Health Emergency Preparedness (PHEP) program for a local health department (LHD) in a frontier community in Montana. Excited to apply the concepts and principles of population-based nursing (see Table 26.1), to improve the well-being of my friends and neighbors, and to be of service to the community that I had called home for over 20 years, I was ready to actualize a long-time career and personal dream. At that point in my 37-year career as a registered nurse (RN), I had accumulated over 15 years of public health nursing (PHN), community health nursing (CHN), and administrative experience in four states and two developing countries. I was ready—or so I thought—to settle into a job where my years of experience and love for my community could be fully integrated and engaged.

TABLE 26.1 Concepts and Principles of Public Health

Concepts	Principles
Levels of PH: • Governance (Boards of Health [BOH], County Commissioners, Governor's Office, and at the national level, the President) • State (State Health Department—SHD) • Local Health Departments (LHD) • Federal (Under the U.S. Department of Health & Human Services [DHHS] and the Centers for Disease Control and Prevention [CDC])	***Healthy People 2020 (HP 2020):*** • Attain high-quality, longer lives without preventable disease, disability, injury, and excess death • Achieve health equity, eliminate disparity, improve the health of all sectors • Create built and natural environments that promote good health for everyone • Promote quality of life, healthy development, and healthy behaviors across the lifespan[1]
Operational Definitions: • "Montana metropolitan" (large) = 40,000 or more • Montana urban = 20,001–39,999 (medium) • Rural = 5,001–20,000 (small) • Frontier = 5,000 or less[2]	**Millennium Development Goals (MDG):** • Eradicate extreme poverty and hunger • Achieve universal primary education • Promote gender equality and empower women • Reduce child mortality • Improve maternal health • Combat HIV/AIDS, malaria, and other diseases • Ensure environmental sustainability • Develop a global partnership for development[3]
PH funding and governance: PH has historically fallen under federal, state, and local governments—being charged with protecting the public—PH is therefore primarily funded through tax dollars and therefore *comes under the authority of elected officials*	**Social Determinants of Health (SDH):** • Inborn features (sex, age, and genetic make-up) • Social and cultural issues (such as social status, gender roles, social support from family, friends, community, social networks, perspectives of health and health care, etc.) • Environment (built and natural) • Education • Health practices, beliefs, and personal habits (such as hygiene, smoking, alcohol consumption, safety, etc.) • Economy—poverty directly correlates to higher rates of excess death and disability • Access to appropriate health care services • Governmental policies and practices • Transportation • Appropriate technology access (communication and information dissemination and equity)[4]

(continued)

TABLE 26.1 Concepts and Principles of Public Health (*Continued*)

Concepts	Principles
Rural: • 20–22% of the U.S. population • According to the U.S. Census Bureau, there are over 314,000,000 Americans[5] • 20% of the U.S. population = 62,800,000 • 22% of the U.S. population = 69,080,000 Whether a person lives in a predominantly rural state or not, millions of Americans live in rural and frontier communities	**10 Essential Public Health Services (EPHS):** • Monitor health status • Diagnose health problems • Inform, educate, and • Mobilize community partnerships • Develop policies and plans • Enforce laws and regulations • Link people to needed personal health services • Assure competent PH workforce • Evaluate effectiveness and quality • Research[6] **3 PH Core Functions:** • Assessment • Policy • Assurance

[1] Adapted from the U.S. Departments of Health and Human Services website at: www.healthypeople.gov/2020/about/default.aspx
[2] See website www.ceic.commerce.state.mt.us/Demog/estimate/pop/City/estplacepop_by county_2007.pdf
[3] Adapted from the United Nations: www.un.org/millenniumgoals/
[4] Adapted from the World Health Organization's SDH: www.who.int/social_determinants/en/
[5] See website www.census.gov/population/www/popclockus.html
[6] Adapted from: www.phf.org/nphpsp/ViewResourceLink.aspx?source=http://www.cdc.gov/nphpsp/essentialServices.html&title=Ten%20Essential%20Public%20Health%20Services

MY JOURNEY IN RURAL AND FRONTIER PH SYSTEM IMPROVEMENT

My community of just 2,000 persons had seen six PH nurses in the six preceding years. The laptop computer that I inherited was blank save for a few personal pictures, and the file cabinets were disorganized and stuffed with obsolete data and materials. The standing orders for immunizations were several years old—signed by a physician who had not been in the county for five years. There were no established systems or processes of any kind; no process for monitoring the temperature in the vaccine refrigerator; no follow-up process for high-risk moms or babies; no communicable disease reporting process; no financial accountability for how PH dollars were being spent; and the Board of Health (BOH) had not met for several years.

Undaunted, I cleaned out the file cabinets, deleted the personal photos from the laptop, and set out to create the best LHD in frontier Montana! It was fun and exciting to create necessary networks, recruit a health officer (HO) who would serve as the medical advisor to the LHD and the BOH, educate the governing board (the County Commissioners), set up operational policies and procedures, and begin to put to use PH evidence-based best practices for our county.

Four months into my new job I attended my first Montana PH conference in several years and was excited to learn all that I could to bridge the gaps in our county's population health. That was when I heard "it." "If you've seen one Montana local health department, you've seen one local health department." That one comment, made by a lead administrator for the Montana State Department of Public Health and Human Services (MDPHHS), had summed up why I had inherited a LHD devoid of systems, processes, or protocols. PH in Montana had no standardized criteria for how an LHD must be operated. Individual programs—like county contracts with the Agency on Aging—held specified deliverables, but standards delineating population-based services did not exist at the county level. Block grant contracts (federal funds dispersed to the State Health Department [SHD] and then allocated to counties based on population) (see Figure 26.1) carried some obligations, and the 10 Essential Public Health Services (EPHS) acted as a guide, but none of these were enforceable (see Table 26.2).

As the months unfolded, the political and economic complexities affecting rural and frontier LHDs grew increasingly evident. The thrill of population-based health care did not lose its luster, and the need for it

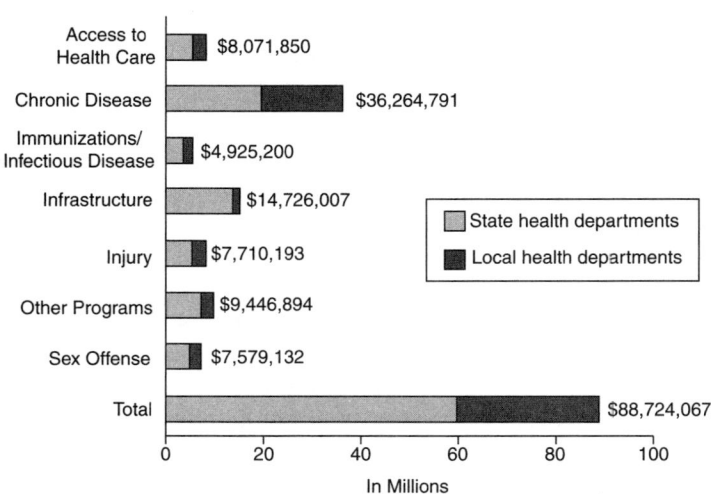

FIGURE 26.1 Preventive Health and Health Services (PHHS) federal block grants. http://www.cdc.gov/chronicdisease/resources/publications/AAG/blockgrant.htm

TABLE 26.2 Essential Public Health Services (EPHS) in Public Health (PH) Language and Common Translation

10 EPHS—PH Version	Common Translation
(1) Monitor health status to identify community health problems	(1) What makes people sick, disabled, causes excess death? How healthy is our community?
(2) Diagnose and investigate health problems and health hazards in the community	(2) Are we ready to respond to health problems or threats in our county? Are we responsive and do we minimize loss, cost, and prevent harm?
(3) Inform, educate, and empower people about health issues	(3) How well do we keep all segments of our community informed about health issues? Do we develop appropriate education materials?
(4) Mobilize community partnerships to identify and solve health problems	(4) How well do we really get people engaged in local health issues?
(5) Develop policies and plans that support individual and community health efforts	(5) What local policies in both government and the private sector promote health in my community?
(6) Enforce laws and regulations that protect health and ensure safety	(6) What local policies in both government and the private sector promote health in my community? How effective are we in setting healthy local policies?
(7) Link people to needed personal health services and assure the provision of health care when otherwise unavailable	(7) Are people in my community receiving the medical and prevention care that they need?
(8) Assure a competent PH and personal health care workforce	(8) Do we have a competent PH staff based on standards, guidelines, and ethics of contemporary PH practice?
(9) Evaluate effectiveness, accessibility, and quality of personal and population-based health services	(9) Are we doing things right? Are we doing the right things?
(10) Research for new insights and innovative solutions to health problems	(10) Are we discovering and using new ways to get the job done and improve outcomes—how do we apply research to improve quality processes and outcomes?

in our community was obvious. The disconnects and a lack of enforceable standards, guidelines, and universally accepted ethics made building a viable, evidence-based, responsive, responsible, and sustainable LHD excruciating—it had become a formidable uphill battle. This scenario was being played out in many frontier and rural LHDs across Montana and across the United States. Some departments had been successful and were thriving, while others were unique LHDs, offering whatever services fell within the skill set, knowledge, and interests of the LHD staff and their governing board, thereby creating person-based LHDs and not standards-based LHDs.

It turned out that I was not alone in looking for the structure for standards-based PH in Montana. I contacted a director of another county health department and together we began the journey to challenge the paradigm of "if you've seen one LHD, you've seen one LHD."

What the Data Told Us

My colleague and I discovered that we faced many of the same challenges when trying to administer a standards-based LHD. To learn more about the challenges facing other administrators, we conducted a review of the literature and a telephone survey of the lead PH official of LHDs serving populations of 5,000 or fewer. We sought to determine the extent of the home health and PH service challenges in these counties, which included 104 incorporated cities and represented 21 or 38% of Montana's 56 counties (average population of the counties surveyed = 2,428.6). With responses from 18 of the 21 counties surveyed (86% response rate),[1] we were able to group the results into three broad categories: (a) availability and access, (b) barriers to PH practice, and (c) resources (see Table 26.3).

Overall, we found PH resources to be inefficiently and—in many instances—ineffectively delivered and utilized as a result of the many challenges and barriers facing PH in frontier and rural communities. The respondents reported being exhausted and frustrated; some even cried—asking us to follow through in our quest to improve LHDs in resource-poor settings in Montana. Indeed, the chasm in the provision of PH across Montana was evident, as was the need for standards and quality-improvement efforts.

Unique characteristics of nursing practice in rural environments have been identified (Bushy, 2012, p. 438):

1. Professional and personal boundaries often overlap
2. Lack of anonymity
3. Requires skills across many disciplines and age groups—a "jack-of-all-trades"
4. Distance
5. Isolation
6. Sparse resources

Pairing these characteristics with the lack of standards and the specificity they bring to an industry adds to rural PHN's many challenges. The science of nursing practice also informs our understanding of the

TABLE 26.3 Results of Literature Search & Survey[1] (n = 18)

(1) Availability and Access to Community/ Public Health Care	(1.1) Average PH Nurse availability = 28.9 hours per week (including grant and county supported)
	(1.2) Four counties (20%) had no PH department; Of the 4 counties without a PH department, 2 had Indian Health Services and 2 were serviced by a neighboring county 1 d/week
	(1.3) 63% had no home health
	(1.4) 37% had "some" home health
	(1.5) 80% reported insufficient time to complete basic PH programs and duties
	(1.6) 40% cited distance challenges/time spent in travel
	(1.7) PH services provided:
	  (a) Immunizations 100%
	  (b) "Minimal" MCH services in all but 2 counties (11%)
	  (c) Tobacco prevention 22%
	  (d) Breast and cervical program 22%
	  (e) Flu clinics 100%
	  (f) Epidemiology 77%
	  (g) School nursing 100% (sole provider or in partnership with school system)
	  (h) PHEP 88%
	  (i) Cancer coalition/grant 44%
	  (j) Agency on Aging senior health programs within the county 22%
	  (k) Well-child 11%
	  (l) Family planning 11%;
	  (m) Some form of home visiting (HV) of the elderly and/or chronic disease management 100% (nonhome health)
	  (n) WIC 22% (Note: WIC is regionalized and some residents must travel to neighboring counties for service)
	(1.8) 100% felt that their county's maternal–child programs were insufficient; few or no parenting classes; little or no high-risk parenting or childhood interventions
	(1.9) When asked how many PH needs they were able to meet in their county (options: none, few, some, most, all) 56% reported meeting "some"; 22% reported "most"; and 22% reported "few"
	(1.10) 49 of Montana's 56 counties are designated Health Professional Shortage Areas (HPSA) (HRSA, 2012)
	(1.11) 53 of Montana's 56 counties are designated Medically Underserved Areas (MUA) (HRSA, 2012)

(2) Barriers to Community/ Public Health Care	(2.1) 90% cited insufficient funding for PH nursing programs (2.2) 100% reported wages below national averages and/or below local hospital pay-scales (one RN with 34 years of experience reported making $10/hr for most of her PH career and only recently began receiving $16/hr) (2.3) 100% reported nursing shortages; retention and recruitment disparities (2.4) 88% stated that they are considering dropping PH programs due to time, human, and fiscal constraints (2.5) 84% reported having poor support from their County Commission (2.6) 88% stated that once they retire from PH they do not think there will be anyone to take on their job: 2 key reasons were cited; unavailable workforce and "no nurse today would take a job with this kind of pay and responsibility"

(continued)

TABLE 26.3 Results of Literature Search & Survey[1] (n = 18) (Continued)

	(2.7) When asked if they could/would offer more PH services 90% stated that they had "enough on my plate ... I don't get everything done as is"
	(2.8) When asked to rank the top barriers to quality and quantity of PH/PH programs in their county, the top four barriers were: (a) money/insufficient budgets, (b) absence of qualified billing personnel, (c) lack of qualified nursing personnel and PH nursing time and, (d) isolation—distance to other services
	(2.9) When asked which PH services are lacking/insufficient due to these barriers the responses were: maternal child health (MCH), teen pregnancy prevention/education, sexually transmitted disease (STD) surveillance and education, family planning, breast feeding, high-risk infant follow-up, diabetes education and follow-up, stroke prevention, better epidemiology, home visiting, case and care management, alcohol and drug prevention, school nursing, and/or improved partnerships, better collaboration with other HC agencies, better health education and disease prevention, and hospice. These were some of the services that the local health jurisdiction (LHJ) felt were needed, but were not provided because of the aforementioned barriers to PH care.
(3) Resource Challenges in Rural and Frontier PH	(3.1) 72% did not have secretarial or administrative support
	(3.2) 76% stated that they were unable to bill for any services because of time, ability, or other barriers—100% of these respondents felt that they could generate revenues for their county if they could bill/bill appropriately
	(3.3) 88% did not attend state or regional meetings because of time, money, and distance, and "no-one to answer the phone when I'm gone"
	(3.4) 100% stated that they could provide improved PH services and perhaps more in-home care if they had more human resources, either as another nurse or secretarial support; preferably both
	(3.5) 12 of the 18 counties employed a nurse: 1% MSN; 60% BSN; 30% ADN; 9% LPN. Note: not all LHD had a nurse on staff)
	(3.6) 40% used federal grant monies to hire secretarial help, but were not able to provide increased direct service tied to the grant funding
	(3.7) 100% felt that the immunization program was a financial liability to the county unless all Vaccines for Children (VFC) is used (related to billing expenses and challenges)
	(3.8) 100% of the counties with the highest poverty rates are rural or frontier
	(3.9) American Indian and Alaska Native race/ethnicity population holds the highest rate of poverty with 24.3% (compared with 12.4% for all US households) of the 2,000 residents living in poverty (MCEE, 2008, p. 459)
	(3.10) Two of the 18 lead PH officials described their county as a "little oil county" (implying that finances were not a significant resource barrier)

[1]The Lead PH Official at 18 LHD was surveyed.

challenges rural and frontier PH nurses face. The metaparadigms of nursing theory—health, environment, person, and nursing—must be considered within the appropriate context (Bushy, 2012). Variables such as environment create a significant impact on nursing practiced in rural settings where distance to clients and to health care are considerable; add winter driving conditions and poor roads in counties that can exceed 5,500 square miles, and the foundations of theory that help to delineate the differences between "rural nursing" and nursing in urban settings become significantly different. One frontier PHN in our survey reported providing PH services to two counties, spending an average of 15 hours per week on the road—traveling at least 200 miles each day of travel. PH nurses in rural and remote settings face myriad complexities that are not modifiable but may be lessened by the adaptation of standards-based practice.

Our next step was to understand what was transpiring nationally. We were relieved and elated to learn about the PH accreditation efforts at the Public Health Accreditation Board (PHAB) (2009). Armed with new evidence and the weight of a national initiative, we took our campaign for PH improvement across Montana and to our legislators. The result of those efforts was House Bill 173 (HB 173, 2009). The purpose of the bill was to conduct a pilot project to assess factors needed to create a sustainable model of standards-based PH for LHDs of every size, in preparation for accreditation. In the Legislative Session of 2009, HB 173 was passed into law.[2]

LESSONS LEARNED

This was by no means a simple effort. Across 18 challenging months, we were able to partner with PH agencies, other LHDs, and our Montana legislators to carry the first local PH bill to a successful outcome. Following are the lessons learned for how rural and frontier LHDs might continue this important legacy for PH quality improvement.

The Journey of HB 173: Ten Rules to Create a Sustainable Model of PH for All of Montana

From our primary research and extensive literature review, my colleague and I had a better understanding of PH quality improvement that could positively affect LPH in Montana. The work to carry a bill forward was tedious and difficult; however, as the saying goes, *"Necessity is the mother of invention"* (Plato, trans. 1955); or said another way, difficult situations inspire ingenious solutions. Our two frontier LHDs were able to pilot a design and a process that led to a coup d'état—the success of HB 173 in the 2009 Montana Legislative session. This bill helped to strengthen the capacity and capability of frontier and rural LHDs across the state to prepare for PH accreditation. From this journey, 10 "rules" of policy change emerged that will need to be continually employed and refined by LHDs in order to cross the quality chasms facing resource-poor settings.

HB 173 was all about "voice"—finding voice, claiming voice, and advocating for the voice of LHDs across Montana.

Rule no. 1: To effect a positive policy change (the foundation for all others), do your best to create a "win-win" situation for all stakeholders.

Policy change requires the action of legislators. *Rule no. 2: To positively influence policy change, recruit your legislative cavalry.*

Become PH advocates and PH experts. *Rule no. 3: Educate, educate, educate!*

Be mindful of the financial landscape. *Rule no. 4: Never consider asking for more money for a program in a poor state that is already awarding money (in sufficient amounts according to the legislators) to a program that sounds an awful lot like what you're trying to do.* No one, anywhere in Montana had ever asked for LHD money specifically to support and address the issue of a lack of standards in local PH departments. PH had been "under" the Montana DPHHS until about 1979, when it was turned over at the behest of LHDs to local commissions and therefore local taxpayers. This bit of history proved to be very important to understanding why LDH like ours were subject to the challenges of providing evidence-based PH, and to understanding the dogma of Montana PH: "If you've seen one LHD, you've seen one LHD"—because each new set of commissioners and lead PH officials (LPHO) "got" to decide what PH was and was not in their county. Asserting that PH is PH, standards are standards, and scope of practice is scope of practice—was an important understanding for all stakeholders as they moved ahead to address the challenges of local PH. *Rule no. 5: Clearly define the roles and responsibilities of stakeholders.*

The next task was to canvas other LHDs to determine the challenges faced by our PH peers. Eighteen HOs from 21 of Montana's frontier and small LHDs were surveyed. The results were sad, alarming, and inspiring. What had started as "let's fix this" became a much larger cause. When all was said and done, the process took about 18 months. *Rule no. 6: Policy change is s-l-o-w. Be patient and thorough and be sure that you are committed to the purpose.*

What had started as a need to understand the state's lack of standards-based LHD for rural and frontier jurisdictions became the answer to our questions. The compelling problem became the solution: We needed a sustainable model of local PH for all Montana. *Rule no. 7: Create a compelling purpose that everyone can understand; "brand" it.*

During our fact-finding mission, we heard cries of desperation and pleas for standards from every one of the 18 LHDs engaged in the study. Other, larger LHDs got wind of the "movement" to create a sustainable model of PH for all Montana and resoundingly said, "Us too!" *Rule no. 8: Create buy-in by making sure that it isn't about "you;" it is about the greater good.*

Finessing and refining the message so that everyone, everywhere "got it" and explaining it *again and again* were necessary tasks to implement this policy change. *Rule no. 9: Be a master communicator and leave no rock un turned when communicating!*

The wave of support that led to the successful legislative adoption of HB 173 came from saying our message; writing about it; and sending briefs to influential PH officials and politicians again and again. *Rule no. 10: Believe in your policy "product" and learn the business of "sales!"*

Following the 10 rules through to a successful conclusion led to an extra rule; personal satisfaction gleaned from a win-win process. Never was the process easy. There were many bumps and hair-pulling sessions along the way. However, the empowerment others felt, the personal power that we discovered, and the many friendships, joy, and knowledge gained along the way were deeply rewarding. *Rule no. 11—the bonus rule— is that the reward is in the process and not necessarily the outcome.*

Summary

A grassroots effort by committed individuals with a passion for excellence and a desire to do the right thing along with strong bipartisan support were critical to the process described in this chapter. As with all bills, many players added their "two cents worth" as the bill progressed through the legislative process. Even so, the intent of the bill remained the same: To determine what it would take to create a sustainable model of standards-based PH for LHDs of every size. Considerations were given to the amount of office space needed for LHDs, the numbers and types of personnel required, and the equipment needed (phones, fax machines, etc.), and directions for meeting the PHAB standards. A review of legal frameworks supporting PH accreditation (Matthews & Markiewicz, 2011) noted the importance of HB173 to the PH accreditation process.

OVERVIEW OF ACCREDITATION

> I had to spend countless hours, above and beyond the basic time, to try and perfect the fundamentals. (Julius "Dr. J" Erving, 1992)

Accreditation is a process that sets and measures fundamental standards of performance across an industry or service and provides users of that industry or service assurance that they can expect that those standards will be met in either the service rendered or from products provided. Accreditation is driven by cost containment and the need for efficiency. The overarching goal of any accreditation process is continuous quality improvement (CQI). Accreditation is always based on best practice and evidence-based practice standards—regardless of the industry. In health care, CQI may be measured in health outcomes, patient satisfaction, cost containment, or other metrics. In addition to hospitals, laboratories, long-term care facilities, clinics, and other health care units can pursue accreditation.

Health care accreditation in the United States can trace its roots back to 1847, when the American Medical Association was formed in response to the poor quality and disorganization of health care in the United States (Luce, Bindman, & Lee, 1994). Hospital conditions continued to be poor into the 20th century and in 1910, Dr. E. Codman presented his ideas about measuring end treatment results as a means of improving the quality of health care (Roberts, Coale, & Redman, 1987). His work led to the formation of the American College of Surgeons and to their subsequent *Hospital Standardization Program*. Health care accreditation was thus born.

The first five standards of the *Hospital Standardization Program* focused on care within hospitals. These were known as the "minimum standards":

1. Organizing hospital medical staffs;
2. Limiting staff membership to well-educated, competent, and licensed physicians and surgeons;
3. Framing rules and regulations to ensure regular staff meetings and clinical review;
4. Keeping medical records that included the history, physical examination, and laboratory results; and
5. Establishing supervised diagnostic and treatment facilities such as clinical laboratories and radiology departments (Luce et al., 1994, p. 263).

Hospitals in the United States have participated in accreditation since 1952, when the American College of Physicians, the American College of Surgeons, the American Medical Association, and the Canadian Medical Association worked together to form The Joint Commission. The Joint Commission (TJC) (2012a) is an independent, not-for-profit organization that accredits and certifies more than 19,000 health care organizations and programs in the United States. In 1966, Avedis Donabedian (as cited in Luce et al., 1994) described three ways to evaluate quality: (a) structure (the operations of patient care—personnel and facilities), (b) process (methods of health care delivery), and (c) outcomes (the end results of health care interventions). This work helped to form the current backbone of quality improvement processes in health care.

Since that time, the "minimum standards" for accreditation have evolved, but the mission of accreditation has remained the same: quality improvement. Today, health care organizations may be accredited through several accrediting bodies; The Joint Commission is just one such entity.

Hospitals and other health care entities with a designated Certification Number (CCN) from the Centers for Medicare and Medicaid Services (CMS) may be accredited by TJC or other approved partners of the CMS. The purpose of TJC accreditation is to "To continuously improve health care for the public, in collaboration with other stakeholders, by evaluating health care organizations and inspiring them to excel in providing safe and effective care of the highest quality and value"[3] (The Joint Commission, 2012b, p. 1).

Government's Role in Accreditation

Accreditation is expensive. Without a means to reimburse accreditation efforts, many rural and frontier counties will most likely not be able to afford the process. The government plays a major role in accreditation through its regulatory and enforcement authority through CMS and its ability to award or withhold Medicare or Medicaid reimbursement. TJC and other accrediting bodies do not have any punitive or regulatory authority outside of granting or denying accreditation. The only funded mandates come through the U.S. Department of Health and Human Services (DHHS)—of which CMS is the health care funding arm. As of this writing, there is no mechanism through CMS, or any other partner, to reimburse accredited LHDs. This important factor—is accreditation financially feasible?—will be a major variable affecting the viability of rural and frontier health department accreditation efforts. Currently, federal funding allocated to LHDs is based on population and not economy of scale or need (see Figure 26.1). This is a national ongoing dialogue: How will we fund PH accreditation?

A new mandate, the Affordable Care Act (ACA) of 2008 (Health Reform.gov, 2008), continues to be played out in the legislative and executive branches of the federal government. Some large third-party payers (insurance companies) have begun adopting the tenets of the ACA. As of this writing, the ACA has not been fully implemented and the "prevention" mandate and its funding are not due to be implemented until 2014. The potential implications and positive financial impact on LHDs are unknown. Will accredited LHDs be awarded financial incentives? How will PH improvement and quality be recognized and compensated? The great confluence of many positive and responsive health care efforts, which hold the potential to address the very chasms that brought about HB 173, are on the horizon.

PH Accreditation Board: Domains, Standards, and Measures

Quality Metrics

PH systems include "all public, private and voluntary entities that contribute to the delivery of essential public health services within a jurisdiction" (Centers for Disease Control and Prevention [CDC], 2010, p. 1). Each of these systems plays a specific role in contributing to the public's health. The governmental PH agency—both at the state and local levels—is a major contributor and leader within this system. The practice of public health has had performance standards since the 1920s (see Table 26.4) and more recently through the CDC when it launched the National Public Health Performance and Standards Program (NPHPSP). The NPHPSP serve as a framework to assess capacity and performance of a PH system and acted as a building block for the development of standards for the newly created Public Health Accreditation Board (PHAB) (2009).

These early CDC standards were only recommendations as there was no existing formal structure within which to manage PH accreditation.

TABLE 26.4 Timeline of Quality Improvement Initiatives in Public Health: From 1850 to 2012

1850	Lemuel Shattack—*Report of the Sanitary Commission of Massachusetts*
1911	First county-based health department
1920	American Public Health Associations (APHA) Commission on Administrative Practices (CAP) releases *Appraisal Form for the City Health Worker*
1927	APHA—CAP releases *Appraisal Form for Rural Health Work*
1988	IOM publishes *The Future of Public Health* (identifies chasms in PH)
1993	Government Performance Results Act (GPRA)
1994	Ten Essential Public Health Services (EPHS) (CDC)
1998–2002	National Public Health Performance Standards Program (NPHPSP)
2002	IOM report *The Future of the Public's Health in the 21st Century*
2005	National Association of City and County Health Officials (NACCHO) publishes *Operational Definition of a Functional Local Health Department*
2007	Public Health Accreditation Board created
2009–2010	Quality Improvement in Public Health defined
2009	House Bill 173 (HB 173) in Montana enacted
2009–2011	HB 173 Pilot Project—assessing what it takes to create sustainable models of accredited PH for jurisdictions of every size
2010	Government Performance and Results Modernization Act of 2010
2010	PHAB Beta-Test Sites reviewed
2011	PHAB Final Standards and Measures released
2012	First applications for PHAB accreditation accepted; site visits began, fall 2012

Accreditation requires the unwavering commitment of a funding body, development of a highly skilled and knowledgeable administrative team, a legal team, and advisory boards, exhaustive research to assess and assure that evidence-based and best practices are appropriately measured and that quality is addressed at both the process levels and in outcome metrics. Essential partnerships must be formed, forged and fully developed, political support garnered and established, and political will sustained (creation of PH champions), sustainable revenue streams created, standards tested and retested for reliability, and stakeholder buy-in developed. Envisioning, designing, implementing, and evaluating an accreditation process was a mammoth project that was successfully launched through the PH accrediting body—PHAB—the Public Health Accreditation Board in Fall 2011. The first applications for PH accreditation were accepted in 2012.

Accreditation criteria are composed of 12 domains that are based on the 10 Essential PH Services (EPHS) (CDC, 1994) (see Table 26.2). LHDs in rural and frontier counties must meet the criteria of the same 12 domains as their larger LHD counterparts in order to become accredited. The domains are composed of standards and each standard is further defined by measures. These standards address quality processes, programs, and interventions germane to the broad range of PH practice.

Accreditation in Rural Jurisdictions

> Variance in the quality and nature of services delivered among rural LHDs and across states was noted as one factor that inhibits progress toward accreditation. (NORC, 2008, p. 18)

Barriers to rural PH accreditation were studied by the National Opinion Research Center (NORC) Walsh Center for Rural Analytics at the University of Chicago (NORC, 2008, pp. 11–13). Their key findings are:

1. Insufficient resources (fiscal, human, facility, education and training, and time).
2. Lack of research to support the benefits of accreditation.
3. Weak PH infrastructure and variable cost–benefit ratios: economy of scale for LHD has not been measured or quantified.
4. Decreased organizational capacity.
5. Deficiencies in workforce skills, knowledge, and professional development as compared to their urban counterparts.
6. Misperception that PH accreditation is only for "the big players," for example, large health departments.
7. Distributed or shared PH authority across counties.

As almost one-quarter of the U.S. population lives in rural and frontier settings, the disparities in health care facing rural dwellers threaten the overall well-being of the population at large. Rural residents have the highest death rates for unintentional injury and motor vehicle accidents; highest death rate among adults for ischemic heart disease and suicide; and highest disability rates in adults with chronic disease. Rural residents have limited access to physician specialists, are least likely to have seen a dentist, and comprise the highest percentage of the population without health insurance (Bushy, 2012).

While there are challenges facing rural and frontier LHDs, it is the very disparities noted above that the EPHS and the PH Core Functions seek to address. In this regard, rural and frontier LHDs are in the greatest need of accreditation, while simultaneously facing the greatest barriers to achieving it. Can rural and frontier LHD be accredited, based on the shortages of human and fiscal resources, infrastructure shortcomings, and skill-mix constraints? Seven Montana counties sought to answer this question through HB 173, and the answer is a guarded yes.

Standardization of LHDs is not intended to increase the workload of PH practitioners; rather, to help them to operate more efficiently in addressing specific county needs while meeting the national standards of PH practice. There is a LHD in all but four of Montana's 56 counties. In some counties, the LHD is the only medical service available in a 60-plus mile radius. With an economy and health care system that is fractured and segmented, people living in these counties depend on their LHD for essential health services. "The underlying premise—and promise—behind improving the performance of a PHD is that doing so results in healthier people and communities" (Riley et al., 2010, p. 5). For LHDs—of every size—the population served deserves and expects the highest standards of practice. To effect the breadth and depth of changes needed to improve the rural public's health, PH stakeholders, management, and leaders must address financial and system inefficiencies and commit to a long-term process to improve population-based outcomes. It is time to create a model of standards-based PH across the state. If the functions of LHDs and the delivery of PH cannot be defined and the scope of practice delineated, it is neither sustainable nor can it be strengthened financially.

SUMMARY

Public health is poised to address the health care disparities in Montana and is charged with improving access to health care for all Montanans. PH services can be cost effective and efficient. PHNs practice prevention; they know the community, and the community members trust and have confidence in them. What better way to provide health care than through strengthened local health departments? Why not invest in the health care that is already established instead of reinventing the wheel? By shoring up the foundation of PH though standardization across the State of Montana, a more functional, sustainable PH practice can be realized that positively affects the well-being of all Montanans.

"The goal of the national accreditation program is to improve and protect the health of the public by advancing the quality and performance of PH departments" (Bialek et al., 2009, pp. 114–115). Through established standards, benchmarks for essential PH services, and ongoing quality-improvement activities at the service level, accreditation demonstrates a commitment to quality while holding PH providers accountable to their governing boards, policy makers, and the community they serve. HB 173 was a beginning step to address challenges facing LHDs in resource-poor settings in Montana. The greatest strength of these combined efforts to enact the legislation is that quality improvement has taken center stage and everyone has been invited to the table to discuss the barriers, challenges, motives, opportunities, and mandates for creating sustainable, responsive, responsible, accredited LHD for communities of every size.

CONCLUSION

While tremendous progress has been made in both public health accreditation and quality improvement in PH, we must not lose momentum as we continue our efforts. (Riley, Beitsch, Parsons, & Moran, 2010, p. 2)

In their commentary *History Will Be Kind*, Turnock and Barnes stated that the accreditation process is on a strong foundation and that "history will indeed be kind to those who helped make it happen" (Turnock & Barnes, 2007, p. 337). It is the hope of this author that the accreditation process will uplift and strengthen every area of PH practice. It seems that the nation is well on the way to improved outcomes and improved processes as a result of the accreditation efforts of the 21st century.

NOTES

1. Survey designed, conducted, and analyzed by Michele Sare on August 18, 2008.
2. See website www.data.opi.mt.gov/bills/2009/billpdf/HB0173.pdf
3. See website www.jointcommission.org/about_us/about_the_joint_commission_main.aspx

REFERENCES

Academy of Achievement. (1992, June). *Julius Erving interview*. Retrieved May 7, 2012, from http://www.achievement.org/autodoc/page/erv0int-1

Bialek, R., Duffy, G. L., & Moran, J. W. (2009). *The public health quality improvement handbook*. Milwaukie: American Society of Quality, Quality Press.

Bushy, A. (2012). Population-centered nursing in rural and urban environments. In M. Stanhope, & J. Lancaster (Eds.), *Public health nursing population-centered health care in the community* (8th ed., pp. 438). Philadelphia, PA: Mosby/Elsevier.

Centers for Disease Control and Prevention (CDC). (2010). *10 Essential public health services*. Retrieved July 24, 2012, from http://www.cdc.gov/nphpsp/essentialservices.html

Centers for Medicare and Medicaid (CMS). (2012). *National health expenditure projections 2010–2020*. Retrieved April 28, 2012, from http://www.cms.gov/Research-Statistics-Data-and-Systems/Statistics-Trends-and-Reports/NationalHealthExpendData/Downloads/proj2010.pdf

Council on Education in Public Health (CEPH). (2012). *History of CEPH*. Retrieved May 21, 2012, from http://www.ceph.org/pg_about_history.htm

Health Resource Services Administration (HRSA). (2012, April). *Primary medical care health professional shortage areas (HPSAs)*; Retrieved May 2, 2012, from http://bhpr.hrsa.gov/shortage/updateddesignations/2012June29/primarycarehpsas06292012.pdf

Health Resource Services Administration (HRSA). (June, 2012). *Shortage designation: Health professional shortage areas & medically underserved areas/populations*. Retrieved July 26, 2012, from http://bhpr.hrsa.gov/shortage/

HealthReform.gov. (2008). *Affordable care act: Laying the foundation for prevention*. Retrieved April 22, 2012, from http://www.healthreform.gov/newsroom/acaprevention.html

House Bill (HB) 173. (2009). *An act creating a pilot project to help local public health agencies undertake activities related to meeting national guidelines; providing for an allocation of funds; and providing an effective date*. Retrieved July 15, 2012, from http://data.opi.mt.gov/bills/2009/billpdf/HB0173.pdf

Luce, J. M., Bindman, A. B., & Lee, P. R. (March 1994). A brief history of health care quality assessment and improvement in the United States. *Western Journal of Medicine, 160*(3), 263–268. Retrieved April 3, 2012, from http://www.ncbi.nlm.nih.gov/pmc/articles/PMC1022402/

Matthews, G., & Markiewicz, M. (2011). *Legal frameworks supporting public health department accreditation: Key findings and lessons learned from ten states*. North Carolina Institute for Public Health, University of North Carolina at Chapel Hill. Retrieved July 14, 2012, from http://www.networkforphl.org/_asset/zpyjq9/Accreditation-Legal-Full-Report.pdf

Montana Council of Economic Education (MCEE). (2008). *The economics of poverty: American Indian reservations in Montana.* Retrieved July 8, 2012, from http://www.econedmontana.org/15_native_american_poverty.pdf

Montana Health Research and Education Foundation (MHREF). (2012). *Critical access hospital.* Retrieved May 5, 2012, from http://www.mtha.org/mhref3.htm

NORC. (2008). *Rural public health agency accreditation final report.* NORC PN No. 6511.01.62; Walsh Center for Rural Analytics, University of Chicago.

Public Health Accreditation Board (PHAB). (2009). *What is PHAB?* Retrieved April 4, 2012, from http://www.exploringaccreditation.org/index.php/about/faq/#history

Public Health Accreditation Board (PHAB). (2012). *Accreditation overview.* Retrieved March 24, 2012, from http://www.phaboard.org/accreditation-overview/

Riley, W. J., Beitsch, L. M., Parsons, H. M., & Moran, J. W. (Jan/Feb 2010). Quality improvement in public health: Where are we now? *Journal of Public Health Management and Practice, 16*(1), 1–2.

Riley, W. J., Moran, J. W., Corso, L. C., Beitsch, L. M., Bialek, R., & Cofsky, A. (2010). Commentary defining quality improvement in public health. *Journal of Public Health Management Practice, 16*(1), 5–7. New York, NY: Wolters Kluwer, Lippincott Williams & Wilkins.

Roberts, J. S., Coale, J. G., & Redman, R. R. (1987). A history of the Joint Commission on Accreditation of Hospitals. *Journal of the American Medical Association, 258*(7), 936–940. doi: 10.1001/jama.1987.03400070074038. Retrieved May 1, 2012, from http://jama.jamanetwork.com/article.aspx?articleid=367766#References

Stanhope, M., & Lancaster, J. (2012). *Public health nursing population-centered health care in the community* (8th ed.). Philadelphia, PA: Mosby/Elsevier.

The Joint Commission (TJC). (2012a). *Joint Commission FAQ page.* Retrieved May 2, 2012, from http://www.jointcommission.org/about/JointCommissionFaqs.aspx?CategoryId=14#81

The Joint Commission (TJC). (2012b). *About the Joint Commission.* Retrieved May 2, 2012, from http://www.jointcommission.org/about_us/about_the_joint_commission_main.aspx

Turnock, B. J., & Barnes, P. A. (2007). Commentary: History will be kind. *Journal of Public Health Management & Practice, 13*(4), 337–341. Retrieved June 2, 2012, from http://www.nursingcenter.com/lnc/journalarticle?Article_ID=728553

Chapter 27

NURSES IN OCCUPATIONAL PRACTICE IN AGRICULTURAL AND RURAL COMMUNITIES IN NEW YORK STATE: PROVIDING OCCUPATIONAL HEALTH AND SAFETY EDUCATION AND PREVENTION SERVICES

Bernadette D. Hodge, Diana E. Gaetano, Susan B. Ackerman, Connie A. Jastremski, and Terry Fulmer

THE BODY OF KNOWLEDGE RELATED to our understanding of rural nursing generally reports on the western and southern areas of the United States. The leading textbook in rural nursing (Winters & Lee, 2010) has been essential to our understanding of rural nursing, and with this edition, the textbook adds a chapter that describes rural nursing in the northeast part of the country and provides an expanded view of rural nursing practice. The purpose of this chapter is to describe the interdisciplinary New York Center for Agricultural Medicine and Health (NYCAMH) and report on the essential services provided by rural occupational health nurses (OHNs) in upstate New York. The population of New York State, as reported by the 2011 estimate of the U.S. Census Bureau, is 19,465,197; 8,175,133 reside in the metropolitan New York City area and over 11 million people live outside this metropolitan area (U.S. Census Bureau State, 2010). The state has a landmass of 47,126.40 square miles (approximately half the size of Colorado). The Adirondack Park comprises over 6 million acres (Adirondack Park 2011 Annual Report, 2011), which is larger than Yellowstone, Yosemite, the Grand Canyon, Glacier National Park, and Great Smoky Mountains National Park combined (Wikipedia, 2012). Further, the southern tier of New York (the area that is geographically below the NY State Thruway) encompasses over 6.8 thousand acres (U.S. Census Bureau State, 2010). The Bassett Healthcare Network is an integrated health care system that provides care and services to people living in an eight-county region covering 5,600 square miles in upstate New York (Bassett Healthcare Network, 2012). Over 400 nurses and 78 nurse practitioners (NPs) are employed in the system. It is in this context that the NYCAMH conducts the important occupational health and safety education and prevention services described here.

RURAL NORTHEAST OCCUPATIONAL CHARACTERISTICS

Geographics and Rural Worksites

New York State averages 411 persons per square mile, but in some of the most rural counties it is as low as two persons. In the central New York region served by NYCAMH, the range is 33 to 124 persons per square mile. The rural nature of large areas of the state is reflected in transportation, communication, and health care challenges that are similar to those experienced in rural areas elsewhere in the United States. Broad swaths of Maine, New York, and Pennsylvania have been designated as health professional shortage areas (HPSAs) by the federal government (Rural Assistance Center [RAC], 2012). Because of the size of these states, the rural population at risk can be considerable. In 2010, over 1.5 million people lived in rural areas in New York State (U.S. Department of Agriculture Economic Research Service [USDA ERS], 2010).

The geography of upstate New York is characterized by rolling hills, river valleys, vast forest-covered mountains, and lakes, making jobs in agriculture, forestry, and fishing prevalent. Typically, the small towns and villages upstate do not have a large manufacturing or business base to provide significant employment or support for the local economies. Schools, health care facilities, county government, and small manufacturers are places of employment for rural residents. County taxes are the main means of providing basic government services such as emergency services and road maintenance. Fire protection is typically provided by community volunteers who essentially are always on call without wage reimbursement. Schools tend to be consolidated districts, centrally located, requiring bus services for large geographic areas, all of which are paid through district taxes. These characteristics taken together tend to support and promote a sense of community among the rural populations, who can manifest a certain pride in the small-town identity and sense of ownership and voice in the decisions about local matters.

THE NEW YORK CENTER FOR AGRICULTURAL MEDICINE AND HEALTH

In the early 1980s, two pulmonologists, Drs. David Pratt and John May, and a nurse researcher, Laura H. Marvel, BSN, RN, at the Mary Imogene Bassett Hospital in Cooperstown, NY, shared an interest in exploring occupational health and safety issues among New York's farming population. In part, they were motivated by the remarkably high rates of occupational fatality, injury, and illness in a large population legislatively exempted from the Occupational Safety and Health Administration's (OSHA) oversight. In 1988, the NY State Legislature established the NYCAMH as a member clinic in the NY State Department of Health's (NYSDOH) eight-member Occupational Health Clinic Network. The addition of this center subsequently granted the NYSDOH support to better understand the causes of agricultural injuries in New York. As a designee in a national project known as Occupational Health Nurses in Agricultural Community (OHNAC), the NYSDOH joined an OHN from NYCAMH with two other agricultural nurses distributed regionally across the state. This collaborative project utilized agricultural health nurses and agricultural engineers to conduct onsite incident investigations and to provide support to farm families following agricultural fatalities.

In 1992, NYCAMH became one of seven agricultural centers designated by the National Institute for Occupational Safety and Health (NIOSH) to be known as the Northeast Center for Agricultural Medicine (NEC). These centers, located in geographically designated regions, act by cooperative agreement to address pertinent and emerging problems related to occupational safety and health in agriculture, forestry, and fishing. Also, in the early 1990s, NYCAMH's "Farm Partners" program was created to identify and address the causes of stress for farm families and their hired workers. Counseling services were provided by a social worker who was often accompanied by a nurse.

In the mid-1990s, NYCAMH began performing annual physical exams and classifications for firefighter and emergency medical service (EMS) personnel. In response to increased requests, the Healthworks occupational health services program was initiated in 1995 to address the health and safety needs of the rural business community.

Organizational Structure, Staff, and Population Served

Federal, state, and private funding are the means by which NYCAMH/NEC provides services to rural and agricultural populations. A combined research team of anthropologists, epidemiologists, statisticians, and public health faculty collaborate with other northeast researchers in agricultural injury and illness surveillance, intervention, and prevention activities. Clinical services are provided by physicians, nurse practitioners

(NPs), social workers, and occupational health nurses (OHNs) within the organizational structure managed by a nurse administrator. A health science librarian with nursing background provides library services and maintains the rural occupational resource collection.

Safety educators provide onsite farm safety and health training to farmers, family members, and farmworkers in English and Spanish languages in New York State and throughout the northeast. Safety training is also made available to the Anabaptist community through collaboration with a nurse educator in Pennsylvania. The population served through the Healthworks service line might be some of those same farmers who are also volunteer firefighters as well as rural business employees throughout much of New York State.

OCCUPATIONAL AND ENVIRONMENTAL HEALTH NURSE PROFESSION

The OHN is utilized in occupational settings to provide health and safety programs and services. These services focus on promotion and restoration of health, prevention of illness and injury, and protection from work-related and environmental hazards. The approach to this type of health care delivery is population focused with the client as an inclusive term, including individual workers, workers' families, worker populations, communities, environments, and employers (American Association of Occupational Health Nurses [AAOHN], 2012).

Because poor employee health costs business about $1 trillion annually (AAOHN, 2012), business executives look to OHNs to maximize employee productivity and reduce costs through lowered disability claims, fewer on-the-job injuries, and improved absentee rates. OHNs possess a combined knowledge of health and business, balancing the requirement for a safe and healthy work environment with a healthy bottom line (Rogers, 2003).

Occupational and environmental health nursing practice maintains a public health model of prevention and an environmental health focus. Typically, OHNs possess a baccalaureate degree in nursing and experience in community health, ambulatory care, critical care, or emergency nursing. Many OHNs have obtained advanced degrees as well as certification in occupational and environmental health nursing. Seven major roles exist in occupational and environmental health nursing: clinician/practitioner, case manager, health promotion specialist, manager, consultant, educator, and researcher (Rogers, 2003).

NYCAMH OHN SERVICES TO RURAL BUSINESSES

The OHNs play a key role in responding to the needs of small rural businesses. Here, the range of services is broad: preplacement and annual employee evaluations; assessments to assure OSHA compliance; and assistance in implementing workplace safety and health programs. For example, in a local pharmaceutical manufacturing worksite, the role of the OHN in support of a blood-borne pathogens program is to ensure that safe working procedures and training are implemented to prevent employee illness. In a nearby science laboratory, the OHN participates in a chemical safety program by ensuring proper management of chemicals present in the facility and by providing employees with necessary safety and health information regarding chemical hazards associated with their jobs. Hearing conservation is another frequently requested service, which ensures that hazardous noise levels are minimized and employees exposed to these noises are properly protected. In varied settings such as a county highway department or a dairy food processor, the OHN provides audiometric testing to document workers' hearing acuity and to monitor the hearing of employees frequently exposed to hazardous noise levels. In addition, the OHN makes referrals to an industrial hygienist for identification and control of workplace exposures to chemical and physical hazards important to worker health. OSHA-mandated respiratory protection programs are another facet of the work with small rural businesses. Recent Healthworks services with a yogurt manufacturer and a construction company ensure that exposures to hazardous air contaminants are minimized and exposed employees are properly protected.

Worksite Wellness Programs

The OHN as a health promotion specialist has a key role in occupational and environmental health nursing. The goal of a worksite health promotion program is improving the overall health status and productivity of the workforce and reducing health care costs (Rogers, 2003). The workplace is where many people spend a third of their life and it can be a unique venue for health promotion activities. The Healthworks OHN administers the worksite wellness program that was initiated in 2011. This fee-for service line is being marketed within an eight-county service area in central New York; it includes assessments of a worksite's readiness to provide support for healthier lifestyles, biometric screenings, and health risk assessments for employees. These wellness programs also assist with the design and delivery of educational, motivational, and self-care programs, and provide support with program evaluation, including return-on-investment data. While the first year was spent in large part on program infrastructure development (educational session development, database building, etc.) and marketing, several important milestones were reached: program staff achieved WELCOA (Wellness Council of America) certification in several areas of worksite wellness programming; educational programming was pilot tested at a training for 100 staff members at a local not-for-profit organization; marketing initiatives enabled relationship building with over 20 separate employers; and initial volunteer biometric screenings to identify risk factors for chronic disease were conducted at one large (500+ employees) public service organization and one large manufacturing plant, with plans to continue the program for each site in 2012 and 2013. A total of 147 employees participated in this first round of screenings.

This effort in worksite wellness builds upon a long-established worksite health promotion program specifically aimed at cardiovascular disease prevention. Administered by an OHN, this program has provided screenings for cholesterol (totals for cholesterol and high-density lipoproteins [HDL] and their ratio), blood pressure, body mass index (BMI), waist/hip ratio, and blood glucose for employees across our region. Recently, at eight area worksites, 208 employees were screened. Each individual received his or her 10-year risk of heart disease assessment (based on the Framingham risk equation), counseling regarding their screening results, and educational information on ways to maintain optimal health and prevent heart disease. One hundred and nineteen individuals were referred for follow-up. These individuals were also screened for blood glucose levels. Two hundred and five employees had normal glucose results; three individuals had impaired fasting glucose or impaired glucose tolerance. Since the inception of this health promotion program in 2001, a total of 15,293 individuals has been screened, of which 9,603 individuals have been referred for medical evaluation.

Volunteer Firefighters and Emergency Service Personnel

Each year, an average of 100 firefighters die while on duty in the United States (Centers for Disease Control and Prevention [CDC], 2012). A leading cause of these fatalities is myocardial infarction (MI) caused by stress and overexertion (Gaetano et al., 2007). As a result of incidents that occurred in 2011, the U.S. Fire Administration (USFA) reported 81 on-duty firefighter fatalities in the United States, and 87 fatalities were reported for 2010 (USFA, 2012). MIs were responsible for the deaths of 48 firefighters (59%) in 2011, nearly the same proportion of firefighter deaths from MI (60%) as in 2010 (USFA, 2012).

The physical demands placed on firefighters can be very high and they often have to go from a state of sleep to near 100% alertness and high physical exertion in a matter of minutes. Further, they must carry heavy equipment through intense heat while wearing heavy gear. Heart rates in this setting often approach 200 beats per minute (Smith, Petruzzello, Kramer, & Misner, 1996). Owing to the physical demands of firefighting, it is recommended that firefighters maintain a high level of physical fitness (Federal, 2002).

The Healthworks program provides health surveillance to rural volunteer firefighters and EMS personnel. According to NY State's 2007–2009 vital statistics data as of March 2011, the cardiovascular disease age-adjusted annual death rate per 100,000 residents is significantly higher in five of the eight counties served by the clinic as compared to the New York State rate (NYSDOH, 2012).

OHNs are uniquely qualified to deliver health and wellness programs to firefighters and EMS personnel at high risk for MI in the line of duty. At the Healthworks onsite screenings, the American College of Cardiology Framingham Coronary Heart Disease Risk Calculations was incorporated into a health evaluation that provides clearance to perform essential emergency job functions. OHNs may utilize cardiac risk profiling to provide an objective measure of coronary heart disease (CHD) risk. These screening clinics have demonstrated that an increase in knowledge of cardiac risk in asymptomatic individuals that are often in the early stages of CHD can result in early health care intervention. The primary focus of health surveillance for rural volunteer fire fighters and EMS personnel is proper job classification. However, surveillance could also encourage primary prevention among individuals who have modifiable risk factors for CHD as well as minimizing liability for a volunteer's cardiovascular disease event in the line of duty. In a 2007 study, 78% of the emergency personnel identified by cardiac risk screening and subsequently referred sought consultation with and initiated treatment of risk factors (Gaetano et al., 2007).

Each year, NYCAMH OHNs and other staff provide over a thousand rural volunteer firefighters and EMS personnel with at least one health surveillance examination and firefighter or EMS classification. The examination includes detailed health and occupational history, vital signs, vision testing, electrocardiogram, spirometry, respirator fit testing, including self-contained breathing apparatus and disposable particulate respirator, as well as physical examination. Volunteers 45 years or older desiring A classification (interior structure firefighter or EMS personnel) or B classification (exterior structure firefighter or EMS personnel) receive a lipid screening and a cardiac risk profile. The Framingham 10-year risk is estimated using established Framingham risk tables and the corresponding point system (Grundy, Pasternak, Greenland, Smith, & Fuster, 1999).

In 2011, a total of 1,617 volunteer firefighters and EMS personnel were evaluated, which included 1,290 men (80%) and 327 women (20%). The mean age of this predominately White, blue-collar population was 42.5 years. Eleven percent of this population were smokers. Cardiac risk profiles were calculated on 197 individuals, with 88% passing. Of the 1,617 volunteers, 264 (16%) had one or more abnormal findings. One hundred and fifty-two (58%) were noted to be hypertensive. Abnormal electrocardiograms were noted in 70 (27%). Abnormal spirometry (predominately obstructive) was noted in 44 (17%). Significant abnormalities in the physical exam were noted in 18 persons (7%). Lipid measurements were available on 55 of the 264 volunteers. Total cholesterol ≥ 200 mg/dL was noted on

30 (55%). Reduced HDL (less than 40 mg/dL) was present in 22 (40%). Unfortunately, a substantial proportion of this middle-aged volunteer population has problems with obesity, hypertension, and indicators of cardiovascular disease.

NYCAMH OCCUPATIONAL SERVICES TO FARMERS AND FARM FARMILIES

Population Demographics

Agriculture is the largest industry in New York State, with a production value of $4.7 billion in 2010. According to the USDA 2007 Census, there are over 36,000 farms in New York State, averaging 200 acres per farm, with an employment total of 100,000 persons. Dairy, nursery, and fruit are the top commodities in NY agriculture (USDA, 2007). In 2007, the average age of the primary farm operator was 56.2 years (up from 52.9 in 1997). Male farm operators have declined from 88% in 1997 to 82% in the 2007 census. In addition, more operators are reporting that farming is not their principal occupation. An aging workforce and part-time farming may imply health- and safety-related challenges such as chronic illness and medication effects, and lower reaction time in elder farmers. Fatigue, inexperience, and child care issues can be relevant to part-time working hours, while gender-related conditions such as pregnancy can be of concern for farm women.

There are also certain characteristics unique to the farming occupation that have health and safety implications: it is the only occupation where families live, work, and play at the worksite; it is where children have a role in the farm operation; there is no retirement age; and in terms of safety and health, the industry is essentially self-regulated. Herein is the framework in which NYCAMH nurses provide clinical, educational, and prevention services to farmers and farm families.

OHN Clinical Services for Farmers

Within the Healthworks program, OHNs provide a major contribution to the NYCAMH mission, which is enhancing agricultural health by preventing and treating occupational injury and illness. The OHN provides clinical consultation to injured or ill farmers through the Farmers' Occupational Health Clinic, a diagnostic clinic that can include a worksite assessment if needed. Owing to the hazardous exposures in their work environments, farmers need to use safe work practices and may need guidance in the identification and selection of appropriate personal protective equipment. Though farmers seldom seek social services, many farm families are in need of referral to such services. The OHN will help to address each of these issues with the farmer.

NURSES IN AGRICULTURAL RESEARCH AND PREVENTION SERVICES

Occupational Health Nurses in Agricultural Communities, and Farm Partners

The OHNAC program allowed for community-based nurses with a farming background to gain the trust of the farming community. This trust was critical both to receiving reports of fatalities and/or serious injuries and to being allowed on the farm to conduct in-depth investigations with the agricultural engineer for serious incidents and fatalities. Reports of injuries and/or fatalities would come through the nurses' networking with local hospitals, veterinarians, extension agents, emergency personnel, sheriff and police departments, and through self-reports. After learning of a case, the nurse would contact the injured farmer and attempt to conduct a site visit along with a safety engineer. Phone contact was attempted following farm fatalities as well, but often an unscheduled visit would be made if phone contact had not occurred. For all case follow-ups, the nurses' goals were to provide support to the injured worker and/or family members, identify the cause of the incident, and develop recommendations for preventing similar incidents. Additionally, OHNAC nurses provided education and outreach, exhibiting at farm shows, educating students and medical providers on traumatic farm injuries and extrication, giving presentations to farm groups, and publishing articles. Papers highlighting some of the more frequent nurse-investigated injuries and fatalities deal with silo gas exposure (Pavelchak et al., 1999), hand injuries (Boyd et al., 1997), bull injuries (Casey et al., 1997a), cow injuries (Casey et al., 1997b), tractor-related fatalities (Roerig et al., 1996), and scalping incidents (Roerig, Melius, & Casey 1992).

In addition to its scientific productivity, this program allowed nurses with a farm background to administer nursing care services to other members of the farm community. Farmers identified with these nurses and were open to assistance that they would not have sought otherwise. Services ranged from removal of stitches to counseling families following the death of a child. For the nurses, this aspect of the OHNAC role was as personally satisfying as the surveillance accomplishments. This unique program allowed interactions for surveillance, intervention, education, and prevention to occur simultaneously, giving the nurses opportunities to concentrate on the essentials of safety and safe practices. An approach consistent with findings in Seiz (2001) was that "Farmers want to know what is important and why; they want essential information uncluttered by matters they perceive as marginal and peripheral to their health and safety" (p. 9).

The Farm Partners program, initiated through W. K. Kellogg Foundation funding, enlisted agribusiness personnel to help identify farmers/

families in social, economic, and emotional crisis and to link them with a social worker for follow-up counseling and referral to community and governmental agencies. If the stressor was perceived as the result of an injury or fatality, the agricultural nurse would assist in the farm visits and subsequent counseling sessions. Often, the Farm Partners cases would be referred by the OHNAC nurse after a farm fatality. Once a relationship had been established with the nurse, the counseling services were more readily accepted, particularly since many farmers are known to express a broad distrust of safety information emanating from professionals with little to no farming experience (Seiz, 2001).

Children and Farm Safety

According to the Childhood Agricultural Injury Survey in the United States between the years 2001 and 2006, an average of 26,655 injury incidences occurred annually to youth under the age of 20 who were working or living on farms. Among youth workers, agriculture has the second highest fatality rate, 21.3 per 100,000 full-time equivalents [FTE] as compared to 3.6 per 100,000 across all industries (National Children's Center, 2011). OHNAC investigations that involved the death of a child were particularly difficult. One sees that these events occur in an instant, where all but one detail goes as planned, and entire families' lives were changed forever. In these situations, the data gathered by the engineer was critically important, but often for the family, the nurse had more impact as she was a farmer and a nurse, listening and comforting.

Farms are a unique industry in that the workplace is the home and so health and safety education often needs to include children as well as adults. What other industry combines the child's home and playground with the parent's workplace and routinely relies upon the labor of preteens and young teenagers? Nurses participate in outreach programs such as Safety Day Camps as a means to provide age-appropriate information for children on important topics such as first aid, animal safety, mechanical hazards, and chemical safety. In 1990, a NYCAMH nurse educator was asked to conduct a 3-hour program on farm safety for a group of rural children ages 7 to 12 years. This was the impetus for the creation of the game named "Play it Safe: The Farm Safety Challenge Game" that could be fun as well as an effective tool for teaching the safety and health concepts relevant to the farm and to rural environments. In 1995, the game was published with NIOSH funding, and 520 games were sold. An evaluation was conducted with adult consumers who used the game with 4H groups, friends, families, and agricultural classes. Since this time, the game has been sold nationally (two nursing programs) and continues to be popular for casual group, family, and classroom farm safety and health learning activities (Marvel, May, & Townsend, 1998).

Another key intervention aimed at child injury prevention is the North American Guidelines for Children's Agricultural Tasks, which was created with guidance from nurses, educators, and farm families to assist parents in deciding if their child was developmentally ready for certain farm chores. NYCAMH nurses participated in the coordination and dissemination of these guidelines as well as a follow-up study to assess the efficacy of the guidelines. Data on childhood injuries, tasks, and hours worked were obtained quarterly for 21 months, on a sampling of NY farms. Injury rates were compared with those of control farms, and the results showed that dissemination of the guidelines reduced rates of work-related childhood agricultural injuries by 50% (Gadomski, Ackerman, Burdick, & Jenkins, 2006).

A Bassett Healthcare Network school-based NP tested the efficacy of another educational intervention, "Keep on Tract," on knowledge levels of farm safety among fifth graders in rural public schools in New York. Her findings revealed that the difference in pre- and posttest mean scores were increased significantly immediately posttest, as well as at 1-month follow-up (Sullivan, 2011).

Skin Cancer Screening

The farming workforce is at risk for the development of skin cancer, particularly because of the long hours of exposure to ultraviolet light, and also because in an aging population, the risk of developing malignancy is increased (Donham & Thelin, 2006). In the past 10 years, NYCAMH nurses have been providing the opportunity for free skin cancer screenings at large northeast farm shows, with participation averaging 188 persons per year. Participants with presumptive diagnoses are followed by the nurses, who give guidance and counsel regarding their medical referral. Over time, the data have demonstrated that approximately one-third of the participants are in need of medical follow-up. The most frequent diagnosis is actinic keratosis, a precancer that warrants early treatment. Few melanomas have been identified and treated over the course of these screenings. Qualitative data consistently show that participants voice positive and appreciative feedback for this service (Gaetano et al., 2009).

Pregnancy and Farm Exposure

An emergency department (ED) report regarding a pregnant farm woman having accidentally injected herself with a hormone she was administering to a cow prompted NYCAMH researchers to compare exposures and risks to pregnant women living and working on farms with the exposures of rural nonfarm pregnant women. Exposures and risks studied included chemicals, heavy lifting, bending, large animals, machinery, veterinarian medications, and long work hours. Comparisons of questionnaire responses from farm and nonfarm pregnant women found that while most exposures for both groups were comparable, for farm women, their exposure and possible skin contamination with such veterinarian medications as oxytocin and antibiotics, as well as exposure to diesel fumes, did represent a possible threat to their pregnancy (Evans et al., 1998).

Migrant Farmworkers

Estimating the migrant farmworker population nationally is an ongoing challenge, primarily due to the seasonal and variable nature of agricultural work. In fact, there is no local, state, or national agency responsible for collecting these data (National Center for Farmworker Health [NCFH], 2012). In New York State, the migrant farm population has changed from working on seasonal crop harvests only to a year-round presence on dairy farms. A NYCAMH nurse coordinated a survey of dairy farms in NY, Pennsylvania, and Vermont to assess the proportion of Spanish-speaking workers employed by these farms. The percentage of Spanish-speaking workers ranged from 20% on large farms to 5% on smaller farms (Stack, Jenkins, Earle-Richardson, Ackerman, & May, 2006). These findings led to the addition of a bilingual safety educator, who conducts farm safety training programs and develops educational materials for Spanish-speaking migrant farmworkers. In the United States, there are 159 federally funded migrant health centers, most of which are not-for-profit corporations operated by community-based organizations or state health departments (NCFH, 2012). NYCAMH has worked with migrant clinics in Maine, Connecticut, and New York on community collaboration-based research projects to address musculoskeletal and ergonomic issues that impact farmworker health and safety.

Nurses who provide occupational health services to the migrant populations in the clinic setting are often required to travel to satellite service sites as well as conduct onsite clinics at farmsteads and field localities. When asked what was unique about her role as a migrant clinic nurse, one nurse responded that being of the same Hispanic cultural origin as her patients helps to develop a trusting relationship and be more effective in her care" (M. Zapata, personal communication, March 22, 2012).

Anabaptist Communities

A nurse educator in Pennsylvania has worked extensively with the Amish community, providing training in cardiopulmonary respiration (CPR), farm emergency response, and first aid for school grades 1 to 8, and for vocational school students 14 years old, adults, and home scholars. She created a training booklet that included information on dental hygiene, hand washing, treatment of colds and flu, hearing loss from noise, burn prevention and treatment, and appropriate responses to animal, insect, and snake bites. This NYCAMH collaborator also provides a program for parents pertaining to safe, healthy children, as well as a farm/home safety and CPR/emergency rescue. Safety and health training includes calculating appropriate dosages for medications; home treatment for diarrhea, vomiting, and thrush; as well as when to see a doctor. Information is shared on where to get low-cost or free immunizations. At health screenings, an NP or college nursing instructor, along with nursing students, conducts physical assessments for each child, including height, weight, vision testing, a dental exam (how many cavities), blood pressure, hearing, and scoliosis check, and advice on various health concerns. Children are referred to a doctor if medically necessary. Since most Amish/Mennonite children are not seen for routine well-baby checkups, they miss all the preventive care and information. In this program, mothers are educated on what to try at home, and when to get medical help. Home-schooled families have as many as 14 children and are very appreciative of this program. When participants have been asked why these programs are so well attended, frequent comments center on the fact that nurses are providing the training and exams.

A rural central NY doctoral dissertation by an NP in rural central New York included examination of the barriers to health care access for the Amish population in a geographic locality in upstate New York and implementation of a collaborative effort to develop a strategic plan of action to address their needs. This Amish group identified cost and transportation to be their largest barriers to accessing health care. Prenatal care, home birthing assistance, and childhood immunizations were identified as priority health needs. The most desired health care provider qualities specified by this group are honesty and trustworthiness. Working collaboratively with the study population, the NP developed an action plan that included reestablishing immunization services and an exploration of independent family practice for this Amish community (McCrea, 2011).

EDUCATIONAL OUTREACH FOR NURSES

Occupational and environmental health topics are a part of the public health curriculum in baccalaureate nursing programs, but they typically receive minimal emphasis. A collaborative effort between faculty in an upper division university nursing program and the occupational nurse staff at NYCAMH resulted in an educational program to assist nurses to gain an understanding of the occupationally related health and safety issues in rural and farming communities. An evaluation by the nurses indicated that they considered the gaining of an awareness of the effects occupational hazards may have on their clients to be a worthwhile use of their program (Hodge, Ackerman, Evans, Erb, & Cook, 2002). This occupational health and safety program has been presented as a lecture every semester for public health nursing students at the university and other area colleges since 1997. In addition to the classroom time, nurses are offered the opportunity to complete clinical hours under the supervision of an OHN.

SUMMARY

Nursing practice in occupational health in agricultural and rural communities encompasses all the traditional nurse functions of patient care, teaching, and research, and may at times be conducted in very nontraditional settings such as farm buildings and fields, village firehouses, highway workshops, community meetings, and even major trade shows. In such settings, nurses can be performing health assessments by checking blood pressure or cholesterol readings, conducting teaching sessions and disseminating health information to a group of rural residents, providing counsel and referral for an injured farm worker, or reviewing medical records for injury surveillance research data. The focus for nurses who practice in public and occupational health is not as much on the individual and a disease state as it is on the group or population and the preservation of health through prevention. This requires the nurse to have a comprehensive understanding of the occupational, environmental, economic, and cultural dimensions of that population, including the risks and hazardous exposures that impact their health and safety. As the nurse utilizes this knowledge in rural and occupational practices, a valuable contribution is being made to advance evidence-based research in the promotion of a healthy and safe working population.

ACKNOWLEDGMENT

The authors gratefully acknowledge the editorial assistance of Dr. Patricia Cabrera and Dr. John May.

REFERENCES

American Association of Occupational Health Nurses (AAOHN). (2012). *The occupational and environmental health nursing profession.* Retrieved March 12, 2010, from https://www.aaohn.org/component/option,com_docman/Itemid,376/task,doc_view/gid,881/

Bassett Healthcare Network. (2012). *Bassett Healthcare Network.* Retrieved April 5, 2012, from http://www.bassett.org/

Boyd, J., Hil, M., Pollock, J., Casey, G., Gelberg, K., Roerig, S. et al. (1997). Epidemiological characteristics of reported hand injuries—New York State 1991–1995. *Journal of Agricultural Safety and Health, 3,* 101–107.

Casey, G., Grant, A. M., Roerig, S., Boyd, J., Hill, M., London, M. et al. (1997a). Farm worker injuries associated with bulls: New York State 1991–1996. *AAOHN Journal, 45*, 393–396.

Casey, G., Grant, A. M., Roerig, S., Boyd, J., London, M., Gelberg, K. et al. (1997b). Farm worker injuries associated with cows. *AAOHN Journal, 45*, 446–450.

Centers for Disease Control and Prevention (CDC). (2012). *Firefighter fatality investigation and prevention program*. Retrieved March 14, 2012, from http://www.cdc.gov/niosh/fire/

Donham, K. J., & Thelin, A. (2006). Agricultural skin diseases and cancer in agricultural populations. In *Agricultural medicine: Occupational and environmental health for the health professions* (pp. 145–172). Ames, IA: Blackwell.

Evans, C., Marvel, L., May, J. J., Erb, T., Jenkins, P., & Townsend, C. (1998, October). *Study of reproductive risks of pregnant farm women*. Presented at the Fourth International Symposium, "Rural Health and Safety in a Changing World". The Center for Agricultural Medicine, Saskatoon, Canada.

Federal Emergency Management Agency, United States Fire Administration, National Data Center. (2002). *Fire fighter fatality retrospective study*. Retrieved March 14, 2012 from http://www.usfa.fema.gov/downloads/pdf/publications/fa-220.pdf

Gadomski, A., Ackerman, S., Burdick, P., & Jenkins, P. (2006). Efficacy of the North American guidelines for children's agricultural injuries. *American Journal of Public Health, 96*, 722–727.

Gaetano, D. E., Ackerman, S., Clark, A., Hodge, B., Hohensee, T., May, J. J. et al. (2007). Health surveillance for rural volunteer firefighters and emergency medical services personnel. *AAOHN Journal, 55*(2), 57–63.

Gaetano, D. E., Hodge, B., Clark, A., Ackerman, S., Burdick, P., & Cook, M. L. (2009). Preventing skin cancer among a farming population: Implementing evidence-based interventions. *AAOHN Journal, 57*(1), 24–33.

Grundy, S. M., Pasternak, R., Greenland, P., Smith, S., Jr., & Fuster, V. (1999). Assessment of cardiovascular risk by use of multiple-risk-factor assessment equations: A statement for healthcare professionals from the American Heart Association and the American College of Cardiology. *Circulation, 100*(13), 1481–1492.

Hodge, B. D., Ackerman, S., Evans, C., Erb, T., & Cook, M. L. W. (2002). An occupational health nursing education program: Relevance to nurses in nonoccupational practice settings. *AAOHN Journal, 50*(6), 257–261.

Marvel, L. H., May, J. J., & Townsend, C. (1998, March). *An evaluation of "Play it Safe: The Farm Safety Challenge Game"*. Poster presented at Health Promotion Across the Lifespan, 9th Annual Art & Science of Health Promotion Conference, Monterey, California.

McCrea, K. L. (2011). *A comprehensive health needs assessment and strategic plan of action for two Amish districts.* Unpublished doctoral dissertation, Frontier School of Midwifery and Family Nursing, Hyden, Kentucky.

National Center for Farmworker Health (NCFH). (2012). *Enumeration and population estimates.* Retrieved March 16, 2012 from http://www.ncfh.org/?pid=23

National Children's Center for Agricultural Health and Safety. (2011). *2011 Fact sheet childhood agricultural injuries.* Retrieved March 26, 2012, from http://www.ncfh.org/?plugin=ecomm&content=item&sku=9267

New York State Adirondack Park Agency. (2011). *Annual report 2011.* Retrieved April 5, 2012, from http://www.apa.ny.gov/Documents/Reports/ADAnnualReport-20120315-KPM-F-AR2011c.pdf

New York State Department of Health (NYSDOH). (2012). *Cardiovascular disease deaths and death rates.* Retrieved March 14, 2012 from http://www.health.ny.gov/statistics/chac/mortality/cardio.htm

Pavelchak, N., Church, L., Roerig, S., London, M., Welles, W., & Casey, G. (1999). Silo gas exposure in New York state following the dry growing season of 1995. *Applied Occupational and Environmental Hygiene, 14,* 34–38.

Roerig, S., Casey, G., London, M., Boyd, J., Hill, M., Anderson, M. et al. (1996). Fatalities associated with improper hitching to farm tractors—New York, 1991–1995. *MMWR, 45,* 307–311.

Roerig, S., Melius, J., & Casey, G. (1992). Scalping incidents involving hay balers—New York. *MMWR, 41,* 489–491.

Rogers, B. (2003). *Occupational and environmental health nursing: Concepts and practice.* (2nd ed.). Philadelphia, PA: Saunders.

Rural Assistance Center, *Health professional shortage areas (HPSAs) & medically underserved areas/populations (MUAs/MUPs).* Retrieved March 22, 2012 from http://www.raconline.org/racmaps/#hpsa

Seiz, R. C. (2001). What farm families tell us that can be useful in educating for health and safety. *Journal of Extension, 39*(6), 1–11.

Smith, D. L., Petruzzello, S. J., Kramer, J. M., & Misner, J. E. (1996). Physiological, psychophysical, and psychological responses of firefighters to firefighting training drills. *Aviation, Space, and Environmental Medicine, 67*(11), 1063–1068.

Stack, S., Jenkins, P., Earle-Richardson, G., Ackerman, S., & May, J. J. (2006). Spanish-speaking dairy workers in New York, Pennsylvania and Vermont: Results from a survey of farm owners. *Journal of Agromedicine, 11,* 37–44.

Sullivan, T. (2011, October). *The efficacy of the 'Keep on Track' educational intervention and its impact on farm safety knowledge levels among rural school age children*. Poster presented at the Biannual International Rural Nursing and Rural Health Conference, Binghamton, New York.

U.S. Census Bureau. (2010). *State and county quick facts 2010*. Retrieved March 22, 2012 from http://quickfacts.census.gov/qfd/states/36000.html

U.S. Census Bureau. (2012). *Census regions and divisions of the United States*. Retrieved March 12, 2012, from http://www.census.gov/geo/www/us_regdiv.pdf

USDA Census of Agriculture. (2007). *State summary highlights 2007*. Retrieved March 26, 2012 from http://www.agcensus.usda.gov/Publications/2007/Full_Report/Volume_1,_Chapter_2_US_State_Level/st99_2_001_001.pdf

USDA Economic Research Service (ERS). (2010). *State fact sheets 2010*. Retrieved March 22, 2012, from http://www.ers.usda.gov/StateFacts/

United States Fire Administration (USFA). (2012). *U.S. Fire Administration announces 2011 on-duty firefighter fatalities*. Retrieved March 14, 2012, from http://www.usfa.fema.gov/media/press/2012releases/010312.shtm

Wikipedia. (2012). Adirondack Park. Retrieved April 5, 2012, from en.wikipedia.org/wiki/Adirondack_Park

Winters, C. A., & Lee, H. J. (2010). *Rural nursing: Concepts, theory and practice*. (3rd ed.). New York, NY: Springer Publishing.

Chapter 28

IMPLICATIONS FOR EDUCATION, PRACTICE, AND POLICY
Jean M. Shreffler-Grant
and Marlene A. Reimer

As an Applied Discipline, Nursing has traditionally measured the relevance of theory by the extent to which it can inform practice, education, and health care policy. Our purpose in this chapter is to make more explicit the relevance of key elements of the rural theory base. We discuss selected educational, practice, and health care policy implications of the key concepts and theoretical statements as reported by Long and Weinert (1989) and Lee and McDonagh (2006). We explore how these implications may need to change as rural nursing theory is revised and extended. We also present exemplars from the United States, Canada, and Australia to illustrate how the key concepts and theoretical statements can inform education, practice, and health care policy that address rural populations and their health across international borders.

IMPLICATIONS OF THE FIRST THEORETICAL STATEMENT

How a group of citizens perceive health, manage their health, and seek health care has broad implications for education, practice, and policy that transcend national borders. The first theoretical statement is "Rural dwellers define health primarily as the ability to work, to be productive, to do usual tasks" (Long & Weinert, 1989, p. 120). The interrelated concepts associated with this statement are work beliefs and health beliefs; health is defined in relation to work, and health needs are secondary to work needs.

Education

On the basis of the original rural nursing theory work, the first theoretical statement suggests that nursing programs should include the concept of role performance as health in curricula so that nurses include actual or potential effects of a health problem on the ability to work and to do usual tasks in their assessments and plans of care. Nursing educators should also offer opportunities for students to learn how clients' definitions of health influence their health and illness management behaviors.

Practice

In the practice arena, the first theoretical statement suggests that rural health services should be oriented, structured, and timed to fit with the rhythm of work and role performance. In addition, the benefits of preventive care may be better communicated by framing them according to what will assist rural dwellers to continue to work and do their usual tasks. Data from both Canada and the United States demonstrate the need to find new ways to approach preventive care among rural dwellers, based on trends in health indicators such as obesity, hypertension, smoking, and frequency of regular health care visits (National Center for Health Statistics, 2012; Pong, Desmeules, & Lagace, 2009; Rural Assistance Center, 2012a).

Policy

Policy implications of the original work include establishing funding mechanisms whereby health services can be offered near where people work that are scheduled around the cycle of rural work. Rural residents may not seek timely health services if work must be delayed or disrupted to seek care (Sellers, Poduska, Propp, & White, 1999).

The original theory development work on definitions of health, as well as beliefs about work and health, was conducted in the United States. Research participants were principally Caucasian rural dwellers, the majority population in the Rocky Mountain and High Plains area in which this work was conducted (89.9% of the current Montana population is Caucasian; U.S. Bureau of the Census, 2012). The original work was not intended to characterize these concepts for American Indians, the primary minority population in the same rural areas (6.4% of the Montana population, U.S. Census). Canadian research on health beliefs of rural dwellers, as reported by Winters et al. (2006), was also drawn primarily from Caucasians living in the western part of the country. Further research is warranted to explore how Native American and Aboriginal people living in rural areas define health and how their conception of health is the same as or different from the dominant population. In any case, it is unlikely that one definition of health or one set of health beliefs would emerge that would characterize health beliefs among different Aboriginal communities or tribes, any more than it is likely that one definition would be true for Caucasian groups of different cultures.

As discussed by Lee and McDonagh (2006), rural dwellers' views of health may now be more diverse across different geographic areas, age and ethnic groups, and occupations than when the original theory development work began, so it may require a reconceptualization of definitions of health, work beliefs, and health beliefs. Of particular note are the subpopulations among rural dwellers.

Discussion

Martin (1997) pointed out that farming and ranching are now experienced more as a lifestyle than as an occupation, thus calling for different approaches to affect behavior change beyond simply appealing to individual's motivations to continue working. Blank (1999) also referred to traditional farming and ranching as a current lifestyle choice. Since many other forms of rural living are available to Americans besides farming and ranching, and also since most food and commodity crops are now produced on large industrial farms, Blank postulated that the American family farm is a lifestyle that many Americans can no longer afford. Another example of a potential need to reframe rural dwellers' definitions of health can be found within rural subpopulations where unemployment has now persisted for multiple generations. Defining health based on ability to work may not be relevant for those who have never had regular work (Long, 1993). Some rural areas are now more racially and ethnically diverse than in the past. Culturally based beliefs about what it means to be healthy are likely to result in different definitions of health among racial and ethnic groups. Migration of urban residents to rural areas has resulted in a subpopulation of exurban rural dwellers who bring their urban values and expectations about health and health care with them (Troughton, 1999). The "graying" of rural areas is well documented in the literature, as people age in place and younger people migrate out for employment and other opportunities (McLaughlin & Jensen, 1998; Ricketts, Johnson-Webb, & Randolph, 1999). With improved health care and healthier lifestyles, people are living many more years postretirement than they once did. How health is defined among this rural population may well have nothing to do with what we traditionally think of as work, but instead may be more consistent with the concept of health as role performance or ability to do usual tasks. Healthy elders may define health as the ability to actively participate in leisure, voluntary activities, and travel. Elders in poor health may define health as nothing more than the ability to complete their activities of daily living. Further research and exploration is warranted to refine the definitions of health for these multiple rural subpopulations.

IMPLICATIONS OF THE SECOND THEORETICAL STATEMENT

The second theoretical statement is "Rural dwellers are self-reliant and resist accepting help or services from those seen as 'outsiders' or from agencies seen as national or regional 'welfare' programs" (Long & Weinert, 1989, p. 120). Related key concepts are self-reliance, outsider, insider, old-timer, and newcomer.

Education

The second theoretical statement underlines the importance of a participative, community development approach in which rural dwellers identify and design health initiatives to fit with their own needs and resources. This approach is consistent with the second theoretical statement as originally conceptualized, as well as with the proposed newer subtheme of symptom-action-timeline (SATL) and the new theme involving choices discussed by Lee and McDonagh (2006). The importance of working in partnership with rural dwellers and communities is an essential content for nursing curricula so that graduates can and will apply the principles of community development and participatory action in rural practice. Skills essential for partnership development and maintenance should also be included in nursing curricula. As a middle-range theory of rural health-seeking behavior evolves, this theory should be derived and validated in partnership with rural residents themselves so that it is consistent with their local needs and beliefs.

Practice

Goeppinger (1993) advocated partnership as a core intervention strategy in health promotion with rural populations at both individual and aggregate levels. Considering the rural tendency to "make do" and what Weissert, Knott, and Stieber (1994) referred to as the "asymmetry of information between citizens and health professionals . . . about what constitutes good care" (p. 366) in traditional care models, empirical testing of the partnership model in promoting the health of rural residents is needed. A Canadian example of a tool to support participative community development for rural citizens is a workbook that was tested in Manitoba, Canada (Ryan-Nicholls, 2004). The workbook was designed to help rural citizens assess the health of their communities and identify goals and strategies to improve the sustainability of rural communities. In the United States, Findholt (2004) studied how rurality influenced community participation in health promotion initiatives. She found that having a structured process for the initiative appeared to compensate for some of the resource and experiential limitations in rural communities. Communities, for example, that had limited experience and success with previous planning efforts were not hindered in their current efforts because they had structured support and resources from a state-level office of rural health.

Policy

The question of what health care resources are necessary and sufficient in rural and remote areas, given the distance to other sources of care, continues as a focus of debate and policy shifts for which evidence for decision making is scarce. The major constraint is the lack of sufficient population to justify a full mix of acute care, long-term care, and supported residential and home care services (Keyzer, 1995). In a study of home care resources for rural families with cancer, Buehler and Lee (1992) found that the more rural the family, the more limited and inadequate the formal resources available to assist them. These investigators also found that the longer the dying trajectory and the greater the deterioration of the person's health, the more resources became inadequate and the greater the caregiver burden. These findings illustrate one of many policy questions that have emerged: the relationship between length of illness and sustainability of resources through the trajectory of illness in rural versus urban environments. It would seem that a mix of formal and informal resources and the resiliency of each to prolonged illness vary, but few studies have systematically addressed this phenomenon.

The Australian Rural Health Strategy adopted in 1994 (Keyzer, 1995) called for "relocation of resources away from services based on existing facilities towards services based on expressed demand" (p. 28). The strategy included changes that would shift power bases from traditional rural primary and hospital care delivery to a system that relied much more on nurse practitioners and interdisciplinary collaboration. However, nearly 20 years later, tension still exists in Australia and elsewhere between the economic arguments for downsizing and closure of rural facilities versus advocacy for aging in place, new life-saving treatments that require pre-transfer interventions at local health care facilities, and other new technologies such as telehealth that minimize the need for travel to urban locations for health care (Mueller, 2001; Ricketts, 2000).

In the United States, the Critical Access Hospital (CAH) has gained broad support as an alternative to closure of local rural hospitals and has been implemented in rural areas across the nation. CAHs must be located in remote areas and are limited to short-stay lower-intensity services in exchange for more flexibility in staffing and other licensure requirements and more favorable Medicare reimbursement as compared with traditional rural hospitals. The underlying goal is to shift the facility's emphasis from inpatient and surgical services to emergency, outpatient, primary, and long-term care, which are services that may be more sustainable in remote rural areas because they better match the needs of area residents (Shreffler, Capalbo, Flaherty, & Heggem, 1999). One of the prototypes for this national model of care was a grassroots effort initiated by a partnership of rural citizens and legislators in a remote rural area in Montana. There are currently 47 CAHs in Montana (Montana Hospital Association, 2012) and 1,327 certified CAHs nationwide (Rural Assistance Center, 2012b).

While the Affordable Care Act (ACA) and its potential to reform the United States health care system are highly controversial, there are many provisions in the ACA that can benefit rural patients and the rural health care system (National Rural Health Care Association, 2012). American rural dwellers are much more likely to be uninsured or underinsured than urban dwellers, which has limited their access to health care. The intent of the ACA is to require coverage for all and to reduce the cost of insurance though purchasing networks, which may be advantageous for those who are self-employed or underemployed. The Act also guarantees renewability of coverage and prohibits preexisting condition exclusions. There are also provisions that address the workforce shortage crisis in rural areas and eliminate payment inequities for rural providers. Although challenges to the constitutionality of ACA have been resolved by the Supreme Court in June 2012, health care reform based on the ACA will be an ongoing process because implementation of many the provisions depend on funding through separate acts of Congress.

IMPLICATIONS OF THE THIRD THEORETICAL STATEMENT

Finally, the third theoretical statement is "Health care providers in rural areas must deal with a lack of anonymity and much greater role diffusion than providers in urban or suburban settings" (Long & Weinert, 1989, p. 120). A related theme mentioned by Long and Weinert that characterizes rural nursing is "a sense of isolation from professional peers" (p. 120).

Education

Implicit in the third theoretical statement is that students planning or potentially interested in rural practice should be given opportunities to develop skills to function in a generalist role or what McLeod, Browne, and Leipert (1998) referred to as a multispecialist role that is characteristic of rural nursing practice. Offering undergraduate students a rural elective experience is one such strategy, particularly when it not only involves placement in a rural site but also seminars on rural health and practice issues. Students with an interest in rural practice should have opportunities to develop strategies to cope with or overcome practice isolation, such as skill development in the use of mentors, consultants, and telehealth applications. Through full engagement with their communities, nurses who are newcomers in rural areas may begin to appreciate the familiarity of life in a rural community and gradually may be seen as insiders rather than outsiders, which may mitigate the negative aspects of lack of anonymity and practice isolation. Some nurses, of course, are already insiders, having come from the particular community. The sense of practice isolation may be less acute for them, but the practical issues of limited access to educational opportunities and ready consultation are nevertheless present to varying degrees.

Practice and Policy

Lack of anonymity, role diffusion, and practice isolation may contribute to recruitment difficulties and high turnover of rural health care professionals and result in shortages of providers in rural practice settings. Here too, policy makers can look to innovative approaches and exchange of best practices. For example, the Rural Physician Action Plan in Alberta recognized that (a) medical students from rural areas were more likely to go into rural practice, but (b) rural applicants were often disadvantaged in the interview and selection processes for medical school because of lack of sophistication in interviewing and preparation of materials (I. Pfeiffer, personal communication, March 4, 2004). An experienced recruiter was hired to help rural applicants prepare for admission interviews. Thus, they went to a root cause with what appear to be positive results.

Stewart et al. (2011) conducted a study to identify factors that predicted intent to leave practice positions among registered nurses (RNs) in rural and remote settings in Canada. The investigators found that some predictors indicated situations that were amenable to interventions that may prevent turnover. Workplace and community predictors relevant to the third relational statement are lower local community satisfaction, higher perceived workplace stress, lower satisfaction with autonomy in the workplace, lower satisfaction with workplace scheduling, and a desire to seek further education. Also, being a "newcomer" to the rural practice setting and community was a significant predictor of intent to leave.

An innovative strategy for addressing shortages of nurses and other health care providers in rural areas can be seen in the growth of educational outreach efforts via distance learning technology to rural areas. Rural residents or insiders who are more likely to select rural practice upon graduation can access all or part of educational programs without leaving their rural communities for significant periods of time. Another successful approach for recruitment of health professionals in rural areas has been educational scholarships for rural residents or "grow your own" programs (Hagopian, Johnson, Fordyce, Blades, & Hart, 2003).

CONCLUSION

The radical changes necessary to shift education, practice, and policy for rural health require a strong theory base and depth of understanding of rural health and practice that can emanate only through experience and research. Those who focus on rural health are used to thinking in terms of local contextual factors and the unique nature of a single rural area, region, or nation. Through engagement in cross-border collaborative research and scholarly work on rural nursing theory, we and our respective teams have deepened our understanding of the extent to which larger issues of health care reform are also shifting. At the end of the day, the relevance of rural nursing theory and concepts as described in this book will likely be measured by its ability to evolve and change as new knowledge shapes it and its ability to positively influence education, practice, and health care policy—and thereby improve the health of rural citizens on both sides of the border.

REFERENCES

Blank, S. C. (1999). The end of the American farm. *The Futurist, 33*(4), 22.

Buehler, J. A., & Lee, H. J. (1992). Exploration of home care resources for rural families with cancer. *Cancer Nursing, 15,* 299–308.

Findholt, N. (2004). *The influence of rurality on community participation in a community health development initiative.* Unpublished doctoral dissertation, Oregon Health & Science University, Portland.

Goeppinger, J. (1993). Health promotion for rural populations: Partnership interventions. *Family and Community Health, 16*(1), 1–10.

Hagopian, A., Johnson, K., Fordyce, M., Blades, S., & Hart, L. G. (2003). Health workforce recruitment and retention in critical access hospitals. *CAH/FLEX National Tracking Project, 3*(5). Retrieved July 20, 2012, from http://www.unmc.edu/ruprihealth/programs/results/vol3num5.pdf

Keyzer, D. M. (1995). Health policy and rural nurses: A time for reflection. *Collegian, 2*(1), 28–35.

Lee, H. J., & McDonagh, M. K. (2006). Further development of the rural nursing base. In H. J. Lee, & C. A. Winters (Eds.). *Rural nursing: Concepts, theory, and practice* (2nd ed., p. 313–321). New York: Springer Publishing.

Long, K. A. (1993). The concept of health: Rural perspectives. *Nursing Clinics of North America, 28*(1), 123–130.

Long, K. A., & Weinert, C. (1989). Rural nursing: Developing the theory base. *Scholarly Inquiry for Nursing Practice: An International Journal, 3,* 113–127.

Martin, S. R. (1997). Agricultural safety and health: Principles and possibilities for nursing education. *Journal of Nursing Education*, 36(2), 74–78.

McLaughlin, D. K., & Jensen, L. (1998). The rural elderly: A demographic portrait. In R. T. Coward, & J. A. Krout (Eds.), *Aging in rural settings: Life circumstances & distinctive features* (pp. 15–43). New York, NY: Springer Publishing.

McLeod, M., Browne, A. J., & Leipert, B. (1998). Issues for nurses in rural and remote Canada. *Australian Journal of Rural Health*, 6, 72–78.

Montana Hospital Association. (2012). *Critical Access Hospital List*. Retrieved July 2, 2012, from http://www.mtha.org/mhref4.htm

Mueller, K. J. (2001). Rural health policy: Past as prelude to the future. In S. Loue, & B. E. Quill (Eds.), *Handbook of rural health* (pp. 1–23). New York, NY: Kluwer Academic/Plenum.

National Center for Health Statistics. (2012). *Health, United States, 2011, with special feature on socioeconomic and health*. Hyattsville, MD: Author.

National Rural Health Care Association. (2012). *Health reform and you*. Retrieved July 5, 2012 from http://ruralhealthweb.org/index.cfm?objectid =57987A08-3048-651A-FE82989BAFF4

Pong, R. W., Desmeules, M., & Lagace, C. (2009). Rural-urban disparities in health: How does Canada fare and how does Canada compare to Australia? *Australian Journal of Rural Health*, 17(1), 58–64.

Ricketts, T. C. (2000). The changing nature of rural health care. *Annual Review of Public Health*, 21, 639–657.

Ricketts, T. C., Johnson-Webb, K. D., & Randolph, R. K. (1999). Populations and places in rural America. In T. C. Ricketts (Ed.), *Rural health in the United States* (pp. 7–24). New York, NY: Oxford University Press.

Rural Assistance Center. (2012a). *Rural health disparities*. Retrieved July 2, 2012 from http://www.raconline.org/topics/disparities

Rural Assistance Center. (2012b). *CAH frequently asked questions*. Retrieved July 2, 2012, from http://www.raconline.org/topics/hospitals/cahfaq.php

Ryan-Nicholls, K. (2004). Rural Canadian community health and quality of life: Testing of a workbook to determine priorities and move to action. (Preliminary Report). *Rural and Remote Health*, 4 (278), 1–10. Retrieved July 20, 2012, from http://www.rrh.org.au/articles/subviewnew.asp? ArticleID=278

Sellers, S. C., Poduska, M. D., Propp, L. H., & White, S. I. (1999). The health care meanings, values, and practices of Anglo-American males in the rural Midwest. *Journal of Transcultural Nursing*, 10, 320–330.

Shreffler, M. J., Capalbo, S. M., Flaherty, R. J., & Heggem, C. (1999). Community decision-making about Critical Access Hospitals: Lessons learned from

Montana's Medical Assistance Facility program. *The Journal of Rural Health, 15*(2), 180–188.

Stewart, N. J., D'Arcy, C., Kosteniuk, J., Andrews, M. E., Morgan, D., Forbes, D. et al. (2011). Moving on? Predictors of intent to leave among rural and remote RNs in Canada. *The Journal of Rural Health, 27*(1), 103–113.

Troughton, M. J. (1999). Redefining "rural" for the twenty-first century. In W. Rampy, J. Kulig, I. Townshend, & V. McGowan (Eds.), *Health in rural settings: Contexts for action* (pp. 21–38). Lethbridge, AB: University of Lethbridge.

U.S. Bureau of the Census. (2012). Retrieved July 5, 2012, from http://quickfacts.census.gov/qfd/states/30000.html

Weissert, C. S., Knott, J. H., & Stieber, B. E. (1994). Education and the health professions: Explaining policy choices among the states. *Journal of Health Politics, Policy and Law, 19*, 361–392.

Winters, C. A., Thomlinson, E. H., O'Lynn, C., Lee, H. J., McDonagh, M. K., Edge, D. S. et al. (2006). Examining rural nursing theory across borders. In H. J. Lee, & C. A. Winters (Eds.). *Rural nursing: Concepts, theory, and practice* (2nd ed., pp. 27–39). New York, NY: Springer Publishing.

Chapter 29

NURSING WORKFORCE DEVELOPMENT, CLINICAL PRACTICE, RESEARCH, AND NURSING THEORY: CONNECTING THE DOTS

Angeline Bushy
and Charlene A. Winters

ACCESS TO HEALTH CARE IN rural underserved areas is often stymied by the success, or the lack thereof, of recruiting and retaining all types of health care providers. In the past decade, concerns about access to health care became a national priority for urban and rural dwellers alike, especially for regions with insufficient numbers of all types of health care providers that are designated as health professional shortage areas (HPSAs). Professional shortages in HPSAs include among others, primary care providers, registered nurses (RNs), physician assistants (PAs), dentists, certified nursing assistants, home care aides, pharmacists, optometrists, public health and behavioral health professionals; laboratory, radiology, and information technicians; and physical, respiratory, and occupational therapists. First, it is important to stress that regardless of the setting, nurses are but one of many members on a team of health professionals. With this in mind, the focus of this chapter is on the state of the rural nurse workforce and its impact on nursing practice, research, and theory development.

BACKGROUND

First and foremost, nurses do not function in isolation! Nurses are one component, albeit major players, of a team of providers in a complex health care system. Before proceeding with a discussion on the nursing workforce, it is important to note that the lack of a standard definition for "rural," as used in federal and state policies, research studies, and workforce data makes comparative analysis problematic (Cromartie, 2008; United States Department of Agriculture [USDA], 2008a, 2008b). Likewise, nursing issues, be they in a rural or urban area, vary with the practice context, the health profile of a given population, and the employing agency or institution. Variances of this nature, coupled with a multitude of other interacting factors, contribute to health professional shortages in a given locale. Factors often cited in the rural literature include the aging workforce; high turnover and vacancy rates, which further hinder recruitment efforts; retirement eligibility; restricted educational and career advancement opportunities; and heavy workloads, along with inequities in salaries and employee benefits (Chipp et al., 2011; Hunsberger, Bauman, & Blythe, 2009).

Workforce needs for RNs in the United States are complex, varying with time and place as well as with local demographic characteristics (Bureau of Health Professions [BHPr], 2010; National Center for Health Workforce Analysis [NCHWA], 2010). Nationally, the number of employed RNs has increased dramatically since 1980 in urban, large rural, small rural, and isolated small rural areas. The National Center for Health Workforce Analysis (NCHWA, 2008) data set offers the most recent comprehensive profile of temporal and spatial trends in nursing availability. Based on NSSRN estimates, the National Center for Health Workforce Analysis report (NCHWA, 2010) reveals there are approximately 3,063,162 licensed RNs living in the United States. These data reflect an increase in the number of nurses from 2004 to 2008. However, the NCHWA report further suggests that 291,000 RNs allowed their licenses to lapse during that time frame. This finding suggests that the projected age-related retirement among nurses has likely started; that trend is expected to continue as baby boomers leave the workforce (NCHWA, 2010). There is inconsistent information on the rural health professional workforce in general and on RNs in particular. The most current information on the rural nursing workforce is provided by Skillman, Palazzo, Hart, and Butterfield (2007) in their study titled "Changes in the Rural Registered Nurse Workforce from 1980 to 2004." While somewhat dated, the findings from this report served as the source for information related to the rural nursing workforce in this chapter.

If we compare the ratio of RNs in rural and urban residence for the general population (RNs per 100,000 population), we see that rural areas consistently have fewer RNs. In 2004, isolated small rural areas only had 369 RNs/100,000 population, small rural areas had 665 RNs/100,000 population, while large rural areas resembled urban areas with 837 RNs/100,000 population. While the ratio of working RNs/100,000 population has increased in many isolated small rural and in small rural areas, the number remains significantly lower than in urban and large rural areas (Skillman et al., 2007; BHPr, 2010). While these patterns of RN employment seem somewhat favorable, other studies suggest that nurses are under great stress, evidenced by self-reported job dissatisfaction and burnout, particularly among direct providers of clinical care (Chipp et al., 2011; Grantmakers in Healthcare [GIH], 2009; Hunsberger et al., 2009; Molinari & Monserud, 2008). Reports of this nature are foreboding relative to retaining and sustaining the nursing workforce, and even more so for rural communities already struggling with inadequate numbers of nurses. Urban, rural, and frontier areas alike confront similar reasons for the nursing shortage, some to a more profound degree than others. Factors often cited in the literature include (LaSala, 2000; NACRHHS, 2011; National Rural Health Association [NRNA], 2005; Rural Assistance Center [RAC], 2011; Roberge, 2009):

- Aging of the nursing workforce
- Shortages and aging of nursing faculty, which hinders educating additional workforce personnel
- Wage disparities and health care economics
- Limited availability of educational scholarships and loans
- Inadequate planning and projection of workforce needs in medically underserved regions
- Failure to sustain an appropriate workforce to meet societal needs

THE NURSING WORKFORCE

The next section presents an overview of demographic characteristics of the nursing workforce in the United States. When available, discussion about variances related to the rural nursing workforce will be included.

Age

In 1988, nationally, half of the RN workforce was under 38 years of age. From 2004 to 2008, the average age of the RN workforce increased to 46 years. Comparing the ages of urban RNs with rural RNs who entered into the workforce since 1980, rural RNs consistently entered the workforce later in life (rural, 28.0 years; urban, 26.8 years). In 2004, about 33% of the RN workforce was 50 years or older. By 2008, nearly half (48%) of the nursing workforce was more than 50 years of age (BHPr, 2010; Skillman et al., 2007). Surprisingly, since 2008, the average age of the nursing workforce has declined somewhat, attributed to an increased number of RNs under 30 years of age who entered the workforce (BHPr, 2010; Skillman et al., 2007). Since 2001, there has been a 62% increase in the number of younger RNs entering the workforce. This workforce trend is noteworthy, given that of the nation's three million nurses, nearly one million are over 50 years of age and nearing retirement. The surge in younger nurses entering the workforce may allay forecasts of projected RN shortages as baby boomers retire, and, hopefully, will meet the growing demands of an aging society (Auerbach, Buerhaus, & Steiger, 2011). One can only speculate as to whether or not this demographic trend is also occurring within the rural nursing workforce, which traditionally has included nurses who are older compared to urban counterparts.

Education

Of all RNs in the workforce, more than one out of five had earned an academic degree prior to their initial nursing degree. Even so, the most prevalent level of nursing education is the Associate Degree in Nursing (ADN, 45%), followed by Baccalaureate of Science in Nursing (BSN) and/or graduate degree (combined, 34%), and hospital-based diploma (20%). In 2008, the majority of rural RNs entered the workforce with an ADN (approximately 50%) or a diploma (20%). Since 1980, rural nurses consistently have had fewer years of formal nursing education compared to urban RNs. Rural RNs are less likely than urban RNs to have a BSN (urban, 51%; rural, 20%) or a master's degree (urban, 14%; rural, 10%) (BHPr, 2010; NCHWA, 2010; Skillman et al., 2007). Increasingly, health care credentialing organizations are requiring that hospitals meet established educational thresholds for staff nurses in order to achieve "Magnet," or "Path to Excellence" status, or some other type of external accreditation (Bushy, 2009; Orsolini-Hain, 2012). Nursing workforce demographics, more specifically, education level, coupled with persistent challenges in recruiting and retaining local nursing talent, may hinder a small rural hospital from obtaining external accreditation or national recognition. Education level is also a factor in rural nurses not having been exposed to content on the research process since such a course is not generally included in the ADN and diploma curriculum. On the one hand, lack of exposure to research content certainly is a factor in the paucity of scholarly activities addressing rural nursing practice. Conversely, this information deficit is an opportunity for urban-based nurse scholars to partner with nurses in rural practice contexts to expand the knowledge and theoretical base for rural nursing.

Diversity

Significant gains in racial/ethnic minority representation in the U.S. population have occurred since 1990. According to recent reports from the Bureau of the Census (2009), of the overall U.S. population, about 33% was minority (nonwhite and/or Hispanic). Correspondingly, since 1990, the proportion of RNs who are non-White and/or Hispanic has grown in both urban and rural areas, but not at the same rate as the overall U.S. population; the number of RNs who were of a minority racial or ethnic background increased from 2000 (333,368 nurses) to 2008 (513,860 nurses) (BHPr, 2010). Diversity is most noted among recently graduated RNs. Still, the current racial and ethnic distribution within the national RN workforce (White non-Hispanic, 83%) is not representative of minorities in the U.S. population as a whole (White, non-Hispanic, 65%) (Auerbach et al., 2011). While these findings probably apply to both urban and rural nurses, precise data on diversity in the rural nursing workforce are not available. Questions emerge as to the impact of persistent homogeneity of the rural nursing workforce on access to culturally and linguistically attuned care for rural residents.

With respect to gender, the proportion of males is gradually increasing in the historically female-dominated nursing profession. Males comprised a very small segment of employed RNs in the national workforce before 2000 (6%), and increased slightly by 2008 (10%). Males continue to be underrepresented in the profession in both urban (6.3%) and rural settings (5.6%). The profile of males in nursing differs from those of females. For instance, males are more likely to be employed as a certified registered nurse anesthetist (CRNA) (BHPr, 2010; NCHWA, 2010; Skillman et al., 2007). Anecdotally, in small rural hospitals that offer surgical services, male RNs most often function in the role of a CRNA as opposed to functioning in a staff nursing position. There is a paucity of evidence-based information related to CRNA practice issues in more remote contexts other than reports describing how they fill a critical health professional void in the rural health care delivery system. How do male nurses' experiences compare to those of females in rural practice? How do those experiences influence recruitment and retention efforts in rural health care facilities? Subsequently, these findings need to be reflected in a theory that guides rural nursing.

Employment Patterns

The National Center for Health Workforce Analysis (NCHWA) indicates that licensed RNs are overwhelmingly employed in nursing (85%) (NCHWA, 2010). This figure represents the highest proportion of RNs in the workforce since the NSSRN commenced tracking the nursing workforce (1977), and hospitals remain their most common employer. Of RNs employed in hospitals, most are under 25 years of age (90%). Of all RNs with a master's degree, less than 50% work in a hospital, 18% function in ambulatory care settings, and more than 12% are employed in academic education. With respect to nurses who are older, in 2008, a smaller percentage were employed in hospital positions, and a greater proportion worked in extended care facilities, academic, and home health settings (BHPr, 2010; NCHWA, 2010). Upon reaching 60 years of age, the number of hours worked by part-time RNs declines steadily with age. Likewise, older RNs are also less likely than their younger counterparts to hold a secondary position in nursing.

Older RNs are more likely to remain in the same position and with the same employer, compared to younger nurses. Comparing RNs less than 50 years old with those who are between 50 and 59 years of age, the latter cohort was less likely to report intent to leave their current nursing position within 3 years. As RNs grow older, especially over the age of 60 years, retirement becomes the dominant consideration for employment changes (BHPr, 2010; NCHWA, 2010). Consistently, over the decades, the rural nursing workforce, along with being older, tends to remain employed in the same setting longer than their urban counterparts (Skillman et al., 2007). The rural expertise of these nurses needs to be sought out by urban-based nurse researchers and scholars in order to design meaningful investigations, validate findings that include a rural perspective, and refine concepts in a theory that is relevant for nursing in diverse rural contexts.

The proportion of RNs working in hospitals has been declining since 1980 for rural as well as urban nurses. However, the more rural the community, the lower is the percentage of RNs who work in hospitals. The percentage was lowest for RNs who live in isolated small rural areas; in 2004, only 37% were employed in hospitals. In contrast, the proportion of RNs working in ambulatory settings and long-term care facilities essentially has remained stable between 1980 and 2004 across all types of rural areas. The percentage of RNs employed in long-term care facilities is highest for those who work in isolated small rural areas (BHPr, 2010; NCHWA, 2010; Skillman et al., 2007). Nursing studies are needed to examine this rural employment trend in long-term care institutions as well as in community-based health care facilities.

Salary

Although there are other factors that contribute to job satisfaction, salary generally is an important consideration most individuals consider when deciding where to work. It is indisputable that there is perceived to be added value associated with rural residence, yet, salary disparities are often identified as a deterrent to recruiting and retaining RNs in rural settings. There are notable differences when comparing (median) full-time salary by highest nursing degree across urban and rural RNs' work area types. Urban-based nurses with a baccalaureate or higher degree earned the highest salary, while those with an associate degree or diploma in rural areas earned the least. However, RNs in rural areas holding a BSN or higher degree generally receive a similar salary to urban-based RNs that are ADN or diploma-prepared (BHPr, 2010; NCHWA, 2010; Skillman et al., 2007). Comparing RN salary gap over time, the urban–rural gap (measured as the percentage difference between highest and lowest salaries) was wider in 2004 (33%) than it was in 1980 (20%). Nonacute care settings fare worst when it comes to urban–rural RN wage disparities. Of particular note in both rural and urban areas, private practice settings, schools, health departments, extended care facilities, community-based institutions, and public health agencies offer even lower salaries than those offered by a local hospital. In regions designated as frontier, salary disparities tend to be more significant. Consequently, recruitment for nurses becomes an even greater challenge for hospital- and community-based providers in these more remote and less populated regions (Skillman et al., 2007; Sumaya, 2012).

Occupational Commuting

In rural contexts, nursing shortages are often exacerbated by rural employers' inability to compete with urban employers in terms of employee wages, benefits, and perhaps enticing financial sign-on bonuses. Another approach to delineate salary disparity among rural nurses is contrasting salaries of RNs who worked within the community to those working outside of the community in which they resided. More specifically, in 1980, the difference in salaries between RNs who lived and worked in the same rural area as opposed to those living in a rural community and working in urban areas was 15%; by 2004, the disparity grew to 22% (Skillman et al., 2007). A common (mis)perception prevails that rural RNs reside in the same community in which they are also employed, but that is not the case. In 1980, of RNs living in isolated small rural areas, 69% worked in the same community; by 2004, it dropped to 36% (Skillman et al., 2007). This finding suggests nearly two-thirds of RNs who lived in isolated small rural areas commuted somewhere else to work—be it to work in a health care facility located in another small rural area, or a large(r) rural are, or in an urban area. Increasingly, nurses residing in all types of rural settings (isolated small, small, and large rural) are commuting to work outside their community of residence. This phenomenon, termed *occupational commuting*, poses even greater challenges to recruiting and retaining RNs in order to meet the nursing needs of rural communities.

Given the aforementioned demographic characteristics of the RN workforce, strategies to address shortages in rural areas may be different from those in urban areas. For instance, one can speculate that rural RNs who commute to work outside of their home community are taking advantage of larger hospitals' recruitment and retention programs. Often, these include flexible or compressed work schedule options (e.g., three 12-hour shifts/week), thereby allowing the nurse to maximize income and minimize time away from home and family. Occupational commuting could also be attributable to an RN's preference for employment in a larger institution that offers an opportunity to work on a specialty unit versus working in a small rural hospital, which requires that a nurse possess generalist stills. Additionally, larger hospitals are more likely to perform procedures or have patient groups that the RN perceives to be more professionally stimulating (Ortiz & Bushy, 2011; Pepper, Sandefer, & Gray, 2010; Roberge, 2009; Skillman et al., 2007).

Little is known or understood about the phenomenon of occupational commuting among nurses who reside in rural communities. Both quantitative and qualitative studies are needed focusing on rural nurses', employment patterns, especially the phenomenon of occupational commuting. Research studies could focus on the lived experience of nurses and their families, and on the impact this has on recruitment and retention efforts of small hospitals, as well as the broader economic impact this has on the rural community. Finally, information needs to be disseminated on factors that contribute to this phenomenon, along with best practices for retaining nurses to work in the communities in which they also reside.

RURAL NURSING PRACTICE

Comprehensive examination of the roles and scope of practice for rural nurses will not be presented in this chapter, due to space constraints. Essentially, there is a wide diversity within and among rural communities with respect to demographic characteristics, economic infrastructures, the health status of the local population, and their nursing care needs. Successful health professionals in general, and RNs in particular, employed in clinics, community agencies, and small hospitals located in rural areas should be "expert generalists." These nurses require a repertoire of skills to meet the nursing care needs of individuals across the life span, who have an array of health concerns and medical diagnoses (see Chapter 16). Essentially, the demographic makeup of a community and the health status of the residents who live there will determine the most often encountered medical conditions. Rural-based RNs must be comfortable and be able to function professionally within the social structure of a small community, which can contribute to diffuse personal–professional boundaries. Nurses in rural facilities must also have the confidence to stabilize a patient for transport to a larger urban-based medical center for complex care with state-of-the-art biomedical interventions not offered in the small hospital (Chipp et al., 2011; Hurme, 2009; Institute of Medicine [IOM], 2005; LaSala, 2000; Winters & Lee, 2010).

Given these practice features, discussions are ongoing among rural nursing scholars as to whether anything is unique about rural nursing practice and whether or not this should be classified as a nursing specialty. Their argument centers on the belief that nursing care is similar regardless of where or when it occurs. Rather, "rural" is perceived to be contextual in nature; there are environmental variances and geographic settings in which a nurse must adapt nursing skills to provide appropriate care. Proponents of this perspective suggest that nursing care is probably no different for rural clients than for individuals in any other setting. They further argue that the knowledge base is lacking and there is no precise theory to support "rural" nursing per se (Molinari & Bushy, 2011).

Nurse scholars holding an opposing view propose that rural practice should be designated a specialty area (or, at least a subspecialty) associated with the need to adapt nursing skills to somewhat unique rural contextual features such as isolation (geographic, professional, educational, social), diffuse personal and professional boundaries, scarce resources, local economic infrastructures, informal social dynamics, and the mandate to care for individual of all ages with a variety of health problems (Molinari & Bushy, 2011). Moreover, there is an emerging theory to support this type of practice (see Chapters 1, 2, and 16), albeit the concepts may need refining in order to fit diverse rural settings and populations (see Chapter 30) (Long & Weinert, 1989; Winters & Lee, 2010). The actual degree to which rural nursing could be defined as a "specialty practice" probably lies somewhere between these two extremes. Research topics focusing on rural nursing in a variety of practice contexts are critical for refining the emerging theory for rural nursing.

INSTITUTE OF MEDICINE RECOMMENDATIONS ON THE FUTURE OF NURSING: RURAL CONSIDERATIONS

The IOM (2011) offers eight recommendations for the advancement of nurses in the emerging model of health care delivery. Although rural nursing is not addressed per se in the IOM document, the following paragraphs will include rural dimensions for each of the eight IOM recommendations.

Recommendation 1: Remove Scope-of-Practice Barriers

The first IOM recommendation is particularly relevant for nurses in advanced practice roles, who should be able to practice to the full extent of their education and training (Newhouse et al., 2011). Of the total nursing workforce, those with advanced degrees in nursing make up about 10% of all RNs. Of rural RNs, about one out of four function in an advance practice role (i.e., certified nurse practitioner [CNP], CRNA, certified nurse midwife [CNM], and clinical nurse specialist [CNS]) (BHPr, 2010; NCHWA, 2010). In rural regions having a federally qualified community health center (FQCHC), one finds an even higher proportion of nurses in advanced practice. Nationwide, nearly half of all the direct care providers in FQCHCs are CNPs, CNMs, and PAs. Currently, FQCHCs employ about 4,000 advanced practice registered nurses (APRNs) and 11,000 RNs, representing an increase from 2010 to 2012 of nearly 20% in nursing staff (Centers for Medicare and Medicaid Services [CMMS], 2011; Wakefield, 2011). Along with varied clinical expertise, rural nurses with advanced education are prepared to implement evidence-based practice, collaborate in research studies, and mentor staff nurses in research activities such as quality improvement initiatives. Urban-based nurse scholars should also consider partnering with these expert clinicians to refine and validate concepts in the emerging theory for rural nursing.

Certified Nurse Practitioners

According to the NCHWA (2010), there were 158,348 APRNs prepared as nurse practitioners and certified in an array of specialties, thus representing the largest group of nurses in advanced practice. Approximately 10% of all CNPs are also prepared as CNSs. About one-third of CNPs are under 45 years of age (35%); most hold a master's degree (85%) or a doctorate degree (4%). Almost all of these CNPs are employed in nursing (89%), with 70% holding a position title of APRN. About 40% are employed in hospital settings, including primary care clinics located in, or owned by, a hospital, and 36% work in other types of ambulatory care settings such as FQCHCs.

Certified Registered Nurse Anesthetists

Of all advanced practice nurses, about 34,821 are prepared as nurse anesthetists; of these, nearly all hold national certification (99%). Most CRNAs are employed in nursing positions (92%); many are below the age of 45 years (40%), of which a high proportion are male (40%). The majority hold a master's or doctorate degree (65%) as their highest nursing or nursing-related degree (BHPr, 2010; NCHWA, 2010). To reiterate, in small rural hospitals, one notes that the advanced practice nurses most often are CRNAs, especially when the facility offers surgical services, albeit for minor surgeries.

Certified Nurse Midwives

The NCHWA (2010) estimates that there are 18,492 CNMs, of which more than half are 50 years of age or older (54%) and hold a graduate degree (51%). Most are employed in nursing positions (84%) but less than half held a job title of "nurse midwife" (42%). The majority of CNMs work in hospital settings (58%) and about a quarter worked in ambulatory care (BHPr, 2010; NCHWA, 2010). Indian Health Service (IHS) facilities, the majority of which are located in rural settings, rely heavily on CNM services. Other than IHS data, precise rural workforce information on nurse midwives was not available.

Clinical Nurse Specialists

Following a marked decline from 2004 to 2008, CNSs still represented the second largest group of APRNs, with an estimated 59,242 nurses prepared as clinical specialists (NCHWA, 2010). A large proportion of CNSs were master's-prepared (92.8%); 7.2% reported a doctorate degree as their CNS preparation; more than 27% also had preparation as CNPs. When dually prepared, nearly 55% worked as nurse practitioners. Eighty-four percent of CNSs were employed in nursing, and nearly one-half worked in hospitals, but only 18.8% had the job title of CNS. Common job titles included administrator, manager, and instructor. Data from the 2008 national survey of registered nurses indicate that 91% of CNSs reported being moderately or extremely satisfied with their position.

Recommendation 2: Expand Opportunities for Nurses to Lead and Diffuse Collaborative Improvement Efforts

Care coordination is crucial to both care quality and safe care, and teams of health professionals are associated with better patient outcomes and improved patient satisfaction. Health care delivery in the United States is increasingly fragmented and episodic. Ideally, new delivery models should include seamless coordination to facilitate the transition of patients and families through their care, over time and in different contexts. Health care delivery in rural settings is at particular risk of fragmentation without care coordination that transcends distance and links different health care systems and providers. When educating the next generation of nurses, interprofessional academic and clinical experiences are essential to advance interprofessional collaboration that facilitates coordinated patient-centered care (IOM, 2005, 2011). In an effort to promote interprofessional models, the Health Resources and Services Administration (HRSA) collaborated with the Robert Wood Johnson Foundation, the Macy Foundation, and the American Board of Internal Medicine Foundation to establish the Interprofessional Education Collaborative (IEC) (Wakefield, 2011). Recently, the IEC (2011) published the following Core Competencies for Interprofessional Collaborative Practice, which are an adjunct to the general competencies of the various health professions:

1. Values/ethics for interprofessional practice
2. Roles/responsibilities for collaborative practice
3. Interprofessional communication
4. Interprofessional teamwork and team-based care

The IEC values can be a stimulus for dialogue and developments of an action plan that facilitates interprofessional practice (Brewer, 2012). It is important for nurse educators and scholars to assume an active role to present the rural nursing perspective in this dialogue, and, subsequently, to integrate the competencies into nursing curricula.

Partnership for Patients (AKA Partners) (Department of Health and Human Services [DHHS], 2011) is another national initiative; it has more than 3,300 partners that have direct and associated connections with health care. Partners support the following goals: providing better care at lower costs, a 40% reduction in preventable treatment errors, and a 20% decline in hospital readmissions. Rural health care facilities and nurses employed in these settings have a critical role in driving the success of the two interprofessional initiatives, especially as providers in underserved areas. How interprofessional and partnering activities play out in rural health care systems remains to be seen, but they are opportunities for nurse innovators and scholars to make nursing care safer and more effective for rural consumers.

The clinical nurse leader (CNL), an emerging role within nursing, is well positioned to address the call for nurses to lead collaborative improvement efforts in health care. CNLs are master's-prepared advanced generalists who coordinate and facilitate care with multiple health care disciplines at the point of care for patients, individuals, families, and communities (American Association of Colleges of Nursing [AACN], 2007). With a primary focus on communication, quality, safety, and evidence-based practice, CNLs assume accountability for client care outcomes across the health care delivery system. As such, the CNL is well suited for practice in rural settings. Early indicators suggest that outcomes improve when CNLs are a part of the health care team (Rosseter, 2009). Additional research is needed to further explicate the role and the outcomes of CNLs in rural practice settings.

Recommendation 3: Implement Nurse Residency Programs

The third IOM (2010) recommendation stresses the importance of strengthening career ladders for nurses. Molinari and Bushy's (2011) publication titled "The Rural Nurse: Transition to Practice" was developed in response to this IOM recommendation. This edited textbook describes national and international rural-focused nurse transition-to-practice strategies for recent graduates/new RNs, and advanced practice nurses, as well as nurses who are entering a new practice setting. Federal initiatives have directed financial resources to institutions of higher education to support nursing faculty and students in an effort to build primary care capacity. While these federal investments are not designed to strengthen rural nursing care exclusively, it is important for nurse educators and scholars to ensure that the initiatives support nurses and health care in rural areas.

Recommendation 4: Increase the Proportion of Nurses with a Baccalaureate Degree to 80% by 2020

In view of the nursing workforce demographics described in the previous paragraphs, the fourth IOM recommendation has particular relevance for rural settings, given the low proportion of BSN-prepared nurses. Academic nursing leaders across all schools of nursing must work together to achieve this goal and also must design curricula that integrate rural content and experiences. Individuals who have a rural background are in a position to offer insights on effective strategies to increase the proportion of BSN-prepared nurses. Nurse leaders in education should partner with accrediting bodies, philanthropic groups, and private and public employers to ensure funding, monitor progress, and increase the number of nurses prepared at the BSN level (Simpson & McDonald, 2011). Ultimately, the nation needs an appropriately educated diverse nursing workforce that is prepared to meet the complex health care needs of a diverse and aging population in rural as well as urban regions. The fact that the nursing shortage in rural communities is strongly influenced by the distribution rather than by the number of available nurses definitely warrants further examination.

Recommendation 5: Double the Number of Nurses With a Doctorate by 2020

The term "doctorate" as used in this IOM recommendation refers to both the research doctorate/doctor of philosophy (PhD) degree and the doctorate in nursing practice (DNP) degree. More specifically, in order to prepare more nurses to enter the nursing workforce, be it rural or urban, there must be an increase in the number of faculty prepared at the PhD level. While positions for PhD-prepared nurses may be limited within a rural community, individuals at this level indirectly organize and deliver curricula that should include a rural component, be it didactic or as clinical experiences. With respect to the DNP, that is the required degree for those pursuing an advanced practice degree. Definitely, nurses prepared at the doctoral level are critical to expand and sustain the rural nursing workforce, as well as providing the expertise to enhance quality clinical practice, implement valid research, and refine theory.

Three federal laws have particular relevance for expanding the health professional workforce in regions defined as HPSAs: Title VII of the Public Health Services Act (enacted in 1963), Title VIII (enacted in 1964), and Title VI (a component of the Affordable Care Act [ACA], 2010) were enacted in response to a shortage of health care providers (Health Professions and Nursing Education Coalition [HPNEC], 2011; Nursing Community, 2011; Office of Rural Health Policy [ORHP], 2011). Title VII was implemented to encourage health care workers to practice in underserved areas by increasing the number of primary care providers as well as increasing the number of minority/disadvantaged students enrolling in health professional programs. Title VIII focuses on preparing advanced practice nurses and increasing the number of minority/disadvantaged students enrolling in these programs (HPNEC, 2011; Nursing Community, 2011;

ORHP, 2011). Title VI (component of the ACA) dedicates financial resources to the National Health Service Corps (NHSC) in the form of student loan-repayment contracts and scholarships for primary care clinicians (NHSC, 2011). Of the 7,500 providers currently serving in NHSC, about 50% serve in rural posts, of which about 1,400 are nurses in advanced practice roles. As with all federal and state initiatives, outcome data are needed to determine whether or not the stated intent was achieved and at what cost, particularly those targeting in rural and underserved regions.

Recommendation 6: Ensure That Nurses Engage in Lifelong Learning

This IOM recommendation reinforces the need for ongoing continuing education by a health profession associated with rapidly emerging knowledge and changing technology to learn new competencies and sustain proficiency in others. The current global, national, and local economic situations impose financial hardships and make it especially difficult for many nurses to continue their education beyond the level for which they were initially licensed. Likewise, nurses living in rural communities, regardless of where they choose to work, must contend with the local economic situation, be it robust or in recession. Rural nurses often do not have the resources, nor is their employer able to offer financial support, to pursue a BSN, an advanced degree or, perhaps even obtain continuing professional education. Technology holds potential for offering educational programs to meet the learning needs of nurses who live some distance from an urban-based university campus. However, evidence is needed to determine the most efficacious approach for distance learning to meet the needs of nurses in rural contexts.

Another dimension of lifelong learning relates to children and adolescents (youth) in small rural communities who have an interest in and the academic ability to pursue a degree in a health profession. It is not uncommon for a rural child to be the first in his or her family to attend college. In these instances, a child is often reared in an environment without any expectation of ever attaining an academic degree. Nor have many children and adolescents who live in a rural area been exposed to or mentored by a health professional or by a nurse in particular. Social determinants of this nature are being addressed in some rural communities with academic "pipelines" that begin in elementary school and continue throughout secondary education. These models are a recruitment and retention strategy to "grow our own" health professionals. With respect to nursing, early on, children should be exposed to local nurses, along with an emphasis on enrolling in the sciences for success in college. Exposure to local role models can reinforce the possibility of nursing as a career option—even if the child is the first in the family to pursue a college degree (NRHA, 2005; RAC, 2011; Skillman et al., 2007). Evidence is needed on effective academic pipeline models and how these contribute to sustaining the nursing workforce. In turn, nurse scholars must disseminate the best information on designing, implementing, and evaluating academic pipelines in concert with recruitment and retention of nurses in historically underserved communities.

Recommendation 7: Prepare and Enable Nurses to Lead Change to Advance Health

The seventh IOM recommendation proposes that nurses, nursing education programs, and nursing professional associations should prepare the nursing workforce to assume leadership positions across all levels. Public, private, and governmental health care decision makers should ensure that leadership positions are available to and filled by nurses. The IOM invites private and public funders, health care organizations, nursing education programs, and nursing associations to expand opportunities for nurses to learn to lead, manage, redesign, and improve practice environments and health systems. As for the rural perspective, in small communities, local nurses tend to be highly esteemed and are deemed an important health care resource by residents. Rural nurses in turn often assume an activist role in local organizations and health-related initiatives. Unfortunately, these same nurses may not be part of the decision-making process within the health care facility in which they are employed (Hurme, 2009; IOM, 2005; Molinari & Monserud, 2008). Given the interpersonal dynamics in small communities, nurses' expertise and leadership are critical when designing, implementing, and evaluating new initiatives that are tailored to advance nursing care in rural health care institutions.

Recommendation 8: Build an Infrastructure for the Collection and Analysis of Interprofessional Health Care Workforce Data

Based on the information presented in this chapter, it becomes obvious that the national nursing workforce data are incomplete, sometimes conflicting, and practically nonexistent for rural nurses; hence, the relevance of the eighth IOM recommendation. In an effort to address the information deficit, the National Health Care Workforce Commission (NHCWC), with oversight from the Government Accountability Office (GAO) and HRSA, are currently collaborating to improve the collection and analysis of data on the health care workforce (Wakefield, 2011). Also, the NHCWC and HRSA are partnering with state licensing boards, state nursing workforce centers, and the Department of Labor, and developing models to ensure that data are timely, relevant, and publicly accessible. Critically needed are complete and reliable regional and state-level workforce data. Health care professionals must serve where they are needed and must have the ability to function in state-of-the-art models of care. Given that mandate, the NCHWA is developing models for projecting supply and demand that include advanced practice nurses. In order to develop a relevant model, HRSA policy decisions on workforce education and equitable distribution requires input from local communities, state offices of Rural Health, state Primary Care Organizations, and Area Health Education Centers (AHEC). In turn, data-driven reports should inform policy deliberations related to the health professional workforce in general and to the nursing workforce in particular.

SUMMARY

Nursing workforce needs have changed with the provision of care shifting from the acute in-patient setting to community-based settings. Current and projected nationwide shortages of RNs threaten access and quality of care in rural and urban communities alike. In rural areas, quality is particularly challenged by an uneven distribution of health care providers—in particular, by a shortage of RNs. Health care can be exciting to deliver in rural areas and informative to study. Nurses living and working in rural environments have an opportunity to meaningfully contribute their expertise and insights to scholars as they design research studies and refine a theory for nursing.

REFERENCES

American Association of Colleges of Nursing. (2007). *White paper on the education and role of the clinical nurse leader.* Retrieved May 15, 2012 from http://www.aacn.nche.edu/publications/white-papers/cnl

Auerbach, D. I., Buerhaus, P. I., & Steiger, D. O. (2011). Registered nurse supply grows faster than projected amid surge in new entrants ages 23–26. *Health Affairs, 30*(12), 2286–2292.

Brewer, K. (2012). Inside ANA—Issues up close. Making interprofessional teams work for nurses, patients. *American Nurse Today, 7*(3), 32–33.

Bureau of the Census. (2009). *Annual estimates of the resident population for incorporated places.* Retrieved March 12, 2012 from http://www.census.gov/popest/cities/SUB-EST2009.html

Bureau of Health Professions (BHPr). (2010). *The registered nurse population: Findings from the 2008 national sample survey of registered nurses.* Retrieved March 12, 2012 from http://bhpr.hrsa.gov/healthworkforce/rnsurveys/rnsurveyfinal.pdf

Bushy, A. (2009). American Nurses Credentialing Center (ANCC) pathway to excellence program: Addressing and meeting the needs of small and rural hospitals. *Online Journal of Rural Nursing and Health Care, 9*(1), 6–10.

Retrieved March 12, 2012 from http://www.rno.org/journal/index.php/online-journal/article/viewFile/171/221

Centers for Medicare and Medicaid Services (CMMS). (2011). *Federally qualified health centers.* Retrieved March 12, 2012 from http://www.cms.gov/center/fqhc.asp

Chipp, C., Dewane, S., Brems, C., Johnson, M., Warner, T. D., & Roberts, L. W. (2011). "If only someone had told me . . ." Lessons from rural providers. *Journal of Rural Health, 27*(2), 122–130.

Cromartie, J. (2008). Defining the "rural" in rural America. *Amber Waves.* Retrieved March 12, 2012 from http://www.ers.usda.gov/AmberWaves/June08/Features/RuralAmerica.htm

Department of Health and Human Services (DHHS). (2011). *Partnership for patients: Better care, lower costs.* Retrieved March 12, 2012 from http://www.healthcare.gov/compare/partnership-for-patients/index.html

Grantmakers in Health (GIH). (2009). *Rural health care: Innovations in policy and practice.* Retrieved March 12, 2012 from http://www.gih.org/files/usrdoc/Rural_Health_Care_March_2009.pdf

Health Professions and Nursing Education Coalition (HPNEC). (2011). *Funding updates.* Retrieved March 12, 2012 from https://www.aamc.org/advocacy/hpnec/

Hunsberger, M., Bauman, A., & Blythe, J. (2009). Sustaining the rural workforce: Nursing perspectives on work life challenges. *Journal of Rural Health, 25*(1), 17–25.

Hurme, E. (2009). Competencies for nursing practice in a rural critical access hospital. *Online Journal of Rural Nursing and Health Care, 9*(2), 67–81. Retrieved March 12, 2012 from http://www.rno.org/journal/index.php/online-journal/article/viewFile/198/256

Interprofessional Education Collaborative (IEC). (2011). *Core competencies for interprofessional collaborative practice.* Retrieved March 12, 2012 from http://www.asph.org/userfiles/CollaborativePractice.pdf

Institute of Medicine (IOM). (2005). *Committee on the Future of Rural Health Care, Board on Health Care Services—Quality through collaboration: The future of rural health.* Washington, DC: National Academies Press. Retrieved March 12, 2012 from http://www.iom.edu/Reports/2004/Quality-Through-Collaboration-The-Future-of-Rural-Health.aspx

Institute of Medicine (IOM). (2011). *The future of nursing: Leading change, advancing health.* Washington, DC: The National Academies Press. Retrieved March 12, 2012 from http://iom.edu/Reports/2010/The-Future-of-Nursing-Leading-Change-Advancing-Health.aspx

LaSala, K. (2000). Nursing workforce issues in rural and urban settings: Looking at the difference in recruitment, retention and distribution. *Online Journal of Rural Nursing and Health Care, 1*(1), 8–17. Retrieved

March 12, 2012 from http://www.rno.org/journal/index.php/online-journal/article/viewFile/63/62

Long, K. A., & Weinert, C. (1989). Rural nursing: Developing a theory base. *Scholarly Inquiry for Nursing Practice, 3*, 113–127.

Molinari, D., & Bushy, A. (2011). *The rural nurse: Transition to practice.* New York, NY: Springer Publishing.

Molinari, D., & Monserud, M. (2008). Rural nurse job satisfaction. *Rural and Remote Health: The Journal of Rural Remote Health.* Retrieved March 12, 2012 from http://www.rrh.org.au/articles/subviewnew.asp?ArticleID=1055

National Advisory Committee on Rural Health and Human Services (NACRHHS). (2011). *The 2011 report to the secretary: Rural health and human services issues.* Retrieved March 12, 2012 from http://www.hrsa.gov/advisorycommittees/rural/2011secreport.pdf

National Center for Health Workforce Analysis (NCHWA). (2010). *The registered nurse population. Findings from the 2008 national sample survey of registered nurses (NSSRN).* Retrieved March 12, 2012 from http://bhpr.hrsa.gov/healthworkforce/rnsurveys/rnsurveyfinal.pdf

National Health Service Corps (NHSC). (2011). *About NHSC.* Retrieved March 12, 2012 from http://nhsc.bhpr.hrsa.gov

National Rural Health Association (NRHA). (2005). *NRHA issue paper: Recruitment and retention of quality health workforce in rural health careers pipeline: Number 2: Nursing.* Retrieved March 12, 2012 from http://www.ruralhealthweb.org/go/left/policy-and-advocacy/policy-documents-and-statements/official-policy-positions

Newhouse, R., Stanik-Hutt, J., White, K. M., Johantgen, M., Bass, E. B., Zangaro, G. et al. (2011). CNE series: Advanced practice nurses outcomes 1990–2008: A systematic review. *Nursing Economics*, 1–21. Retrieved March 12, 2012 from http://s3.amazonaws.com/enp-network-assets/attachments/3559/original.pdf?1314047839

Nursing Community. (2011). *Title VIII of the Public Health Service Act: Nursing workforce development programs.* Retrieved March 12, 2012 from http://www.thenursingcommunity.org/#/advocacy/4542346557

Office of Rural Health Policy (ORHP). (2011). *Rural guide to federal health professions funding.* Retrieved March 12, 2012 from http://www.hrsa.gov/ruralhealth/pdf/ruralhealthfundingguidance.pdf

Orsolini-Hain, L. (2012). Mixed messages: Hospital practices that serve as disincentives for associate degree-prepared nurses to return to school. *Nursing Outlook, 60*(20), 81–90.

Ortiz, J., & Bushy, A. (2011). A focus group study on rural health clinic performance. *Family & Community Health, 34*(2), 111–118.

Pepper, C., Sandefer, R., & Gray, M. (2010). Recruiting and retaining physicians in very rural areas. *Journal of Rural Health, 26*(2), 196–200.

Roberge, C. (2009). Who stays in rural nursing practice? An international review of the literature on factors influencing rural nurse retention. *Online Journal of Rural Nursing and Health Care, 9*(12), 82–93. Retrieved March 12, 2012 from http://www.rno.org/journal/index.php/online-journal/article/viewFile/180/230

Rosseter, R. (2009). A new role for nurses: Making room for clinical nurse leaders. *The Joint Commission Perspectives on Patient Safety, 9*(8), 5–7.

Rural Assistance Center (RAC). (2011). *Rural health care workforce: Frequently asked questions.* Retrieved March 12, 2012 from http://www.raconline.org/topics/hc_providers/workforcefaq.php

Simpson, C., & McDonald, F. (2011). "Any body is better than nobody?" Ethical questions around recruiting and/or retaining health professionals in rural areas. *Rural and Remote Health.* Retrieved March 12, 2012 from http://www.rrh.org.au/articles/subviewnew.asp?ArticleID=1867

Skillman, S., Palazzo, L., Hart, G., & Butterfield, P. (2007). *Changes in the rural registered nurse workforce from 1980 to 2004.* WWAMI Rural Health Research Center. Retrieved March 12, 2012 from http://depts.washington.edu/uwrhrc/uploads/RHRC%20FR115%20Skillman.pdf

Sumaya, C. (2012). Enumeration and composition of the public health workforce: Challenges and strategies. *American Journal of Public Health, 102*(3), 469–474.

United States Department of Agriculture (USDA). (2008a). *Rural America at a glance: 2010 edition.* Retrieved March 12, 2012 from http://www.ers.usda.gov/Publications/EIB59/EIB59.pdf

United States Department of Agriculture (USDA). (2008b). *What is rural?* Retrieved March 12, 2012 from http://www.nal.usda.gov/ric/ricpubs/what_is_rural.shtml#character

Wakefield, M. (2011, June 13). *HRSA speech: Remarks to the joint forum on rural health and nursing solutions.* Retrieved March 12, 2012 from http://www.hrsa.gov/about/news/speeches/2011/06132011ruralhealth.html

Winters, C. A., & Lee, H. J. (Eds.). (2010). *Rural nursing: Concepts, theory and practice* (3rd ed.). New York, NY: Springer Publishing.

Chapter 30

AN ANALYSIS OF KEY CONCEPTS FOR RURAL NURSING

Helen J. Lee, Charlene A. Winters,
Robin L. Boland, Susan J. Raph, and
Janice A. Buehler

LONG AND WEINERT (1989) NOTED that during the initial "process of data organization ... some concepts appeared repeatedly in the ethnographic data collected in several different areas of the state" (p. 118). Following the initial publication of their article in 1989, faculty in the Rural Nursing Theory Special Committee within the Montana State University-Bozeman College of Nursing embarked on a plan to analyze identified concepts. The committee's efforts were enhanced through course work involvement of graduate nursing students enrolled in Montana State University College of Nursing's rural generalist program. The purpose of this chapter is to summarize the analyzed concepts contained in the first edition of *Conceptual Basis of Rural Nursing* (Lee, 1998) and other conducted relevant research (Boland & Lee, 2006; Raph & Buehler, 2006). The summary provides a quick reference of the analyzed concepts and allows for easy identification of areas needing further work.

The concepts are organized according to the framework provided in the rural nursing theory base. Following each theoretical statement are concept summaries pertinent to that particular statement. Each concept summary is presented using the analysis framework selected by the chapter authors from *Conceptual Basis of Rural Nursing* (Lee, 1998). Elements of the framework, whether explicit or implicit, contained in the chapters are presented; elements not evident are indicated by statements such as "none given" or "not identified."

FIRST STATEMENT: HOW RURAL DWELLERS DEFINE HEALTH

The first statement indicates that "rural dwellers define health primarily as the ability to work, to be productive, to do usual tasks" (Long & Weinert, 1989, p. 120). Work beliefs and health beliefs were key concepts; isolation and distance were identified as related concepts. Health beliefs, isolation, and distance were three of the four concepts analyzed.

Health Beliefs (Long, 1993)

Method of analysis: Smith's (1983) four models of health—clinical, role performance, adaptive, eudemonistic.
 Definition: Rural dwellers often conceptualize health within the role performance model (Long, 1993).
 Defining attributes:

1. "Ability to work . . . [and] perform one's daily activities" (p. 124).
2. "Determine health needs primarily in relation to work activities" (p. 124).
3. "As a result of their environment, rural dwellers are more frequently called upon to be independent and self-reliant" (p. 124).

Antecedents: Beliefs held will affect "health-promotion behaviors, health care seeking, and acceptance of preventive and treatment interventions" (p. 123).
 Consequences: Knowledge of client's concept of health is important for development of relevant and acceptable assessment approaches and intervention strategies (p. 123).
 Empirical referents: none identified.

Isolation (Lee, Hollis, & McClain, 1998)

Method of analysis: Wilson's method (Walker & Avant, 1995).
 Definition: None given.
 Essential attributes:

1. Separation—"Being divided from the rest" (Lee et al., 1998, p. 69).
2. Relativeness—"Something dependent on external conditions for its specific nature . . . existing or having its specific nature only by relation to something else; not absolute or independent" (p. 69).
3. Perception—"Consciousness or awareness" (p. 69).

Antecedents: "Presence of an indicator directing attention to the condition of isolation (geographical terrain, distance, changes imposed by weather, economic costs, time or personal preference)" (p. 69).

Consequences: "Decreased communication or interaction with other individuals that results in social or professional isolation" (p. 70).

Empirical referents: None identified.

Distance (Henson, Sadler, & Walton, 1998)

Method of analysis: Wilson's method (Walker & Avant, 1988).

Definition: "Implies a degree of separation between two or more entities.... The nature of separation may be in space, time or behavior" (Henson et al., 1998, p. 51).

Essential attributes:

1. Mileage—"Total number of miles traveled" (p. 56).
2. Time—"Measurement in minutes it takes to travel from one place to another" (p. 56).
3. Perception—"Variation in awareness of data that is different from others' awareness" (p. 56).

Antecedent: "Access to health care" (p. 58).
Consequence: "Potential for compromised health care" (p. 58).
Empirical referents:

1. Objective:
   (a) "Distance" (miles, kilometers) (p. 58).
   (b) "Travel time" (p. 58).
   (c) MSU Rurality Index (county of residence population, distance to emergency care) (Weinert & Boik, 1995).
2. Subjective:
   (a) "Perception" (Henson et al., 1998, p. 58).

SECOND STATEMENT: SELF-RELIANCE

The second statement is "... rural dwellers are self-reliant and resist accepting help or services from those seen as 'outsiders' or from agencies seen as national or regional 'welfare' programs. A corollary to this statement is that help, including needed health care, is usually sought through an informal rather than a formal system" (Long & Weinert, 1989, p. 120). Key concepts analyzed were self-reliance, outsider, insider, old-timer, newcomer, resources, informal networks, and lay care network.

Self-Reliance (Chafey, Sullivan, & Shannon, 1998)

Method of analysis: Qualitative research inquiry (Morse, 1995).
Definition:

1. "The capacity to provide for one's own needs" (Agich, 1993, as cited in Chafey et al., 1998, p. 158).
2. "The desire to do for oneself and care for oneself" (Long & Weinert, 1989, p. 119).

Sample: Cohort of nine women between 70 and 85 years of age, living in small rural towns.

Data collection: Interview using structured guide developed to elicit participants' perceptions of self-reliance (Chafey et al., 1998, p. 160).
Characteristics:

1. Primary
   (a) Learned—"A skill emanating from previous learning events that started in their youth (family chores and assumption of responsibilities), continued into adulthood, and was reinforced by later life events (retirement, death of a parent or spouse)" (p. 162).
   (b) Decisional choice—"Making one's own decisions and choices" (p. 164).
   (c) Independence—"Independence or dependence on self, dependence on others, self-assertion or freedom of action, and self-identity" (p. 166).
2. Secondary—Embodied an aspect of their self-reliance experience.
   (a) Self-confidence (p. 170).
   (b) Self-competence (pp. 170–171).

Outsider (Bailey, 1998)

Method of analysis: Wilson's method (Walker & Avant, 1988).

Definition: "Being exterior to the group, matter, or boundary in question" (Bailey, 1998, p. 140).
Defining attributes:

1. Differentness—"In terms of cultural orientation, standards, lifestyle, education, religion, occupation, social status, worldview, interests, or experience"; "the quality or state of being different" (pp. 143–144).
2. Unfamiliarity—With the matter in question (p. 144).
3. Unconnectedness—"Having no family of personal ties" (p. 144).

Antecedents: "Lacking understanding or knowledge of the social context, beliefs, rituals, customs and history of the community" (p. 144).

Consequences: "One may be excluded from access to knowledge and information, not be accepted, not be recognized, be isolated, and be distrusted" (p. 144).

Empirical referents: None identified.

Insider (Myers, 1998)

Method of analysis: Wilson's method (Walker & Avant, 1995).

Definition: "Someone who is a member of a group and has access to special or privileged information" (Myers, 1998, p. 127).

Defining attributes:

1. "Member of a group" (p. 132).
2. "Having access to privileged information" (p. 132).
3. "An awareness of implicit assumptions and social context" (p. 132).
4. "A long-time occupant" (p. 132).

Antecedents: "Acceptance by the group" (p. 135).
Consequences:

1. "Power ... because of having information that others lack" (p. 135).
2. "Reserved social position ... that is unavailable to others" (p. 135).
3. "Lack of objectivity" (p. 135).
4. "Committed to the group" (p. 135).

Empirical referents: None identified.

Old-Timer (Caniparoli, 1998)

Method of analysis: Wilson's method (Walker & Avant, 1995).
Definition:

1. "One who is long established in a place or position" (Caniparoli, 1998, p. 103).
2. "A man who has lived in the county a long time" (American slang, 1968, as cited in Caniparoli, 1998, p. 103).

Defining attributes:

1. "Age" (p. 108).
2. "Length of time spent in a community" (p. 108).
3. "Establishment of a relationship within the community" (p. 108).

Antecedents: "Identification as an old-timer" (p. 110).

Consequences: "Establishes a relationship within the community . . . [that] can be viewed as positive or negative depending on the role of the viewer" (p. 110).

Empirical referents: None identified.

Concept Verification Research

Boland conducted a qualitative study with a convenience sample of nine participants living in small rural communities in central Montana (Boland & Lee, 2006). The study findings confirmed the three defining attributes for old-timer and identified land ownership as the key element of the third attribute. The old-timers spoke of their functions within the community as working together for survival, holding social events to accomplish work and play, to share traditions, and act as historians.

Most participants identified themselves as "old-timers" despite earlier historical literature describing "old-timers" as persons who were "mysterious, unusual and fiercely independent" (Caniparoli, 1998, p. 106). These study participants expressed doubt about their level of influence within the communities, originally attributed to them in the earlier rural nursing theory development. Loss of influence was attributed to changing times (fewer farms and ranches, increased identification with the nearby larger towns and cities) and "the loss of respect for elderly people in today's society" (Boland & Lee, 2006, p. 50).

Newcomer (Sutermaster, 1998)

Method of analysis: Wilson's method (Walker & Avant, 1995).
    Definition: "One that has recently arrived" (Sutermaster, 1998, p. 113).
    Defining attributes:

1. "Newly arrived" (p. 120).
2. "Unaware of the history of the area/institution" (p. 120).
3. "Their existence may result in change" (p. 120).

Antecedents: "Individuals or families would have had a need or desire to move" (p. 121).

Consequences: "There is a new individual or family living in the community" (p. 121).

Empirical referents: None identified.

Resources (Ballantyne, 1998)

Method of analysis: Wilson's method (Walker & Avant, 1995).

Definition: "Resources are properties, resorts, or assets that are finite by nature and are made available for use by populations through an allocation process. Resources are accessed and used in response to a population's or individual's motivation for need satisfaction. ... Furthermore, these three elements can be visualized in a circle with the flow of energy between the allocated resource, accessibility of the resource, and use of the resource" (Ballantyne, 1998, p. 181).

Defining attributes:

1. Property—"Resource is a property or an asset that has value for consumption by populations in need of that property" (p. 181).

2. Expedient—"Continuance or plan for solution of a particular problem" (p. 181).

3. Resort—"Turning inward to one's resources" (p. 181).

Antecedents: Knowledge of "local, regional, and national availability" (p. 187).
Consequences: "Allocation, accessibility, and use" (p. 187).
Empirical referents: None identified.

Informal Networks (Grossman & McNerney, 1998)

Method of analysis: Wilson's method (Walker & Avant, 1995).

Definition: "Networks are interconnected relationships, durable patterns of interactions, and interpersonal threads that comprise a social fabric" (Grossman & McNerney, 1998, pp. 201–202).

Defining attributes:

1. Volunteer—includes family members, coworkers, and neighbors who offer assistance free of charge (p. 204).

2. Information exchange (p. 204).

3. Support—has two components: Emotional component (being a friend, listening) and physical (assistance with daily living, health promotion, and maintenance activities) (p. 204).

4. Guidance—"May be given as advice, consultation (availability of resources, referral to health care providers, sources of alternative treatments), and information" (p. 204).

Antecedents:

1. "A bond ... the tie that exists among ... the core of the informal network (family, friends, neighbors, and coworkers)" (p. 206).

2. "Are generated in response to a perceived need" (p. 206).

Consequences: "The perceived need is met or not met" (p. 206).
Empirical referents: None identified.

Lay Care Network (Turnbull, 1998)

Method of analysis: Wilson's method (Walker & Avant, 1988).
Definition: None given.
Defining attributes:

1. Interconnection or net—"An interconnection is the means by which one thing connects with another, whereas a net consists of fibers woven together for catching something" (Turnbull, 1998, p. 195).
2. Of the people—"Belonging to, concerned with, or performed by the 'people' in a nonprofessional capacity" (p. 195).
3. Sense of concern—"The idea that one develops or maintains an interest in the well-being of a person or object, to oversee with the intent to protect" (Oxford, 1989 as cited in Turnbull, 1998, p. 195).

Antecedents: None identified.
Consequences: None identified.
Empirical referents: None identified.
Conclusion: Turnbull recommended "further refinement of the concept, 'lay care provider,' and suggests a change in the wording of the concept itself" (p. 198). The literature review clearly delineates between lay providers and informal care providers, whereas the wording "lay care providers" combines two different concepts.

THIRD STATEMENT: LACK OF ANONYMITY AND ROLE DIFFUSION

The third statement is "Health care providers in rural areas must deal with a lack of anonymity and much greater role diffusion than providers in urban or suburban settings" (Long & Weinert, 1989, p. 120). The key concepts are lack of anonymity and role diffusion. Related concepts are familiarity and professional isolation. Analyzed were anonymity, familiarity, and professional isolation.

Lack of Anonymity (Lee, 1998)

Method of analysis: Wilson's method (Walker & Avant, 1995).
Definition: "A condition in which one cannot remain nameless or unknown" (Lee, 1998, p. 77).

Defining attributes:

1. Visible—"That which can be seen, is apparent or obvious" (p. 83).
2. Identifiable—"Being able to recognize or establish the condition or character of a person" (p. 83).
3. Diminished personal/professional boundaries: "Borders or perimeters through which one functions are smaller, more circumscribed" (p. 83).

Antecedents: "Lack of anonymity occurs in an environmental context characterized by a low level of stimulation. It contains fewer number of individuals and/or objects (e.g., automobiles, buildings) needing to be considered in the normal deliberation of one's activities" (pp. 83–84).

Consequences: "A relationship [in which] one's actions are visible and readily observed" (p. 84). Greater difficulty in maintaining personal and professional privacy exists because of the relationship.

Empirical referents: None identified.

Concept Verification Research

Raph conducted a pilot study focusing on the phenomenon "lack of anonymity" with four informants employed in a western rural "frontier" county health department (Raph & Buehler, 2006). Using grounded theory technique, four differing interactive categories emerged through the data analysis: (a) Personally affirming interactions were defined as "friendly encounters that did not place the informant in a professional role" (p. 199); (b) professional affirming interactions were those seeking clarification on "general information about vaccines, appointments, or needed after-hour services.... usually (taking place in) public places in the community" (pp. 199–200); (c) professionally threatening interactions "placed health care providers in a position of potentially doing harm if not handled correctly" (p. 200); and (d) personally threatening encounters were those that "provoked fear and anger" (p. 201). The four categories, placed in a continuum from positive to negative, extend the second and third defining attributes of the lack of anonymity (see above) and verify the consequences of the "greater difficulty in maintaining personal and professional privacy" (Lee, 1998, p. 84).

Familiarity (McNeely & Shreffler, 1998)

Method of analysis: Wilson's method (Walker & Avant, 1995).

Definition: "An antithetical concept that includes the positive ideas of thorough knowledge of or an acquaintance with [someone] and closeness and intimacy, such as one would find in a family or deep friendship, and the contrasting perspective of offensive, unwarranted, intimate conduct that might include behaviors such as flirting, sexual harassment, domestic violence, abusive relationships, or incest" (McNeely & Shreffler, 1998, p. 91).

Defining attributes:

1. "Friendly relationship or close acquaintance" (p. 98).
2. "Intimacy" (p. 98).
3. "Informality" (p. 98).
4. "The exhibited familiarity is welcome or unwelcome depending on the perceptions of the receiver" (p. 98).

Antecedents: None identified.
Consequences: None identified.
Empirical referents: None identified.

Professional Isolation (Shreffler, 1998)

Method of analysis: Wilson's method (Walker & Avant, 1988).
Definition: None given.
Defining attributes: "An actual separation from or a deficiency in a resource needed to fulfill one's professional responsibilities or needs (objective component)" (Shreffler, 1998, p. 426); "professional need is perceived as partially or wholly unmet (subjective component)" (p. 426); "the actual separation or deficiency is on a continuum" (p. 426); "the individual is not voluntarily separating herself/himself from an available professional resource" (p. 426); and "the objective component is more likely to be present in rural areas" (p. 426).

Antecedents: The individuals experience "separation from or deficiency in resources needed to fulfill professional responsibilities" and have "needs for resources to fulfill their professional responsibilities," "can make choices about the use of available resources," and "are able to perceive whether professional needs are met" (p. 429).

Consequences: They "are specific to the need that is unmet and the vulnerabilities of the individual in the occupation or job position" (p. 429).

Empirical referents:

1. "The availability of the needed resource is measured and found deficient" (p. 429).
2. "Individuals.... express awareness of an unmet need or exhibit signs of the consequence of the unmet need" (pp. 429–430).

CONCLUSION

In this chapter, we summarized the concepts found in *Conceptual Basis of Rural Nursing* (Lee, 1998). Most of the analyses were conducted using the Wilson method (Walker & Avant, 1988, 1995). However, some of the elements (e.g., definitions, antecedents, consequences, and empirical referents) were not addressed. Furthermore, some key concepts were not analyzed (e.g., work beliefs, role diffusion). Further development of the concepts is needed. Paramount is the need for validation of concepts with rural dwellers.

REFERENCES

Bailey, M. C. (1998). Outsider. In H. J. Lee (Ed.), *Conceptual basis for rural nursing* (pp. 139–148). New York, NY: Springer Publishing.

Ballantyne, J. (1998). Health resources and the rural client. In H. J. Lee (Ed.), *Conceptual basis for rural nursing* (pp. 178–198). New York, NY: Springer.

Boland, R., & Lee, H. (2006). Old-timers. In H. J. Lee, & C. A. Winters (Ed.), *Rural nursing: Concepts, theory, and practice* (2nd ed., pp. 43–52). New York, NY: Springer Publishing.

Caniparoli, C. D. (1998). Old-timer. In H. J. Lee (Ed.), *Conceptual basis for rural nursing* (pp. 102–112). New York, NY: Springer Publishing.

Chafey, K., Sullivan, T., & Shannon, A. (1998). Self-reliance: Characteristics of their own autonomy by elderly rural women. In H. J. Lee (Ed.), *Conceptual basis for rural nursing* (pp. 156–177). New York, NY: Springer Publishing.

Grossman, L. L., & McNerney, S. (1998). Informal networks. In H. J. Lee (Ed.), *Conceptual basis for rural nursing* (pp. 200–208). New York, NY: Springer Publishing.

Henson, D., Sadler, T., & Walton, S. (1998). Distance. In H. J. Lee (Ed.), *Conceptual basis for rural nursing* (pp. 51–60). New York, NY: Springer Publishing.

Lee, H. J. (1998). Lack of anonymity. In H. J. Lee (Ed.), *Conceptual basis for rural nursing* (pp. 76–88). New York, NY: Springer Publishing.

Lee, H. J., Hollis, B. R., & McClain, K. A. (1998). Isolation. In H. J. Lee (Ed.), *Conceptual basis for rural nursing* (pp. 139–148). New York, NY: Springer Publishing.

Long, K. A. (1993). The concept of health: Rural perspectives. *Nursing Clinics of North America, 28*, 123–130. Philadelphia, PA: Saunders.

Long, K. A., & Weinert, C. (1989). Rural nursing: Developing the theory base. *Scholarly Inquiry for Nursing Practice: An International Journal, 3*(2), 113–132.

McNeely, A. G., & Shreffler, M. J. (1998). Familiarity. In H. J. Lee (Ed.), *Conceptual basis for rural nursing* (pp. 89–101). New York, NY: Springer Publishing.

Morse, M. J. (1995). Exploring the theoretical basis of nursing using advanced techniques of concept analysis. *Advances in Nursing Science, 17*(3), 31–46.

Myers, D. D. (1998). Insider. In H. J. Lee (Ed.), *Conceptual basis for rural nursing* (pp. 125–138). New York, NY: Springer Publishing.

Raph, S., & Buehler, J. A. (2006). Rural health professionals' perceptions of lack of anonymity. In H. J. Lee, & C. A. Winters (Ed.), *Rural nursing: Concepts, theory, & practice* (2nd ed., pp. 197–204). New York, NY: Springer Publishing.

Shreffler, M. J. (1998). Professional isolation: A concept analysis. In H. J. Lee (Ed.), *Conceptual basis for rural nursing* (pp. 420–432). New York, NY: Springer Publishing.

Smith, J. A. (1983). *The idea of health: Implications for the nursing profession.* New York, NY: Teachers College Press.

Sutermaster, D. J. (1998). Newcomer. In H. J. Lee (Ed.), *Conceptual basis for rural nursing* (pp. 113–124). New York, NY: Springer Publishing.

Turnbull, T. S. (1998). Lay care network. In H. J. Lee (Ed.), *Conceptual basis for rural nursing* (pp. 189–199). New York, NY: Springer Publishing.

Walker, L., & Avant, K. (1988). *Strategies for theory construction in nursing* (2nd ed.). Norwalk, CT: Appleton-Century-Crofts.

Walker, L., & Avant, K. (1995). *Strategies for theory construction in nursing* (3rd ed.). Norwalk, CT: Appleton-Century-Crofts.

Weinert, C., & Boik, R. (1995). MSU rurality index: Development and evaluation. *Research in Nursing and Health, 18,* 453–464.

INDEX

A-B-C. *See* airway, breathing, circulation
A&I Database. *See* Abstracting and Indexing Database
AACN. *See* American Association of Colleges of Nursing
Abstracting and Indexing Database (A&I Database), 52, 53
ACA. *See* Affordable Care Act
Acceptability Scale, 216, 218
    frequencies of dependent variables, 220
    households, 221
    individual items in, 217, 219
    local rural health care, 222
    qualitative comments, 219
    rural residents, 223
    score computation, 219, 220
    willingness to use, 222
accessibility, 216
accommodation, 186, 216
accreditation, 411. *See also* public health (PH)
    CQI, 411
    government's role in, 413
    health care, 412
    minimum standards, 412
    PHAB, 411, 414–415
    in rural jurisdictions, 415–416
    TJC accreditation, 413
aces, 251
acquired immune deficiency syndrome (AIDS), 237, 318
activities of daily living (ADL), 120
ADL. *See* activities of daily living

advanced practice registered nurse (APRN), 27, 315, 457
affordability, 217
Affordable Care Act (ACA), 413
aging, 80, 87, 114
agrarian myth, 357
AHEC. *See* Area Health Education Centers
AIDS. *See* acquired immune deficiency syndrome
airway, breathing, circulation (A-B-C), 250
American Association of Colleges of Nursing (AACN), 259, 293, 460
American Nurse Association (ANA), 244
ANA. *See* American Nurse Association
Anabaptist communities, 432–433
ADN. *See* Associate Degree in Nursing
APRN. *See* advanced practice registered nurse
Area Health Education Centers (AHEC), 464
Associate Degree in Nursing (ADN), 452
Australian Rural Health Strategy, 443
autonomy, 266
availability, 216

Baccalaureate of Science in Nursing (BSN), 452, 462
bar [tavern] family, 181
basic social process (BSP), 133
Behavioral Risk Factor Surveillance System (BRFSS), 316

481

BMI. *See* body mass index
Board of Health (BOH), 403
body mass index (BMI), 316, 426
Border TB Photovoice Project, 319
Border Youth Alcohol Project
 (BYAP), 322
 in El Paso, 323
 SBIRT model, 322–323
boredom, 252
BRFSS. *See* Behavioral Risk Factor
 Surveillance System
BSN. *See* Baccalaureate of Science in
 Nursing
BYAP. *See* Border Youth Alcohol
 Project

CAH. *See* critical access hospital
CAM. *See* complementary alternative
 medicine and treatments;
 Complementary and
 alternative methods caregiver
 challenges, 185
 primary, 237
 rural, 24
caregiving
 burden and strain, 174, 175
 care recipient's emotional, 174
 caring for family members, 174
 challenges, 193–194
 family, 173
 gender-cultural model, 188, 189
 using Lazarus' Stress Theory, 175
 literature of male, 175
 NINR, 174
 physical needs, 174
 requirements, 185
 rural, 173
 services, 190
CDC. *See* Centers for Disease Control
 and Prevention
CE. *See* continuing education
Center for Research on Chronic Health
 Conditions in Rural Dwellers
 (CRCHC), 209
Centers for Disease Control and
 Prevention (CDC), 80
 monitoring health disparities, 229
 recommendations, 414
 T2D study, 317

Centers for Medicare and Medicaid
 Services (CMS), 412, 413
certified nurse midwife (CNM), 457, 458
certified nurse practitioner (CNP),
 457, 458
certified registered nurse anesthetist
 (CRNA), 453, 457, 458
CHD. *See* coronary heart disease
CHIP. *See* Head Start, Children's Health
 Insurance Program
chronic illness, 159
 access to care, 24
 in America, 159–160
 findings, 167
 health care providers, 168
 implications, 167–168
 role nurses play, 169
 rural/urban health differences, 160
 rural women with, 26
 self-management, 160–161
church family, 181
CHW. *See* community health worker
CINAHL. *See* Cumulative Index to
 Nursing and Allied Health
 Literature
clinical experiences
 evaluation of, 296
 involving nursing students in, 299
 in rural setting, 298
 SDSU nursing program with, 294
 use of rural facilities for, 296
clinical instructors
 clinical group, 294
 experiences, 300
 responsibilities, 295–296
 selection, 295
clinical nurse leader (CNL), 460
clinical nurse specialist (CNS), 457,
 458–459
CMS. *See* Centers for Medicare and
 Medicaid Services
CNL. *See* clinical nurse leader
CNM. *See* certified nurse midwife
CNP. *See* certified nurse practitioner
CNS. *See* clinical nurse specialist
CO. *See* radon, carbon monoxide
Cochrane Database of Systematic
 Reviews (CDSR), 52–53
Cochrane library, 52–53

Commission on Social Determinants of
    Health (CSDH), 339
community, 65–66
    advocacy activities, 103
    members facing problem, 319
    membership impact, 58
    participation in characteristic
        study, 370–371
    support, 73, 75–76, 180, 190
community health worker (CHW),
    308, 320
    for CAM, 308
    sustainability issue, 321–322
    utilization, 317, 318
community resiliency, 377. *See also* rural
        communities
    Australian case studies, 381–382
    Canadian and U. S. Exemplars
        studies, 379–381
    central Alberta pilot study, 383–384
    characteristics, 385
    community action, 387
    future research
        recommendations, 388
    interactions as collective unit, 386
    nursing education
        recommendations, 387–388
    original community resiliency
        model, 382
    research background, 378
    research studies, 378–379
    revised resiliency model, 382, 383
    rural RN's role, 385–386
    sense of community
        development, 386–387
    study in Barriere and La Ronge, 385
    updated resiliency model, 384
complementary alternative medicine
        and treatments (CAM), 146,
        205. *See also* health literacy
    acute health conditions, 206
    among older rural adults, 211
    among older rural women, 208–209
    chronic illness, 206, 209
    communication, 205
    IOM, 207
    MSU CAM health literacy
        scale, 210–211
    products and treatments, 206

providers in rural locations,
    209–210
in rural dwellers, 207
in United States, 205–206
Complementary and alternative
    methods (CAM), 307
cross-border service utilization,
    308–309
promotores, 308
protective factors, 309
connectedness, 125
conscientious consumer, 71, 75
continuing education (CE),
    126, 276
    ensuring nurses in lifelong
        learning, 462–463
    out-of-town workshops, 249
continuous quality improvement
    (CQI), 411
coronary heart disease (CHD), 427
CQI. *See* continuous quality
    improvement
CRCHC. *See* Center for Research on
    Chronic Health Conditions in
    Rural Dwellers
critical access hospital (CAH), 215,
    262, 443
    acceptability, 216, 217
    Acceptability Scale scores, 219, 220
    cost-based Medicare
        reimbursement, 215
    dependent variables, 218, 220
    households and residents, 221
    independent variables, 218
    local providers, 221
    location, 215
    Medicare, 215
    multivariate logistic regression
        models, 220
    qualitative comments, 221–222
    in rural areas, 215–216
CRNA. *See* certified registered nurse
    anesthetist
CSDH. *See* Commission on Social
    Determinants of Health
Cumulative Index to Nursing and
    Allied Health Literature
    (CINAHL), 52, 53, 146
cyber friends, 163

DHHS. *See* U. S. Department of Health and Human Services
diabetes mellitus (DM), 160
Diagnostic and Statistical Manual (DSM-IV), 309
Direct Relief International (DRI), 351
disenfranchisement, 237–238
Dissertations and Theses, A&I, 53
DM. *See* diabetes mellitus
doctorate in nursing practice (DNP), 461
DRI. *See* Direct Relief International
DSM-IV. *See Diagnostic and Statistical Manual*

EBP. *See* evidence-based practice
Economic Research Service (ERS), 278
ED. *See* emergency department
Education Research Complete, 53
EHR. *See* Electronic health records
EKG. *See* electrocardiography
electrocardiography (EKG), 10
Electronic health records (EHR), 298
emergency department (ED), 262, 317, 322
emergency medical service (EMS), 67, 423
emergency medical technician (EMT), 67
emergency room (ER), 322
emergency service personnel, 426–427
EMS. *See* emergency medical service
EMT. *See* emergency medical technician
environmental risk-reduction (ERR), 359
Environmental Risk Reduction through Nursing Intervention and Education (ERRNIE), 359
  behavioral determinants, 363–364
  design, 361
  efficacy of ERR interventions, 363
  measurement, 361
  Precaution Adoption Process Model, 361–362
  sample description, 362
  self-efficacy and precaution adoption, 362–363
  TERRA model, 359, 360
environmental tobacco smoke (ETS), 359

EPHS. *See* Essential Public Health Services
equanimity, 81, 86–87
ER. *See* emergency room
ERR. *See* environmental risk-reduction
ERRNIE. *See* Environmental Risk Reduction through Nursing Intervention and Education
ERS. *See* Economic Research Service
Essential Public Health Services (EPHS), 404
  accreditation criteria, 415
  in PH language and common translation, 405
ethnographic data, 5. *See also* rural nursing theory (RNT)
  health care providers, 8
  isolation and distance, 6
  old-timer/newcomer, 7
  ordering scheme, 6
  Personal Resource Questionnaire, 7–8
  rural dwellers, 7
  self-reliance and independence, 6
  welfare programs, 7
ETS. *See* environmental tobacco smoke
evidence-based practice (EBP), 275
  attitudes of tenure cohorts, 282
  implementation, 276
  nurses' attitudes and beliefs, 276
  role diffusion, 277
existential aloneness, 81, 87
expert generalists, 247

family caregivers, 173–174
family health navigator (FHN), 321, 322
Family Health Navigator Resource Center program (FHNRC program), 321, 322
family stressors, 226
farming and ranching, traditional, 441
farming occupation characteristics, 428
farming workforce, 431
Farm Partners program, 429–430
federally qualified community health center (FQCHC), 457
FHN. *See* family health navigator

FHNRC program. *See* Family Health Navigator Resource Center program
fibromyalgia (FM), 80, 82
first theoretical statement. *See* rural dwellers defining health
FM. *See* fibromyalgia
formal health care system, 11
FQCHC. *See* federally qualified community health center
frontier, 132, 176, 178
frustration, 252
FTE. *See* full-time equivalents
full-time equivalents (FTE), 430
functional doers, 338

GAO. *See* Government Accountability Office
gardening, 397, 398
gender role negotiation, 185–186
    compromise, 186
    conflict preservation, 186–187
    reconstruction, 187–188
    rural male caregivers, 188, 189
geographic isolation, 179, 189–190
GNI. *See* gross national income
Google Scholar, 53, 56
Government Accountability Office (GAO), 463
gross national income (GNI), 338
grounded theory, 54, 178
    BSP and SATL process, 133
    convenience sample, 132
    emerging interactive categories, 477
    face-to-face focused interviews, 133
    individual health insurance, 132
    NBC study using, 96
    qualitative method, 132

Haiti. *See also* rural nursing theory (RNT)
    built environment, 340–341
    CSDH, 339
    economy, 342
    education, 343–344
    genetics and historical factors, 341–342
    health care services, 344–345
    individual lifestyle, 346–347
    leading causes of death, 345
    policy and politics, 345, 346
hardiness, 70, 75
HB 173. *See* House Bill 173
HB program. *See* Healthy Border program
HDI. *See* human development index
HDL. *See* high-density lipoproteins
Head Start, Children's Health Insurance Program (CHIP), 233
HEAL approach. *See* Health Education and Action for Latinas approach
Health-Needs–Action Process model (HNAP model), 142, 153. *See also* Symptom–Action–Timeline process (SATL process)
    actions types, 153, 154
    limitations, 154
    for psychological symptomatology, 152
    SATL process model, 154
    studies of men in rural communities, 151
    symptom with health needs, 153
health-promoting lifestyle profile (HPLP), 83, 84
health-seeking behaviors, 24–25, 42
health, 8–9, 42
health care, 215
    actual or realized access, 215
    5A's, 216, 217, 218
    individual items, 217
    in local communities, 219
    potential access, 215
    resources, 67–68
    rural residents, 218, 222–223
    services, 11
Health Care Choices study, 207–208. *See also* health literacy
    CAM providers in rural locations, 209–210
    chronic illness, 209
    MSU CAM Health Literacy Scale, 210–211
    older rural women, 208–209

health disparities, 299
  air pollution, 230
  attributes and place-bound features, 229–230
  DC routinely publishes rates, 299
  in life expectancy, 229
  poverty, 232–235
  racial and ethnic minority groups, 230–232
  rural populations, 232
  social determinants, 299
Health Education and Action for Latinas approach (HEAL approach), 320–321
health literacy, 205
  CAM, 205–206, 210
  chronic illness, 206
  MSU CAM Health Literacy Scale, 210–211
health officer (HO), 404
health professional shortage area (HPSA), 422, 449
  federal laws, 461
  professional shortages in, 449
Health Resources and Services Administration (HRSA), 308, 459, 463
Healthworks program, 426–427
Healthy Border program (HB program), 310
Healthy People 2020 (*HP2020*), 310
  epidemiological realities of border region, 311–314
  HB program, 310
  health literacy, 205
  leading health indicators, 311–314
  social determinants of health, 228
hearing conservation, 425
hermeneutic phenomenology, 261. *See also* rural male nurses
  data collection and analysis, 262–263
  procedure, 261–262
high-density lipoproteins (HDL), 426
Hispanic or Latino health paradox, 309
Hispanics, 304
  CAM of health care, 307
  earning, 306
  T2D effect, 316

HIV. *See* human immunodeficiency virus
HNAP model. *See* Health-Needs–Action Process model
HO. *See* health officer
hospital demographics, 246–247
Hospital Standardization Program, 412
House Bill 173 (HB 173), 409. *See also* public health (PH)
  policy change rules, 410–411
  standards-based PH model, 409
HP2020. *See Healthy People 2020*
HPLP. *See* health-promoting lifestyle profile
HPSA. *See* health professional shortage area
HRSA. *See* Health Resources and Services Administration
human development index (HDI), 338
human immunodeficiency virus (HIV), 229, 307
hunting, 397, 398

ICN. *See* International Council of Nursing
IEC. *See* Interprofessional Education Collaborative
ILO. *See* intensive livestock operation
immigrant advantage, 309
informal networks, 475–476
informant demographics, 245–246
information literacy, 285
informed risk, 71–73, 75, 76
insider, 7, 473
  community support, 181, 190
  differentiation with outsider, 368, 369, 372, 373
Institute of Medicine (IOM), 58, 205. *See also* nursing workforce
  doubling number of nurses, 461–462
  ensuring nurses in lifelong learning, 462–463
  increasing proportion of nurses, 460–461
  infrastructure for data collection and analysis, 463–464
  nurse residency program implementation, 460

opportunity expansion for nurses, 459–460
preparing nurses to leadership positions, 463
primary sources of information, 207
scope-of-practice barriers removal, 457–459
intensive livestock operation (ILO), 380
International Council of Nursing (ICN), 28, 350
Interprofessional Education Collaborative (IEC), 459
IOM. *See* Institute of Medicine

Joint Commission, The (TJC), 275, 412. *See also* Joint Commission on Accreditation of Healthcare Organizations (JCAHO)
Joint Commission on Accreditation of Healthcare Organizations (JCAHO), 246. *See also* Joint Commission, The (TJC)

lack of anonymity and role diffusion, 7, 16, 444, 476–477. *See also* rural nursing theory (RNT)
 educational implications, 444–445
 familiarity, 477–478
 implying ability for rural people, 36
 nurse responsibilities, 9–10
 policy implications, 445
 practice implications, 445
 professional isolation, 478
 rural men actions and reputations, 177
La Frontera. *See* U. S.–Mexico border
lay care network, 476
lay resources stage, 135–136
leading health indicators (LHI), 310
lead PH officials (LPHO), 410
Léogâne, 336, 337, 339
LHD. *See* local health department
LHI. *See* leading health indicators
local health care
 acceptability, 222

Acceptability Scale score, 221
frequencies of dependent variables, 220
keeping or maintaining, 222
multivariate logistic regression models, 220
predictors, 218
local health department (LHD), 401
 rural and frontier, 404, 405, 415, 416
 standardization of, 416
 standards-based, 406, 409
logistic regression analysis, 208
LPHO. *See* lead PH officials

MDPHHS. *See* Montana Department of Public Health and Human Services
Medicare reimbursement, 215
MI. *See* myocardial infarction
migrant farmworkers, 432
Ministry of Public Health and Population (MSPP), 343, 344, 350
Montana City, 37, 65, 66
 community support, 73
 conscientious consumer, 71
 hardiness, 70, 75
 health care, 67–68
 health status, 68
 informed risk, 71–73
 self-reliance, 69–70
 themes, 69
Montana Department of Public Health and Human Services (MDPHHS), 404
Montana State University-Bozeman (MSU-B), 15
Montana State University (MSU), 207
MS. *See* multiple sclerosis
MSPP. *See* Ministry of Public Health and Population
MSU-B. *See* Montana State University-Bozeman
MSU. *See* Montana State University
MSU CAM Health Literacy Scale, 210–211

multi-disciplinary palliative care teams, 123
multiple sclerosis (MS), 159, 160
multispecialist role, 444
myocardial infarction (MI), 426

NAC & AARP. *See* National Alliance for Caregiving & American Association of Retired Persons
NAFTA. *See* North American Free Trade Agreement
NANIH. *See* National Association of Nurses Licensed in Haiti
NAS. *See* North American Study
National Alliance for Caregiving & American Association of Retired Persons (NAC & AARP), 173
National Association of Nurses Licensed in Haiti (NANIH), 350
National Center for Complementary and Alternative Medicine (NCCAM), 206
National Center for Health Workforce Analysis (NCHWA), 450
  APRNs, 458
  CNMs, 458
  for projecting supply and demand, 463–464
National Consensus Project (NCP), 119
National Council Licensure Examination for Registered Nurses (NCLEX®), 346
National Health Care Workforce Commission (NHCWC), 463
National Health Service Corps (NHSC), 461–462
National Institute for Occupational Safety and Health (NIOSH), 423
National Opinion Research Center (NORC), 415
National Prevention and Promotion Strategy (NPHPS), 228
National Public Health Performance and Standards Program (NPHPSP), 414

National Rural Health Association (NRHA), 176
NBC study. *See* northern British Columbia study
NCHWA. *See* National Center for Health Workforce Analysis
NCLEX®. *See* National Council Licensure Examination for Registered Nurses
NCP. *See* National Consensus Project
newcomer, 7, 36, 474
  nurses, 248
  old-timer versus, 373
  physicians, 251
  practicing rural nursing, 257
  in rural areas, 444–445
New York Center for Agricultural Medicine and Health (NYCAMH), 421, 423
  clinical services, 423–424
  occupational services to farmers, 428
  rural northeast occupational characteristics, 422
  safety and health training, 433
  services to rural and agricultural populations, 423–424
NGO. *See* nongovernmental organization
NHCWC. *See* National Health Care Workforce Commission
NHSC. *See* National Health Service Corps
NIOSH. *See* National Institute for Occupational Safety and Health
nongovernmental organization (NGO), 320
  in Haiti's development, 345
  improving nursing practice quality, 343
  medications through, 344, 345
NORC. *See* National Opinion Research Center
North American Free Trade Agreement (NAFTA), 306
North American Guidelines for Children's Agricultural Tasks, 431

North American Study (NAS), 28–29
northern British Columbia study (NBC study), 95
  becoming hardy, 100–101
  data analysis, 98–99
  data collection, 97–98
  findings and theory, 99
  limitations, 99
  making best of north, 101–102
  methods, 96
  political action, 103–104
  purposes, 96
  resilience development, 99, 100
  rural women in, 95
  sample, 97
  setting, 96–97
  vulnerability management, 100
NPHPSP. *See* National Public Health Performance and Standards Program
NRHA. *See* National Rural Health Association
nursing education
  challenges in U. S.–Mexico border region, 315
  men, experience in, 260
  recommendations for, 387–388
  use of rural hospitals, 298
nursing education reestablishment. *See also* Haiti
  after 2010 Haitian earthquake, 351
  functional doers, 338
  Haiti's demographics, 338–339
  health data, 339
  Léogâne, 336, 337
  NANIH and ICN work, 350
  nursing aid organization's work, 349–350
  students and nurses skills, 337–338
nursing literature
  corollary to relational statement, 19–20
  descriptive theoretical statement, 17–18
  relational theoretical statement, 18–19, 20–21
  RNT article, 17

nursing opportunity. *See also* rural male nurses
  for autonomy, 266
  for challenge, 268–269
  for expanded practice, 264–265
  and gender for recruitment, 270
  for meaningful relationships, 266–268
  for rural rewards, 269
nursing practice implications
  community support, 77
  conscientious consumers, 76–77
  hardiness, 77
  health care practitioners, 76
  health care services, 11
  informed risk effects, 76
  rural nurses, 11–12
  self-reliance, 11, 77
nursing staff tenure, 248
nursing workforce, 449–450
  age, 451–452
  diversity, 452–453
  education, 452
  employment patterns, 453–454
  needs for RNs, 450–451
  occupational commuting, 455–456
  rural nursing practice in, 456–457
  salary, 454–455
NYCAMH. *See* New York Center for Agricultural Medicine and Health
NYSDOH. *See* NY State Department of Health
NY State Department of Health (NYSDOH), 423

occupational commuting, 455–456
occupational health nurse (OHN), 421. *See also* New York Center for Agricultural Medicine and Health (NYCAMH)
  in agricultural research, 429
  Anabaptist communities, 432–433
  children safety, 431
  clinical services for farmers, 428
  educational outreach for, 433–434
  emergency service personnel, 426–427
  Farm Partners program, 429–430

occupational health nurse (OHN) (*Contd.*)
    farm safety, 430
    health and safety programs and services, 424
    migrant farmworkers, 432
    OHNAC role, 429
    pregnancy and farm exposure, 431–432
    services to rural businesses, 424–425
    skin cancer screening, 431
    volunteer firefighters, 427–428
    worksite wellness programs, 425–426
Occupational Health Nurses in Agricultural Community (OHNAC), 423, 429, 430
Occupational Safety and Health Administration (OSHA), 423
Office of Rural Health (ORH), 369
OHN. *See* occupational health nurse
OHNAC. *See* Occupational Health Nurses in Agricultural Community
old-timer, 7, 249, 473–474
    anonymity nonexistent for, 254
    nurses, 248
    responsibilities, 250
    versus newcomer, 373
older rural adult, 152
online support group conversations, 163–164
    maintaining balance, 165
    others first, 165
    physical and emotional isolation, 164
    uncertainty/searching, 164
    vigilance, 165–166
    ways of coping, 166–167
ORH. *See* Office of Rural Health
OSHA. *See* Occupational Safety and Health Administration
Out-of-town workshops, 249–250
outdoor activities, 101, 269
outsider, 7, 9, 16, 122, 123, 472–473
    differentiation, 368–369
    insider versus, 373

PA. *See* physician assistant
palliative care, 119. *See also* rural palliative care
Partners in Health (PIH), 344
PCI. *See* Project Concern International
PE. *See* physical education
perseverance, 81, 85
PH. *See* public health
PHAB. *See* Public Health Accreditation Board
PHEP program. *See* Public Health Emergency Preparedness program
PHHS. *See* Public Health and Human Services
PHN. *See* public health nursing
photovoice method, 96, 318–319
    adaptations of initiative, 319–320
    Border TB Photovoice Project, 319
physical education (PE), 395
physician assistant (PA), 317
PIH. *See* Partners in Health
pinch hitters, 251–252
poverty, 232
    barriers to access to care, 234–235
    communities, 234
    correlates of, 232–233
    demographic features, 234
    disciplines, 233
    index, 233–234
    near or working poor families, 233
Precaution Adoption Process Model, 361–362
prediabetes, 316
predictors, 218
    Acceptability Scale score, 221
    use and willingness, 219
    workplace and community, 445
professional resources stage, 136
    medicine man, 136–137
    symptoms, 136
    timeline variations, 136
Programa Compañeros, 320
Project Concern International (PCI), 319. *See also* U. S.–Mexico border
    BYAP, 322–323
    FHNs, 321

financial support security, 320
global experience with CHWs, 320
HEAL approach, 320–321
sustainability issue, 321–322
promotores. See community health worker (CHW)
Psychology and Behavioral Sciences Collection, 53
PsycINFO database, 53
public health (PH), 401, 402
   data analysis results, 406
   EPHS in, 403, 404, 405
   literature search and survey results, 407–408
   nursing practice characteristics, 406
   PHHS federal block grants, 404
   quality improvement initiatives, 414
   rural and frontier LHDs, 404, 409
   system improvement, 403, 404
Public Health Accreditation Board (PHAB), 409, 414
   CDC standards, 414–415
   EPHS, 414
   quality improvement initiatives, 414
   quality metrics, 413–414
Public Health and Human Services (PHHS), 404
Public Health Emergency Preparedness program (PHEP program), 401
public health nursing (PHN), 336
PubMed database, 53, 56

QSR NUD*IST software program, 163

RAC. *See* Rural Assistance Center
radon, carbon monoxide (CO), 359
regional health care center, 59
registered nurse (RN), 120, 135, 245
   age, 451–452
   diversity, 452–453
   education, 452
   employment patterns, 453–454
   occupational commuting, 455–456
   salary, 454–455
   workforce needs for, 450–451
resilience, 79, 84, 228
   adaptation, 84–85
   in adulthood, 81

aging adults, 80
   characteristics, 81
   contribution of early life, 88
   data comparison, 88–89
   demographic profile, 84
   development process, 100
   equanimity, 86–87
   existential aloneness, 87
   fibromyalgia, 80
   hardiness theory, 228–229
   and healthy aging, 81–82
   HIV infection, 299
   meaningfulness, 85–86
   networks and services, 299
   older frontier women, 80–81
   perseverance, 85
   physical and mental health, 80
   research method, 82–84
   RS and HPLP scores, 84
   self-reliance, 86
   success and support, 87–88
Resilience Scale (RS), 82, 84
resilient aging role models, 89
resilient women, 81
revised rural nursing theory structure
   choice, 25–26
   descriptive theoretical statement, 22
   distance, 23–24
   environmental context, 26
   health-seeking behaviors, 24–25
   listserv members, 29
   NAS, 28, 29
   relational theoretical statement, 22–23
   resources, 24
   social capital, 26–27
   vision, 28
RN. *See* registered nurse
RNT. *See* rural nursing theory
role diffusion, 10, 21. *See also* lack of anonymity and role diffusion
RS. *See* Resilience Scale
RUCA scale. *See* Rural–Urban Commuting Area scale
Rural Assistance Center (RAC), 216, 422, 451

rural children. *See also* Environmental
    Risk Reduction through
    Nursing Intervention and
    Education (ERRNIE)
  barriers to healthy food choices,
      396–397
  barriers to physical activity, 395
  healthy food choice supporting
      factors, 397
  physical activity supporting factors,
      395–396, 398
  research study, 394
  rural environment effects on,
      393–394, 397–398
rural communities, 215, 247, 367
  acceptance of health development
      leader, 374–375
  adolescents, 235–236
  children, 235–236
  community characteristics effects,
      367–368
  community participation, 369
  confidence in ability, 374
  data analysis, 370
  demographic characteristics,
      371–372
  disenfranchisement, 237–238
  efficacy of collective action,
      368, 372
  elderly, 236
  health development, 374
  insider or outsider differentiation,
      368–369, 372–373
  interviews, 369–370
  isolation and distance, 373–374
  lack of anonymity, 373, 375
  priority given to health, 368,
      371–372
  women, 237
rural dwellers, 36, 65, 207
  CAM, 211
  CRCHC in, 209
  data analysis, 178–179
rural dwellers defining health, 439, 470.
    See also rural nursing theory
    (RNT)
  distance, 471
  educational implications, 440
  health beliefs, 470

isolation, 470–471
  policy implications, 440–441
  practice implications, 440
rural hospitals
  benefits, 296–297
  challenges, 297–298
  evaluation, 296
  implementation, 294–296
  implications for education, 298–299
  implications for practice and
      research, 299–300
  nurses, 247–248
  nursing shortage in, 293
  opportunities for, 294
rurality, 176–177, 179
  challenges, 181–182
  communities, 181
  good neighborliness, 180–181
  paradoxical to self-reliance, 180
  participants, 180
  subcutaneous pump, 179–180
rural living, 357
  contaminant patterns, 358
  distance, 168
  environmental exposures, 359
  exposure risks to children, 357
  risks for local residents, 358
  rural nursing practice
      requirements, 358
rural male caregivers, 174
  findings, 194
  gender-cultural model, 188, 189
  gender role negotiation in, 189
  implications, 195–196
  limitations, 194–195
rural male nurses, 259–260
  limitations, 260, 271–272
  recommendations, 271–272
  results, 263–264
  in rural nursing practice, 270–271
  significance, 260
rural masculinity
  attributes, 191
  common sense, 184–185
  emotional needs, 184
  masculine self-reliance, 182
  participants, 182, 183
  provider role, 185
  relinquish control, 182–183

rural northeast occupational characteristics, 422
rural nurses, 7, 10
  boredom, 252
  educational preparation, 12
  embracing ethic of openness and honesty, 256
  frustration, 252
  functions, 50, 277, 386, 463
  identification, 249
  interpersonal closeness, 250
  practicing medicine, 250–251, 255
  treat generations of families, 268
rural nurses' attitudes and beliefs, 276, 287. *See also* evidence-based practice (EBP)
  attitudes of tenure cohorts, 282
  barriers, 286
  connecting nurses with research experts, 286
  data analysis, 280
  data collection, 278
  education level effect, 283, 285
  information literacy, 285
  instrument, 278–279
  positive attitudes, 285
  practice setting effect, 283
  questionnaire items, 279
  research questions, 279
  RNT, 277
  role diffusion, 277–278
  role effect, 283, 284
  rural nurses finding research, 280
  sample demographics, 281
  sample result, 280
  study limitations, 287–288
  study purpose, 276–277
  years of experience effect, 282, 286–287
rural nursing, 1–2, 35–36, 257, 277
  boundaries, 256–257
  Canadian study, 40, 41
  demographics, 39–40
  describing methods, 245
  health care providers, 36
  human responses, 256
  investigators, 58
  lack of anonymity, 9–10
  methods and procedures, 37
  Montana study, 37–38, 40
  nature, 244, 255
  qualitative data, 2–4
  quantitative data, 4–5
  retroductive theory generation, 3–4
  rigorous data collection, 10–11
  role diffusion, 10
  rural dwellers, 36
  scope, 244–245, 255–256
  themes and sub-themes, 40
  theory-building process, 2, 36–37
  updating, 15
rural nursing practice, 241
  being rural, 242–243
  education and professional development, 249–250
  group acceptance, 248–249
  hospital demographics, 246–247
  informant demographics, 245–246
  interpersonal relationships and, 250
  knowing patients personally, 254–255
  knowing rural, 243–244
  nature, 244
  nursing staff tenure, 248
  in nursing workforce, 456–457
  practicing medicine, 250–251
  requirements of, 358
  rural communities, 247
  rural expertise, 251–253
  rural hospital nurses, 247–248
  scope, 244–245
rural nursing theory (RNT), 45, 277, 347–348
  aims, 49
  articles, 54–55
  choices, 43, 44–45
  communities, 58–59
  data analysis, 41
  databases, 52–53, 54
  definition of health, 42, 42–44
  descriptive, 35
  distance, 43–44, 45
  functionality, 50–51
  health-seeking behaviors, 41, 42–44
  health care-seeking behavior, 16
  intervention, 49–50
  methodology, 52
  middle range theory, 16

rural nursing theory (RNT) (*Contd.*)
  MSU-B nursing researchers, 16
  nurse and health, 55–56
  person and environment, 55–56
  primary health care source, 17
  qualitative data, 2–4, 16–17
  quantitative data, 4–5
  and relevance to Haiti, 348
  research designs, 50
  resources, 42–43, 44–45
  rural definitions, 57–58
  self-reliance, 41, 43, 44
  theoretical statements, 16
rural palliative care
  case study, 120–122
  challenges, 122–123
  connectedness, 125
  emotional and physical isolation, 124–125
  health care professionals, 124–125
  health care provider shortages, 124
  multi-disciplinary team, 123
  opportunities, 125–126
  outsiders, 123
  rural residents, 123–124
  in rural settings, 124
  themes, 124
rural residents, 22, 123–124, 232, 259
  death rates, 416
  rural practice selection, 445
  sense of community, 126
  travelling outside, 210
Rural–Urban Commuting Area scale (RUCA scale), 369

SAP model. *See* Symptom Action Process model
SATL process. *See* Symptom–Action–Timeline process
SBIRT model. *See* screening, brief intervention, referral, and treatment model
SciVerse Scopus database, 52, 53
screening, brief intervention, referral, and treatment model (SBIRT model), 322–323

SD. *See* standard deviation
SDSU. *See* South Dakota State University
second theoretical statement. *See* self-reliance
self-care activities, 143
self-care stage, 134
  initiating and evaluation, 135
  Native American woman, 134–135
  using self-care tools, 134
  symptoms, 134
self-reliance, 9, 43, 69–70, 442, 471–472. *See also* rural nursing theory (RNT)
  characteristics, 74–75, 191
  depending on, 86
  educational implications, 442
  informal networks, 475–476
  insider, 473
  lay care network, 476
  newcomer, 474
  old-timer, 473–474
  outsider, 472–473
  pervasive in overlap, 190–191
  policy implications, 443–444
  practice implications, 442–443
  resources, 474–475
self-reported health status, 83–84
  demographics, 39–40
Serving the Underserved: Cultural Competence Enhancing Success (SUCCESS), 315
SES. *See* socioeconomic status
SHD. *See* State Health Department
skin cancer screening, 431
social capital, 26–27
  agencies, 377
  community infrastructure, 378
  professional nurse, 55
  RNT and relevance, 348–349
  suggestions, 388
  theories and models, 54
social determinants, 225
  health-related disparity, 228
  place-related, 227–228
  policies, 228
  positive influence, 227
  social engagement, 227

socioeconomic status (SES), 232, 309
  air pollution, 230
  cumulative effects, 310
  disadvantages, 228
  education, 310
South Dakota State University (SDSU), 294
  campus of, 295
  nursing instructors, 294–295
  nursing program, 294
  using rural hospitals, 298
  semesters in nursing program, 294
southwest Ontario study (SWO study), 95
  data analysis, 98–99
  data collection, 97–98
  drug dealers not welcome, 104
  limitations, 99
  making best of north, 101–102, 110
  methods, 96
  older rural women in, 105
  physical health and safety risks, 104
  psychosocial health risks, 105
  resilience development, 106–108
  rural church, 105, 106
  rural communities, 110, 111–112
  setting, 96–97
standard deviation (SD), 82
State Health Department (SHD), 402, 404
SUCCESS. *See* Serving the Underserved: Cultural Competence Enhancing Success
SWO study. *See* southwest Ontario study
Symptom Action Process model (SAP model), 141
  chronic conditions, 145
  decision-making process, 145–146
  health care providers, 147
  health need concept, 144
  HNAP model, 146, 152–153
  psychological symptoms, 144
  rural dwellers, 151
  self-care action, 145
  self-efficacy and health behavior, 151

Symptom–Action–Timeline process (SATL process), 23, 133, 141, 145, 442. *See also* Symptom Action Process model (SAP model)
  actual or potential health problems, 137
  CAM and CINAHL, 146
  characteristic variables, 150
  facilitate rural residents responses, 137
  four phases, 142, 143
  health needs identification and actions, 148
  HNAP model, 142, 152–153
  using keyword, 146
  using lay resources, 148–149
  lay resources stage, 135–136, 143–144
  limitations, 151
  participants' demographic characteristics, 147, 148
  perceived barriers, 151
  using professional resources, 144, 149–150
  professional resources stage, 136–137
  recommendations, 142
  rural dwellers, 151
  rural health care, 146
  self-care stage, 134–135
  using self-care strategies, 148
  symptom identification, 133–134, 142
  timeline aspect, 151–152
symptom identification stage, 133
  participants, 133
  properties, 133–134
  variation, 134

T2D. *See* type 2 diabetes
TB. *See* tuberculosis
TDH. *See* Texas Department of Health
TERRA model. *See* Translational Environmental Research in Rural Area Model
Texas Department of Health (TDH), 308–309
theory-building process, 2, 36

third theoretical statement. *See* lack of anonymity and role diffusion
tight-knit families, 181
translational environmental research in rural area model (TERRA model), 359, 360
trauma-related events, 226
tuberculosis (TB), 306
   border and rural health care, 325
   border TB photovoice project, 319–320
   HP2020 leading health indicators, 314
   morbidity and mortality, 318
type 2 diabetes (T2D), 315
   cost of long-term treatment, 317–318
   disproportionate effect, 316
   health state of participants with, 317
   promotores utilization, 317
   risk factors for, 316
   in U.S.–Mexico border, 316

UNDP. *See* United Nations Development Program
United Nations Development Program (UNDP), 338
United States (U.S.), 173
   CAM, 205–206
   federal government, 233
   population, 452–453
   RN, 260
   USFA, 426
United States Department of Agriculture (USDA), 227, 278, 450
University of Texas at El Paso (UTEP), 324
   simulation with standardized patients, 324–325
USDA. *See* United States Department of Agriculture
USDA ERS. *See* U.S. Department of Agriculture Economic Research Service
U.S. Department of Agriculture Economic Research Service (USDA ERS), 422

U.S. Department of Health and Human Services (DHHS), 310, 413
   concepts and principles, 402
   family health navigators, 321
   national initiative, 460
USFA. *See* U.S. Fire Administration
U.S. Fire Administration (USFA), 426
USMBCC. *See* U.S.–Mexico Border Counties Coalition
USMBHC. *See* U.S.–Mexico Border Health Commission
U.S.–Mexico border, 303–304
   APRN shortage in, 315–316
   BRFSS, 316–317
   CAM, 307–309
   colonias juxtaposes rural realities, 304, 306
   cross-border networks, 307
   demography, 304
   disparities, 306
   educational attainment and poverty rates, 307
   geography, 304
   health care practitioner's challenges, 315
   HP2020, 310, 311–314
   opportunities, 315
   photovoice method, 318–320
   promotores utilization, 317
   simulation and training, 323–324
   social determinants, 309–310
   standardized patient scenarios, 325
   T2D, 316, 317–318
   unemployment rates, 306–307
   USMBHC, 303–304, 305
   UTEP, 324–325
U.S.–Mexico Border Counties Coalition (USMBCC), 304
U.S.–Mexico Border Health Commission (USMBHC), 303–304, 310
UTEP. *See* University of Texas at El Paso

vigilance, 165–166
   caretaker, 363
volunteer firefighters, 427–428

vulnerability, 225
    communities or neighborhoods, 226–227
    coping abilities, 226
    family stressors, 226
    to less than optimal conditions, 225–226
    spiraling snowball, 226
    trauma-related events, 226
vulnerare, 225

Web of Science database, 52, 56
WELCOA. *See* Wellness Council of America
Wellness Council of America (WELCOA), 425
WIC. *See* Women, Infants, and Children
Wilson's method of analysis
    distance, 471
    familiarity, 477–478
    informal networks, 475–476
    insider, 473
    isolation, 470–471
    lack of anonymity, 476–477
    lay care network, 476
    newcomer, 474
    old-timer, 473
    outsider, 472
    professional isolation, 478
    resources, 474–475
Women, Infants, and Children (WIC), 233, 359
women, resilience in rural and remote Canada, 95. *See also* northern British Columbia study (NBC study); southwest Ontario study (SWO study)
Women to Women Project (WTW), 161
    computer group, 162
    cyber friends, 163
    data analysis, 162–163
    participants eligibility in, 161
    qualitative and demographic data, 162
    quantitative data, 162
worksite wellness programs, 425–426
WTW. *See* Women to Women Project